Medical Encounters in British India

Contents

Medical Encounters in British India

Edited by

Deepak Kumar
and
Raj Sekhar Basu

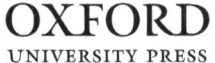
OXFORD
UNIVERSITY PRESS

OXFORD
UNIVERSITY PRESS

Oxford University Press is a department of the University of Oxford.
It furthers the University's objective of excellence in research, scholarship,
and education by publishing worldwide. Oxford is a registered trademark of
Oxford University Press in the UK and in certain other countries

Published in India by
Oxford University Press
YMCA Library Building, 1 Jai Singh Road, New Delhi 110 001, India

ISBN 13: 978-0-19-808921-6
ISBN 10: 0-19-808921-X

Typeset in Minion Pro 10.5/13.72,
at MAP Systems, Bengaluru 560 082, India

for
Michael Worboys

Tables and Figures

Tables

Figures

Acknowledgements

An edited volume is by definition a collaborative project. Our greatest debt is to the contributors who originally presented these essays at the third conference of the Asian Society for History of Medicine hosted by Jawaharlal Nehru University with support from the Indian Council of Medical Research. When the idea to bring some thematically connected articles specific to colonial India came up, they agreed to revise and always responded to the queries promptly. We are grateful to the anonymous referees for incisive comments. Madhuri Sharma helped in preparing a comprehensive bibliography. We also acknowledge the help received from Srilata Chatterjee, Dhrub Kumar Singh, Manas Dutta, and Malay Das. Our heartfelt thanks to the editorial team at the Oxford University Press, New Delhi, for taking such meticulous care and the elegant production.

The volume is dedicated to long-time friend and colleague Professor Michael Worboys, who, through his researches and publications, has enriched our understanding of the theories and practices in the realm of tropical and colonial medicine.

Abbreviations

AIWC	All India Women's Conference
ARMCB	Administrative Report of the Municipal Commissioner for the City of Bombay
BLC	Bombay Legislative Council Debates
CMARS	Calcutta Medical Aid and Research Society
CMS	Church Missionary Society
GD	General Department Volumes, Maharashtra State Archives, Mumbai
GR	Government Resolution
IMS	Indian Medical Service
LMS	London Missionary Society
NTI	National Tuberculosis Institute
NTP	National Tuberculosis Programme
RAC	Rockefeller Archive Centre, Tarrytown, New York, USA
RF	Rockefeller Foundation
RG	Records Group
RMS	Records of the Malaria Survey of India
RN	Report on Native Papers, Bombay Presidency
RSC	Report of Sanitary Commissioner, Bombay
SOAS	School of Oriental and African Studies
STD	Sexually Transmitted Diseases
TB	Tuberculosis
WHO	World Health Organization

Introduction

Deepak Kumar and Raj Sekhar Basu

> This was the age of science—goodbye to luck and fate. Man will fight death and disease. When he was helpless he saw immortality in death, now he is looking for immortality in life...Modern medical science is forging ahead; with the discovery of the microscope, the inner eye has opened, germs are being identified. The entire idea about causes of diseases is fast changing...
>
> *Arogyaniketan* (a novel in Bengali)[1]

Not very long ago, medicine was believed to have addressed a world without boundaries, more of 'a primeval space characterized by the shifting humors and movements of cold and damp'.[2] It was indeed thought that long periods of drought, excessive heat, hot burning winds, clouds of suffocating dust, and heavy downpour paved the way for epidemic pestilence and outbreaks. Thus, the origins of diseases came to be situated either in meteoric phenomenon or in the low, marshy, and alluvial soil content of the earth. This inhospitable physical space of the earth and the sky proved to be ideal breeding ground for the diseases.[3]

However, the word disease has always been what society had chosen it to mean, nothing more, nothing less. In fact, the definition of disease has differed with time and its place in history. For Foucault, disease is a 'deviation within life'.[4] The names assigned to diseases have been more of abstractions, although at times they acted as real entities. Last but not least, the definition of disease in diagnostic terms has also not been accurate and able to satisfy all. The relationships between disease and medicine have also differed in terms of geography, culture, traditions, and ideas about the natural space. The majority of studies on disease and medicine have often ignored the non-Western concepts of disease and the possible ways of providing succour to the affected humanity. Such studies seemed to have focused more on the tensions between those who believed that diseases were real entities with an existence of their own (ontologists) and the others who believed that disease should be perceived as illness, as a unique process in one person over time (physiologists).[5] These tensions persisted over a long period of time, because physicians believed that they as professionals must have a reasonably precise definition of what they meant by disease.

Interestingly, the late 19th and 20th centuries witnessed conflicts over the usage of terms such as Western and non-Western medical systems. In the past several decades, non-Western has been interpreted as a dubious concept, because, historically, Western medicine has long influenced regions outside the West.[6] The same might also hold true for the non-Western, since the interchange of ideas between the cultural zones was not simply a one-way movement and they may have increased in terms of intensity over a period of time. But how can the boundaries of the system be determined? How can changes in the system be analysed?

The usages of terms like Western and non-Western are to be seen as symbols of a definite form of ethnocentrisms, which always privileged one form of tradition over another. In medical parlance, it is almost unacceptable to think that treating bodily ills can take place within a certain 'metamedical' framework of thought. As it has been observed, 'The biomechanistic model within which the professional formation and deformation of the doctor takes place in our culture, one such "metamedical" framework, is by no means universal'.[7] The degree of systematicity prevalent in different forms of medical treatment is not only problematic but something which is also culturally variable.

In 19th century Europe, the idea of a disease was seen as deviation from normal. This idea existed as early as Plato's *Timaeus* and was basic to the enduring humoral pathology. The word normal had a number of meanings, two of which were of great importance. The first was of conforming to a type, to an ideal or object of desire. It was thus something which was open to a value judgment.[8] The second did refer to something that was usual and could be determined by enumeration. The medical practitioners not only had to deal with the problems of fixing the ranges of normality but in reaching a consensus as to the magnitude of departure from these ranges, which could be ultimately labelled as disease. Thus, throughout the 19th century, the physicians were involved in developing methods of quantifying physiological functions.

By the last decade of the 19th century, the concept of specific etiology was firmly established. This paved the way for the final vindication of the

germ theory of human disease. It was believed that not only were there specific diseases but each apparently had a specific cause. Thus, disease was no
longer viewed as deviation from the normal, determined by vague and un-
quantifiable etiologic agents such as the four humours or nervous energy.
A number of social forces added strength to the tradition of ontology. The
emergence of the hospital system brought together many patients, whose
ailments for all practical purposes seemed to be identical. These developments strengthened the ontological view at the turn of the 20th century.[9]

The myth of the Western superiority in medicine exploded when it
was reported that mastoidectomies, open heart surgeries, and similar
other surgical invasions were routinely performed in China on the basis
of acupunctural analgesia. The biomechanistic model of the West came
to be seriously challenged. The anthropological researches in Africa and
South America also revealed interesting information. In such societies,
abnormal physical illnesses were not explained within a biomechanistic framework which separates nature from the supernatural, the social
world from the world of nature, and the physical individual from his
social ambience. In fact, there seemed to be an interdependence of all
the four—nature, super nature, society, and person. Physical illness was
therefore interpreted within a framework that was not naturalistic, but
cosmic. The participation of the 'significant others', mainly the primary
groups and networks based on extended family, kin, and neighbours,
were also important in the treatment process. Thus, it is clear that the
model of 'non-Western' medicine was by no means universally valid.[10]

However, despite the criticism of universalism, it needs to be stressed
that certain medical traditions did symbolize attempts on part of different systems to come close to one another. The pre-Islamic Arab folk
medicine, practised over a large part of present Middle East Asia, was
tightly bound up with magic. The major historical importance of this pre-
Islamic medicine lay in the fact that by the end of the Umayyad period, it
was presented as 'Prophetic Medicine', supposedly based on a part of the
Prophet's corpus of writings. This undoubtedly was a strategy which was
devised by the more religious elements to build up a medical tradition
which was opposed to the Greek medicine, then viewed as something
heathen.[11] But soon it was the influence of Galen which proved to be the
foremost in the nascent Islamic world. The doctrine of humours, the concept of the three digestions, and the movement of blood and the teleologi-
cal thinking which sought to recognize and explain each organ and each
natural process in terms of its purpose were all derived from his ideas.

But more importantly, by the end of the 8th century, the main corpus of Greek medicine had been translated into Persian and Arabic and several medical texts from India also had reached the Caliph's Court. In the middle of the 10th century, an Arab physician, Ali Ibn-Sahl al-Tabari, described the Indian medical system in the appendix of his main work concerning Hippocratic and Galenic traditions of medicine. In his work *Kitab Firdaws al-Hikma*, he did refer to the Indian works available in Persian and highlighted the significant differences between the systems.[12]

Incidentally, this period also witnessed the arrival of Western medical knowledge in India. Western medical knowledge had travelled to India via the Arabs and this was possibly the reason for the popularity of the term *Unani* (the very name being derived from Ionian). In the succeeding years, Unani competed and complemented the older Ayurvedic system in the treatment of diseases. 'The practitioners of the two systems seem to have collaborated because each had much to learn from the other and we have no record of any animosity between Hindu and Muslim in the field of medicine'.[13] Both systems interacted and borrowed from each other. Remarkable, however, is the absence of changes in the theory. The borrowings that can be detected are restricted to the practice of medicine. A number of drugs used by the hakims were adopted by the Indian *vaidya*s, while the reverse process took place as well. These developments have not been studied in detail. The texts edited so far convey the impression that it was more widespread in northern than in southern India, and that the followers of Vagbhatta were rather immune to it.[14] At about this time, Chinese medicine constituted another influential school and it shared with Unani the fundamental theory of the humours. But each of these systems had developed their own internal logic. In the case of China, alongside Taoism and Buddhism, Confucian materialism with its this-worldly emphasis on earthly duty, provided a metamedical context which was entirely different from the other-worldly Hindu cosmology. Undoubtedly, to interpret these distinctions, the purely spiritual nature of Hinduism came to be questioned. Marxist historians of Hindu thought have emphasized that the Brahmanical interpretation of Hinduism had not always been influential, though some anthropologists have argued that Brahmanism acted as a brutal force in preserving the order.[15]

It has often been argued that the interactions between the West and the East essentially form a part of a long historical process. Some scholars have tried to understand medical history in terms of cross-currents

which flowed across 'Oikumene' of the world constituted by the great
civilizations stretching across the continents of Europe and Asia. The
exchange of ideas was not one-way traffic and it was not all from the
West to the East. In the case of America, concepts such as 'hot and cold'
had been an important part of medical theory which pre-dated Columbus' conquest of the continent. In the case of India, any discussions on
the interactions of the West and the East in medical terms would definitely bring out the coherence and contradictions which were present
within the different medical traditions. While it is true that there were
distinct systems of medical knowledge based on the ancient Sanskrit
classical texts, Unani medicine based on classic Arabic-Persian texts,
there was also a syncretic tradition which tended to cut across the
boundaries of culture and social systems. Over more than six centuries,
spanning between the 13th and the 19th centuries, different systems
of medical knowledge interacted with each other, disagreed with one
another, and also assimilated ideas and concepts from each other. This
process of assimilation took various forms which included various types
of folk medicine, popular medicine of the mass, market, and society. In
fact, similar to that of the West, there was also reliance on magico-religious forms which undoubtedly proved the popularity of cult-culture.[16]

However, the discussions on the interactions between the East and
the West, in the context of medicine, do also bring into focus several
other issues. In the West, the rise of scientific authority and the claims of
achieving spectacular success did lead to the limited nature of Western
medicine. It also led to a narrowing of the range of alternative systems of
treatment. In the East, despite the prevalence of traditional cultures there
was awareness of alternative traditions. In these traditions, the domination of Western medicine has not been that overwhelming as it is often
believed to be. In countries like India and China, Western medicine, till
date, continues to be expensive for the vast majority of the population,
whose survival depends largely on the fortunes of the agrarian economy.
This tradition of medicine also has an urban orientation and this is primarily responsible as to why the health institutions built along Western
lines are considered to be remote by the rural population. The traditional
medical system seems to dominate the primary level of health care, but
Western medicine increasingly gains importance as one moves up to the
higher levels. Indian medicine is largely pluralistic in nature. As late as
the 1970s and 1980s, national and state health services provided only

10 per cent of all medical treatment and the city based allopathic medical practitioners treated only 10 per cent of the suffering humanity. The vast majority of people depended upon what has been referred to as the underground systems, ranging from home treatment to the 'drug detailmen' who sell a variety of medicines, including Western medicine, on a massive scale. But interaction between the traditional medical systems such as Ayurveda and Western allopathic medicine has been far from anything smooth. The Ayurveda practitioners often complained that Western educated allopathic medical practitioners treated their knowledge as inferior and considered them to be second class doctors. This sort of conflict was not simply confined within the borders of India. In countries like China, the early decades of the 20th century witnessed a clash between traditional medicine which was viewed as a 'particularly noxious symbol' of conservatism and the supporters of Western medicine who were often seen as modernizers. Yet, within five years of the revolution, the Communist government in China opted for a pluralist policy, whereby traditional systems proved to be predominant in the countryside and Western medicine gained popularity in the cities.[17]

This interaction between the West and the East also brought into purview several other issues which are of great importance. In Asia, medicine was not viewed simply as a biological phenomenon. The concept of treatment relied on a number of factors, which included accounts of the societal standing of the patients and their relationship with the therapists. In the eastern cultures, there was a belief that there were invisible agents of disease. Though this might have differed from the Western germ theory, there was enough space for the different kinds of medicine to flourish and interact in the field of diagnosis and treatment of the ailments. How did the vaidyas react to the introduction of bacteriology? The reply was—germs attack only when the *Tridosha*'s (the three humours) balance goes wrong.

They believed that the germ theory and the humoral theory are independent, equally valid theories of disease causation. Syncretism indeed takes curious forms.

INTERROGATING THE INTERACTIONS

In fact, for a fairly long period of time, it was believed that East-West encounter was essentially a clash of civilizations. It was argued that Western Europe advanced and changed in a paradigmatic way, while

Asia did not. 'At the most, Asia kept doing what it had been doing for centuries; Europe changed basically'.[18] But in recent times, academic projects aimed towards the writing of new global histories have provided new ways of understanding such encounters without being confined to the parochial boundaries defined on the basis of religion or the nation-state. New global histories offer a number of explanations which go much beyond the binaries of one ideological doctrine or the other. Scholars like Arjun Appadurai are inclined to believe that what is essentially defined as 'global' is actually a conglomeration of many 'local' interchanges instead of the colossal blocks which go in the names of nations, cultures, and civilizations.[19] French historians, in presenting their own researches on global history, had always insisted on the inherent links between history and geography and argued that migration of people essentially has to be understood as movements between ecological zones distinct from national borders.

However, there have been very few attempts to write history of medicine and health from a global perspective. The exchange of peoples' practices, information, goods, as well as diseases, through the trading companies as well as the missionary denominations, bring into focus the relevance of the global history/histories. But there are certain barriers which have impeded the adoption of the networked view of global history vis-à-vis the history of medicine. In recent times, the concepts associated with culture often present a number of complexities. As Harold Cook argues, cultures have tended to remain rooted in language and upbringing and so some very important elements of the medical behaviours of one region do not get exchanged with other regions.[20] Therefore, despite the importance of new global histories, there has been a propensity to reject the essentialist comparisons involving different cultures and civilizations. The dominant opinion seems to be in favour of the view that there are different groups of people across the world, culturally different, but they do remain connected with one another. These connections are to be understood more in terms of the contours of local histories rather than totalities. Therefore, if these ideas are to be borrowed by historians of medicine, they would be forced to consider the more intricate and complicated patterns of interactions pertaining to health and diseases and may gradually lead to a breaking down of unified medical traditions which have defined themselves as either Eastern or Western medicine.

None can deny that medical ideas and interactions need to be analysed in the context of socio-historical background. What has essentially been believed as medical knowledge is not something which is static; rather, it was constantly incorporating new features, thereby presenting a new form or appearance in course of history. In other words, the emphasis seems to be more on the diffusionist models of knowledge transmission. In the context of the East-West encounter, it undoubtedly brings into focus the relations between the centre and the periphery and the areas of contestation. Recent scholarship seems to uphold the idea that transmission should no longer be seen as one emanating from a powerful centre. The exchange and adoption of ideas are not always something which should be thought of as something imposed from above forcibly nor as osmotic transfers, rather they come from the logic of the interactions between the global and the local. The value of exchange can never be underestimated; it can be as productive and creative as the production of knowledge *per se*. But, as the very first chapter in this volume argues, 'transmission', 'exchange', or 'negotiations' do not negate the equations of power. 'Domination and marginalization lurk in the background and mostly appear as the two sides of the same coin'. In Foucauldian terms—

> With the new 'micro-physics' of power in which the individual body be-
> came the target and effect of a ubiquitous and calculating gaze, the field of
> knowledge and human understanding was reformulated. It became pos-
> sible to imagine a docile workforce, a disciplined army, a growing child,
> and a medicine that analysed and investigated bodies.[21]

In late 19th century, the colonial arteries had hardened and the practitioners of modern medicine felt genuinely assured of their superior scientific knowledge.[22] Later, the rising tides of nationalism also posed obstacles to the exchange of ideas in the realm of medicine. The indigenous medical practitioners raised their voices against the dominant medical discourse which favoured the large scale intrusion of Western allopathic medicine. These indigenous practitioners stoutly defended their knowledge system and did not believe that their tradition was confined under the veils of unscientific or irrational thoughts. However, they did strongly believe that there was nothing wrong in learning and benefiting from the new knowledge.[23]

The East-West exchange encompassed both elements of difference and sameness. In the field of medicine, this exchange, Jayanta Bhattacharya says, had a long past stretching back to the 16th century. This interation ranged from assimilation to experimentation to transformation and finally dissemination. In the course of this tortuous trajectory, there were moments when the West hegemonically talked to the East.[24] The East tried to preserve its presence by locating the fissures within the hegemonic discourses of modern medicine and by differentiating practical therapeutics from the wider issues of health.

A LONG HISTORY

Historians too often believed that the earliest interactions between Indian and European practitioners of medicine came through the spice trade. The cargoes of spices always contained a large number of substances, which had their use in the treatment of diseases. In the early centuries of interactions, brought through the operation of the European trading companies, there seemed to be an eagerness in understanding the techniques and strategies of the indigenous practitioners of medicine.[25] The early Jesuit writers in Goa characterized the vaidyas as the Goa Brahmins who were gifted with keen intellect and cured 'with simple remedies unlike European physicians'. However, even before the arrival of the Portuguese in Goa, there had been a flow of Indian medical knowledge to the West via the Arab merchants. By the 13th century, several Indian medical texts had been translated into Latin and had become standard texts for medical practitioners in Europe. The descriptions of Indian medical practitioners and their treatment of patients in the Portuguese texts reveal that Portuguese medical practitioners had tried to understand the working of the Indian medical traditions in great details. However, with the passage of time, the assimilationist approach gave way to one of conflict, leading to obstacles in the flow of ideas.

Mark Harrison, in his chapter, takes up the colonies as repositories to a wide range of drugs that were not commonly available in Europe. In his view, the use of the calomel or mercurous chloride, which had been pioneered in the hospitals of the East India Company, had an important impact on medicine in 19th century Britain. At the same time, the insistence on the part of the Company's surgeons that tropical diseases were distinctive led to the development of a distinct branch of Western medicine, which was believed to be the medicine of hot or warm climates. Interestingly, in the use of mercury, the Company's surgeons made a clear distinction in terms of the locale and geography. In the case of Britain, physicians were instructed to be more moderate in the quantity they generally administered against fever and other related ailments. However, this growing sense of distinctiveness, which was reflected in British medical practice, did not prove to be a barrier to the transmission of ideas and practices from the colony to the homeland.

David Arnold in his chapter points out that changing 'cross cultural fortunes' possibly provides one of the many ways of understanding the issues of health in Asian medical history. But he is a little sceptical about the idea of the East-West exchange. To him the process of exchange was by no means defined by the exigencies of modernity, rather this process had an ancient past, preceding the arrival of the Europeans in the East. Nonetheless, the idea of exchange could certainly be a powerful strategy in countering the 'facile assumptions about the simple imposition (or uncontested hegemony) of Western medicine over South Asian societies'. Arnold stresses the point that there were significant exchanges between European medicine and Ayurveda, since the time of the arrival of the Portuguese, and it later intensified in the late 18th and early 19th centuries. However, the 'colonial knowledge' favoured an asymmetrical power relationship and this possibly explains the intention of the British colonist to override Ayurveda's remarkably rich tradition of dietetics. This undoubtedly led a section of Ayurvedic practitioners to initiate changes possibly to justify their claims of equal status with the practitioners of Western medicine.[26] But, this did have important implications for Ayurveda since the entire scheme of dietetics was downplayed, if not marginalized.

In the 1930s, as Sunil Amrith has pointed out in his chapter, there was the emergence of an optimistic narrative which emphasized that technology, knowledge, and education could essentially challenge the traditional ideas relating to 'tropicality' (a vision that tropical Asia was an area of heat and humidity and naturally poor). This shift in the realm of ideas led to linking of bio-medical sciences to the wider discourse on social citizenship. A large number of observers, ranging from colonial medical officers to Asian social reformers, felt that the new system of education could transform the human characteristics and practices which had essentially been produced by the tropical condition. Interestingly, this emphasis on education was also responsible for the emergence of a new nutritional discourse, particularly in South Asia. A number of colonial medical scientists argued that the preponderance of highly milled rice in the South Indian diet accounted for a wide range of nutritional deficiencies and apart from this, the lack of leafy vegetables and protein foods was also responsible for the poor physical conditions of the people in that region. Such views were contradicted by Gandhi, who believed that changes in dietary habits could be directly related to the impact of the economic policies of the colonial state. Gandhi also believed that overt mechanization in the sphere of agriculture had also led to the economic and moral impoverishment of the rural localities in India.

However, despite the nationalist critique of the 'new knowledge of nutrition', the colonial discourses of tropicality could rarely be obliterated in terms of the post-colonial visions of development. While the notion of tropical development had a clear link with the 19th century colonial views, the discourses about tropical nature in the mid-20th century within Asia revealed that the colonial discourse had not really lost its importance. In other words, the growing emphasis on the whims of nature revealed the fact that post-colonial states suffered from an element of indecision when it came to encountering the changing aspects of their physical environment.

CULTURE, COLONIALISM, AND DISEASE

Throughout the 19th century, Indian physicians tried to understand and contextualize Western medical traditions in accordance to their own cultures and ideas. In Bengal, people like Mahendra Lal Sarkar, a product of modern medical education, who shifted to homoeopathy and still, unlike its founder Hahnemann, did not accept that homoeopathy was an absolute system of medicine. He did not believe in Hahnemann's idea that there was only one law of cure. Dhrub Kumar Singh in his little long chapter has argued that apart from such ideas, Sarkar also envisioned a plural culture of medicine. This softness towards the plurality of therapeutic science led him to believe in the ideal of 'cultivation of science'—an intellectual tradition in which specialization would not be akin to something like parochialism and the utilitarian goal would be the most important.

Madhuri Sharma in her case study of Benaras does accept the fact that the intrusion of Western allopathic medicine influenced the Ayurvedic practitioners to identify themselves with new world of modern science. These practitioners also tried to avoid the humiliation from the allopathic practitioners by acquainting themselves with the new techniques of diagnosis.[27] The application of these techniques did not bring about the overwhelming domination of modernity; rather they operated within a situation in which there was no real breach of the old order. This strange situation born out of a symbiosis between modernity and indignity was responsible for the framing of the modern notion of sanitation and municipality in accordance with religious codes. In that sense, despite the growing influence of Western science, the educated sections of the Indian society tried to locate science in the Vedic past and invoked the intellectual supremacy of the Vedic scriptures. Sharma thus argues that the educated sections were not just passive recipients, but tried to explicate them in their own terms, possibly to enable them to secure a space within the newly created professional structure and to attain a privileged social status.

The colonial state's attempt to regulate and erase many of the 'native' medical practices received wholehearted support from the Western medical missionaries who form the subject of Basu's chapter. The missionaries defined the cultural terrain of India in terms of their own understanding of the 'cultured' and the 'uncivilized'. To most missionaries, India resembled Africa in terms of ignorance and backwardness. Such bizarre portrayals of India as a strange land reverberating with stories of mysteries and of deaths and horrors lent strength to Europe's civilizing mission in India. The Western missionaries worked with the European colonial powers to bring Western medical science to the doorstep of the unfortunate nations. In India, the British official classes often justified the Christian missionary claims that medical mission was one of the ways of civilizing the ignorant and uneducated masses. However, the medical missionaries failed to eliminate the 'heathen' ritual and practices which their Christian converts practised during the times of illness. Despite their success in some parts of south India, the medical missionaries hardly succeeded in their aims to be the catalysts of mass conversion and their activities remained confined to peripheries of the Indian society.[28]

Disease control lay not in the hands of the ordinary people or the missionaries or the social reformers; responsibility lay with the government. Mridula Ramanna's chapter delineates the different approaches and responses to malaria control in the urban and rural regions of western India. Her chapter is based on the contemporary accounts, especially the Indian press reports. She shows how in small cities like Surat and Broach malaria was rampant while in Bombay malaria could be controlled thanks to the collaborative efforts of malariologists, doctors (both Indian and British), community leaders, and the vigilant press. For rural regions, the less said the better. Individual members of the legislature and local bodies, even of the elite Indian Medical Service (IMS), asked for state support but in vain. Paucity of funds remained the main excuse. As Rogers argued, 'with sufficient foresight and organisation, the greater part of the loss could have been prevented'.[29] But the blame was put on the insanitary habits and culture of the people.

Government's apathy was aided by the colonial sociologists and ethnographers who, in their study of the Indian populations, were often responsible for stereotyping certain communities as 'virile' and 'healthy' and some others as 'weak' and susceptible to diseases. The epidemiological data was also clearly built around the premise of privileging the health standard of certain social groups as well as exposing the weak physical and health standards of some other communities. All these were also integrated into the general colonial discourse which made a distinction between the colony and the metropolis. In fact, as late as the 1930s, the British medical journals emphatically stated that the Indian population, as a whole, was more susceptible to tuberculosis than the population of England or Scotland. Consequently, there was an attempt to establish the fact that once the virgin population and virgin region was exposed to the disease, the vulnerability to bacillus greatly increased.

However, it was often found that in explaining incidence of diseases, there was a propensity on the part of the official classes to fall back upon the disproportionate male–female sex ratio. In fact, the susceptibility of women to infections was not only noticed in the East but also in the West. Bikram Kumar Choudhary in his chapter argues that in course of the 19th and 20th centuries, the colonial understanding of diseases like tuberculosis from the perspective of gender underwent a change. While in the West women's specific physiological characteristic was blamed for the incidence of tuberculosis, the British medical practitioners in India tried to locate the incidence of diseases within certain cultural practices and traditions. In other words, the higher prevalence of tuberculosis among Indian women was linked to issues like purdah, child marriage, early pregnancy, and unhealthy practices during childbirth. Yet, the understanding of the social dimension of the disease was by no means complete, and inconsistencies remain. In the rural areas, both during and after the colonial period, the hegemony of patriarchy prevented the collection of information as to why diseases like tuberculosis affected women, particularly from the lower strata of the society. This possibly explains the reasons behind the branding of women as carriers of disease and the linking of gender identity to a culture of 'victim blaming'.

Arabinda Samanta in his chapter on the social construction of tuberculosis in colonial and post-colonial India argues that in most societies there existed little dialogue between the patient and the doctor. While the patients had their own notions of the disease, which was often informed by certain value-loaded cultural specificities, the doctors had their own project of therapeutic intervention. In the long run, the technological intervention was responsible for generating a belief in certain sections of society that the idealized self-image of the tuberculosis would be subverted, and this naturally led to what may be defined as a situation of extremes—symbolized by the patient's insularity from the outside world or the patient's freedom to move around as they expected. Thus, tuberculosis remained no longer a private or a personal problem but became clearly public. Yet, culture-driven knowledge about disease causations was constantly weighed against knowledge derived from the West.

However, it needs to be stressed that the missionary as well as the colonial discourses on the lax morals of the Hindus presented an entirely new picture on sexuality and sexual behaviour in India. In fact, this was opposed by the nationalists who strongly stated that while the Indians did have a glorious past, their moral and physical weaknesses were of recent origin and had been induced by changes brought about by colonialism. For Indira Chowdhury, more important are the ways through which 'a certain domain of knowledge about Indian sexual practices came to be hegemonically established within a colonial framework and how this domain implicitly incorporated selected information about Indian culture'. In other words, the colonial state and its advocates employed a wide range of epistemological networks to build up their own ideas about sexuality and population control in India.

Interestingly, the responses of the Indian elites towards population control in the early 20th century were not very different from that of the Western birth controllers. Most of them believed that the rigid social system was responsible for 'unbalanced' marriage practices. The constraints that the matrimonial system placed on women resulted in the prevalence of abortions and forced the young widows to turn to prostitution. But what is interesting is that the debates around population and birth control in the 1930s brought into the centre stage the 19th century domain of knowledge that had identified Indians as possessing 'depraved' bodily practices and claimed that the institution of marriage in India had always lacked the fundamental ingredients of sexual hygiene. Thus, the notion of the body, its pleasures and functions as they were known to the Indians were replaced by a different epistemic domain 'that tended to interpret experiential knowledge through laws of what was permitted and forbidden'. In other words, the colonial state sought to bring under its control the esoteric practices of the 'native' system of medicine and tried to restrain their functioning by the imposition of a certain disciplinary mode.

REFLECTIONS

It needs to be stressed that most historians are still caught within the parochialism of nationalist approach and this thereby inhibits cross fertilization of ideas and principles. We must recognize—there is no 'pure' East, no 'pure' West. A good deal of confusion and prejudice seems to arise from a false antithesis between 'Western' and 'Eastern' or 'indigenous' medicine. The true contrast is between 'rational' and 'traditional'.[30] The word 'Western' in relation to medicine has, correctly speaking, no meaning. Science knows no geographical limitations. We do not speak of 'Western' mathematics or of 'Western' chemistry. The science of medicine is indebted to Eastern nations for some notable advances. It was, for example, a Japanese scientist who discovered the organism of plague. The distinction should be made, therefore, not between 'Western' and 'Indian' but between 'Modern' and 'Ancient' medicine.[31] The seeds of the 'modern' can be seen also in the 'ancient'. There were many who wanted 'to develop the study of both the Western and Eastern systems of medical science side by side and make them serve as complements to each other'.[32] These interlocutors did not want to throw the baby with the bathwater! As an Indian practitioner of modern medicine wrote in 1876—

> the Yunani system of medicine as contained in Persian and Arabic literature, though very inferior and in some respects absurd and ridiculous, presents several useful hints of practical suggestion which should not be lost sight of; we should not throw off the roses because they are surrounded with thorns. We can pick out and learn a few good things even from savages.[33]

Superb defence, no doubt! This brings to fore the cultural dimensions of the encounter. It is only in recent times that the field of medicine, which had traditionally been limited to studies emphasizing the internal development of medicine, has undergone significant changes. The recent studies tend to emphasize more on the changing patterns of the diseases, their impact on the society, and the socio-cultural ways in which people relate to health issues.[34]

But more interestingly, studies have questioned the logic of equating Western medicine with higher standard of health. In fact, now the trend is to understand the interactions that had taken place between the Western and the non-Western counterparts in terms of disease, healing, and medicine. There has been a growing emphasis on culture and following the anthropologists, many social historians of medicine are trying to understand the non-Western medical practices within the wider orbit of tribal ethno medicine. As a consequence, there is now an intense search to understand the traditional health maintenance crafts of the non-Western medical systems. In other words, what had long been considered as scientific may lose out in terms of logic and this undoubtedly is bringing the Eastern botanical knowledge into prominence.[35]

This volume essentially explores the nature of interactions between the East and the West in the field of medicine. It brings into focus a whole range of historical processes through which this exchange gained a great deal of importance. It also brings into play the condition and ambience in which there was an interaction between the social and medical domains, particularly under the rubric of colonialism. The exchange of ideas and that of tradition was not a simple journey but rather a long and tortuous trajectory which was characterized by both assimilation as well as initiative which sought to differentiate one set of ideas from another. The level of interaction was seldom smooth and it was often ridden with the languages of dominance and hegemony. This entire story of conflicts, differences, and aggression rarely finds a place in most of the articles. The clash of cultures was too real to be totally brushed aside and there were constant intellectual discords which threatened to hegemonize human bodies and also construct complex discourses over issues of individual and private health. The narrative on this contest would have been further enriched had there been an attempt to understand the nature of the exchanges in terms of the interactions between the practitioners of Unani and those of modern Western medicine. The other noticeable miss which characterizes most of these studies on the history of medicine, including the ones in the present volume, lies in the inability to project the resistance of the East in real terms. While there are critiques of the hegemonic discourse of colonialism, the East is often seen as condescending and weak vis-à-vis the Western intrusion shaped by power and knowledge. Even within the indigenous traditions, one needs to probe what constitutes the indigenous and bring out the hitherto neglected local or specific flavours. This pedagogical weakness needs to be overcome and the theoretical frame has to be more diversified. It is the narratives of difference and exclusion which should have figured more extensively in the encounter discourse. The recent works by David Hardiman, Neshat Quaiser, J. S. Alter, Projit Bihari Mukharji, Madhulika Banerjee, and Madhuri Sharma are significant contributions in this direction.[36]

It needs, however, to be stressed that the colonial situation proved to be the background of a number of encounters, which often had moral and political dimensions. The emphasis on bacteriology and laboratories, as introduced in British India, appeared something as a moral force and this enabled it to maintain a distance from any alternative moral critique of its methods. There is no doubt that the indigenous non-European medical practices (if not theories) changed over the course of colonial/global encounters. To what extent the indigenous European practices were influenced calls for more research. To conclude with Schiebinger, 'what knowledge was picked up and what discarded, what knowledge was assimilated or transmuted... is an exciting area open for further exploration'.[37]

NOTES

1. Bandyopadhyaya (1996:162–297).
2. Armstrong (2002:5).
3. Ibid.
4. Foucault (1975).
5. Kiple (1993:45).
6. Worsley (1982:315).
7. Ibid.
8. Kiple, *op. cit.* (1993:48–50).
9. Ibid., pp. 48–50
10. Worsley, *op. cit.* (1982:316).

11. Bellemy and Pfister (1992:88).

12. Ibid., p. 91.

13. Basham (1976:18–43).

14. Meulenbeld (1995:1–9).

15. Worsley, *op.cit.* (1982:318).

16. Ibid., p. 320.

17. Ibid., pp. 341–2.

18. Pearson, 'The Thin End of the Wedge: Medical Relativities as a Paradigm of Early Modern Indian–European Relations, *Modern Asian Studies*, 29, 1, (1995:141–70).

19. Appadurai (1996).

20. Cook (2007).

21. Armstrong (1985:4).

22. In 1925, a British doctor in Madras lamented—'What they (Madras Government) really need is an altered scientific outlook, they need to understand the difference between metaphysical and positive knowledge, between the study of facts through the coloured glass of theological dogma and their study in the plain daylight of sciences...Western medicine has nothing to learn from than that it has not long ago learnt, classified, and standardized...now that medicine is a transferred subject under an Indian Minister, the latter has the last word is such decisions and his European colleagues are powerless'. Letter by R. H. Elliot, *British Medical Journal*, 25 October 1924.

23. The questions of reform and science within Unani have been discussed by Neshat Quaiser in the context of a 'critical anti-colonial public sphere'. See, Quaiser in Uma Das Gupta (ed.) (2011). Guy Attewell has argued that the Unani practitioners sometimes emulated colonial medical practices, such as sanitation or diagnostic technologies, but they were also careful to integrate them with the pre-existing categories. For more details, see, Attewell (2007:236–7).

24. The hegemony of the West was clearly visible after the revolt of 1857, when the Victorians sought to define India's 'difference' in accordance with scientific systems of knowing. But, as they constructed their 'India', the British had always to negotiate a disjuncture based on two contradictory paradigms, one insisting on the acknowledgement of similarity, the other insisting upon difference. For more details, see, Metcalf (1998:66–7).

25. The East-West interaction in the field of medicine can also be understood in terms of the trading operations of the English East India Company and Vereenighde Oostindische Companie in Asia and Africa. In 1588, only 15 per cent of drugs had come from outside Europe and by 1621, it had increased to 48 per cent, and by 1669, it had attained 70 per cent, the majority coming from India and the East Indies, with an import value of £6000. For more details, see, Bellemy and Pfister, *op.cit.* (1992:140).

26. Kavita Sivaramakrishnan has argued that in the early 20th century, *vaid* publicists, in the face of attacks launched by the doctors associated with the Indian Medical Services, argued that Ayurvedic learning was based on legitimate and rationalized tradition and on scholarly texts which dealt with the branches of physiology, pathology, and anatomy. Ayurvedic learning, according to the vaids was also based on theories such as Tridosha which were not outdated humoral theories but rivaled the Western germ theory. Thus, Ayurvedic knowledge was scientific and was in every way at par with Western medicine. For more details, see, Sivaramakrishnan (2006:136–40).

27. In 1920s, the Banaras Hindu University developed a medical course which had both Ayurveda and modern medicine. An American visitor was puzzled; he was told, 'When these are once installed, the principal said, the students will see how ridiculous Ayurvedic medicine is and it will die a natural death. If it were opposed it would occupy a martyr's place and be much more likely to continue'. Rockefeller Archive Centre, RG 12.1, Heiser Diaries (1925–6:423).

28. 'Any kind of hospital may be a great power for the Gospel if it has the right staff. Indians as well as Europeans, and of course it is equally true that the best equipped hospital may fail lamentably if the Christian sprit is not permeating its work'. National Library of Scotland, Acc. 7548, B55, Papers on Kamla Hospital, Burdwan (1938).

29. Rogers Papers, PP/ROG/C.18, Wellcome Trust, London.

30. S. K. Brown Papers, Minute dt. 23.12.1924, IOR/L/E/7/1150.

31. Note by J. N. Smith, Medical Advisor to Govt. of India, dt. 19.12.1924. IOR/L/E/7/1150.

32. *Bombay Samachar*, 24 August 1911, *Native Newspaper Reports*, No. 34 (1911:27–8).

33. Chetan Shah, 1876, 'Hakims are not so ignorant as doctors believe them to be', *Indian Medical Gazette*, April 1, pp. 95–6.

34. For more details, see, Branca (1977:2).

35. Bellemy and Pfister, *op.cit.* (1992:xviii–xx).

36. Hardiman (2009); Quaiser in B. Pati and Harrison (eds) (2001); Alter (2004); Mukharji (2009); Banerjee (2009); Sharma (2012).

37. Schiebinger, 'The European Colonial Science Complex', *ISIS*, 96, 1, (2005:52–5).

I

The Multiplicity of Domains

1 Probing History of Medicine and Public Health in India

A Study of Encounters at Multiple Sites[†]

DEEPAK KUMAR

Medical knowledge is at the centre of history of medicine and public health. It, basically, consists of systematic knowledge of body and its surroundings. Medicine is behaviour as well as cognition; it is in the everyday life of village apothecaries as well as in the lectures and experiments of professors. To this the social scientists have provided a new edge, that of critical contextualism. Ideas would be lame without context. Medical ideas and clinical interactions need to be viewed in a socio-historical context. During the civilizational progress, what medical knowledge was picked up and what was discarded, what knowledge was assimilated or transmuted, therefore, is an interesting and relevant area of research.

Diffusionist models of knowledge transmission have had a long sway. These were probably useful in the context of centre-periphery explanations. Recent scholarship has moved ahead. Transmission is no longer seen as emanating from a powerful centre. Now more attention is paid to the changes and adaptations that occur in the process. Adoption and adaptation are not always imposed or induced from above or outside; these can come from within and on their own.

[†] Originally published in *Indian Historical Review*, Vol. 34, No. 1, 2011, Copyright ©Indian Council of Historical Research, New Delhi. All rights reserved. Reproduced with the permission of the copyright holders and the publishers, Sage Publications India Pvt. Ltd, New Delhi.

As post-colonial theorists argue, these could be both multi-sited and hybrid. To quote a contemporary critique—

> A postcolonial perspective suggests fresh ways to study the changing po-
> litical economies of capitalism and science, the mutual reorganisation of
> the global and the local, the increasing trans-national traffic of people,
> practices, technologies, and contemporary contests over 'intellectual
> property'.[1]

What could be the nature of post-colonial histories of medicine? Should it focus on 'decentred diasporic or global rewriting' of earlier 'nation-centred imperial grand narratives'? There is no doubt that we need multi-sited histories of medicine as Sigerist had argued in the 1930s and as Warwick Anderson does now. Here it is important to emphasize the value of 'dialogues' and 'conversations'. But these alone do not explain knowledge 'production' or 'dissemination'. It is much more complex a process. It could be socio-cultural as well as politico-economic. 'Dialogues' or 'negotiations' do not negate the equation of power. Analyses do not always lead to synthesis; similarly negotiation does not necessarily mean integration. Domination and marginalization lurk in the background and mostly appear as the two sides of the same coin.

To illustrate the above arguments, this chapter would focus on the examples from India's medical tradition and the challenges it faced when modern medical system entered the country as colonial luggage. Though the Indian society has always been 'knowledge-oriented', and never a xenophobic one, it seldom saw paradigmatic changes. Here, knowledge revolved round canonical texts and advanced, albeit slowly, through commentaries and discussions. *Ayurveda* as 'science of (living to a ripe) age' originated in a magico-religious milieu but gradually progressed with Buddhist rationalism.[2] Its protagonist might have been inaccurate in their knowledge of human physiology but they were extremely good at plant morphology, its medical functions, and therapeutics.[3]

MEDICINE IN PRE-COLONIAL INDIA

The canonical texts like the *Samhita*s of *Charak* and *Sushruta* were there to guide but knowledge advanced through commentaries and even replications.[4] In the deep South, the *Siddha*s (a Tamil variant of Ayurveda) had developed knowledge of pulse and methods of diagnosis by eight kinds of clinical examination.[5] By the end of the 13th century, thanks to the works of Chakrapanidata, Vangasena, and Sarangdhara, a new change had come in the shape of the blending of Ayurveda and *Rasashastra* (medicine and alchemy). These developments have been mostly internal but the possibilities of external influences from other cultures can not be ruled out.[6] But unfortunately these texts and later commentaries have no anatomical or surgical illustration.[7] Dissection became a taboo and knowledge became secretive, confined to one's own son or the Brahmanas. *Todarananda* (a 16th century encyclopaedic work), for example, says that *rasavidya* (alchemy) is to be kept 'as secret as mother's genitals'.[8] Even mineral classification reflected the caste divisions. For example, the diamonds are described as of four types, Brahmana, Kshatriya, Vaisya, and Sudra; they are also male, female, or *napunsaka* (the third gender).[9] The *Anandakanda* (The Root of Bliss) encompasses almost the entire Hindu alchemical tradition in six thousand verses. It is the sole attempt to fuse *rasa siddhas* (alchemists) with the *nath siddhas* (spiritual tantrics/yogis).[10]

Apart from attempts for synthesization, there may be some examples of total repudiation or departure. Dominik Wujastyk has recently brought to notice one such rare example, a text titled *Rogarogvada* (Debate on Illness and Health) composed by Viresvara in 1669. This text explains systematically the principal theories of Ayurveda and then refutes them one by one. For example, the authorities define disease as identical to an inequality in the humors and yet they accept that the humors may naturally exist in different quantities without causing illness. Phlegm predominates at the start of the day or after a meal but one is not always ill after a meal! And so the central doctrine that humoral imbalance is identical with disease must be wrong.[11] Thereafter, Viresvara gives a curious explanation; diseases come and go for no apparent reason. Just like the rising and setting of stars, disease is the pain of the mind, body, or sense organs and it arises for no reason. This explanation may appear quixotic but it is nevertheless offered in 'a spirit of intellectual rigour and debate which speaks of an original if impulsive mind'.[12]

The scenario becomes even more interesting when the Islamic medical men introduced the Galenic tradition. There gradually appeared a hybrid of Muslim-Hindu system known as the *Tibb*. They differed in theory, but in practice both traditions seem to have interacted and borrowed from each other. A fine example of this interaction is *Ma'din al-shifa-I-Sikan-darshahi* AD 1512, which was authored by Miyan Bhuwah.[13] He leaned heavily on the Sanskrit sources and even thought that the Greek system was not suitable for the Indian constitution and climate. From the Islamic side, the concept of *arka* (distillation) entered Ayurveda. Several Sanskrit medical texts were translated into Arabic and Persian, but instances of Islamic works being translated into Sanskrit are rare. The 18th century is significant because of the appearance of two Sanskrit texts *Hikmatprakasa* and *Hikmatparadipa* which refer to the Islamic system and use numerous Arabic and Persian medical terms.[14] The concept of individual case studies and hospitals (*bimaristans*) also came from the *Unani* practitioners.[15] In 1595, Quli Shah had built a huge *Dar-us-Shifa* (House of Cures) in Hyderabad.[16] During the reign of Muhammad Shah (1719–48) a large hospital was constructed in Delhi, and its annual expenditure was more than Rs 300,000. Numerous medical texts, mostly commentaries, were written during this century, for example, Akbar Arzani's *Tibb-I-Akbari* (1700), Jafar Yar Khan's *Talim-I-Ilaj* (1719–25), Madhava's *Ayurveda Prakasha* (1734), and *Bhaisajya Ratnavali* of Govind Das. A Christian Mughal, Dominic Gregory, wrote *Tuhafatul-Masiha* (1749), which, along with the descriptions of diseases, anatomy, and surgery, contains important notes in Persian and Portuguese on alchemy and the properties of various plants, along with drawings of instruments, and interestingly, a horoscope.[17] An outstanding physician of this century, Mirza Alavi Khan, wrote seven texts of which *Jami-ul-Jawami* is a masterpiece embodying all the branches of medicine then known in India.[18] Another great physician during the period of Shah Alam II (1759–1806) was Hakim Sharif Khan who wrote ten important texts and enriched unani medicines and indigenous Ayurvedic herbs.[19] Some works were unique and ahead of their time. For example, Nurul Haq's *Ainul-Hayat* (1691) is a rare Persian text on plague, and Pandit Mahadeva's *Rajsimhasudhasindhu* (1787) refers to cowpox and inoculation.[20]

Caravans of men and streams of thought constantly moved and flowed between India, Iran, and Central Asia resulting in intimate cultural relations. The Mughal court patronized notable hakims. Shams-al-din-Gilani was *Hakim al-Mulk* during Akbar's reign (1556–1605), Abul Qasim under Jehangir (1605–27), Mir Muhammad Hashim during Aurangzeb's period (1658–1707) and Mir Muhammad Jafar under Muhammad Shah (1719–48). Hakim Gilani had authored the famous commentary (4 volumes) in Arabic on Ibn Sina' *Qanun* called *Sharh-I-Gilani*.[21] As for the Mughal translations and compositions, a recent critic says—

there is a pathos in their efforts and waste in their labours. The system of medicine on which they spent hours and hours translating and transcribing was already dying and outdated. Discoveries were being made everyday which rendered their views obsolete. Had they looked outside their circle, had they listened to the strangers who were coming to their country in such large numbers, they could have learnt that their physiology had been proved by practical experiment to be full of error, that their pathology was being overturned by such new inventions as the microscope and the test tube, and that most of their anatomy was pure imagination...[22]

A number of European physicians visited Mughal India. Francois Bernier, Niocolao Manucci, Garcia d'Orta, and John Ovington wrote extensively on Indian medical practices. The Western medical episteme was not radically different from that of Indian physicians; both were humoral, but their practices differed greatly. Neither of them was able to develop a comprehensive theory of disease causation, but there seems to be a general agreement that the Indian diseases were environmentally determined and should be treated by Indian methods. Europeans, however, continued to look at the Indian practices with curiosity and disdain.[23] They preferred bloodletting whereas the *vaidyas* prescribed urine analysis and urine therapy. But in the use of drugs, Europeans and Indians learned from each other, as the works of van Rheede, Sassetti, and d'Orta would testify.[24] The Europeans introduced new plants in India that were gradually incorporated into the Indian pharmacopoeia. They had brought venereal diseases such as syphilis which was noticed as early as the 16th century by Bhava Misra, a noted vaidya in Benaras, who called it *Firangi roga* (disease of the Europeans). Indian diseases received graphic description in Ovington's travelogue.[25] The best account of smallpox and the Indian method of variolation was given by J. Z. Holwell in 1767. To him, this method although quasi-religious, still appeared 'rational enough and well-founded'.[26] The travellers depicted Indian medical practices more as a craft and one that was governed by caste rules and wrapped in superstition. Yet, they could not help admiring the wonder called rhinoplasty (on which modern plastic surgery is founded), nor could they deny the efficacy of Indian drugs. The Indians on their part did not completely insulate themselves from the 'other' practices. This was reflected in a 19th century text *Brhannighanturatnakara*. Other examples of the impact of the West on the Indian nosology are Govindadasa's *Bhaisajyaratnavali* (18th century) and Binod Lal Sen's

Ayurvedavijnana (19th century). This reference to Ayurveda as *vijnana* (science) is significant. As the interaction grew in the 18th century, the vaidyas even took to bleeding in a large number of cases. Yet, while the European medical men were gradually moving, thanks to the works of Vesalius and Harvey, from a humoral to a chemical or mechanical view of the body, Indians remained faithful to their texts. Asia kept doing what it had been doing for centuries; Europe changed basically.[27]

THE COLONIAL WATERSHED

As for the use of the prefix colonial, post-colonial theorists and diaspora scholars have tried to challenge, even reject, the binary division between the colonizer and the colonized. A recent work talks of the 'tensions of empire' based on the universalizing claims of European ideology and the limitation faced by the rulers.[28] This is smart subterfuge. The meaning of 'colonial' is neither elusive nor shifting. What makes colonization real is that even in its rejection there is an implicit acceptance of the standards set by the colonizer. By arguing that the colonial power and discourse is shared by both the colonizer and the colonized, and by putting emphasis on 'ambivalence' and 'indeterminacy' in this relationship, are the post-colonial critics trying to take the (political and economic) sting out of colonialism?[29]

Western medical discourse functioned in several ways—as an instrument of control which would swing between coercion and persuasion, as the exigencies demanded, and as a site for interaction and often resistance. This discourse was mediated not only by consideration of political economy but also by several other factors. Polity, biology, ecology, the circumstances of material life, and new knowledge interacted and produced this discourse. The emergence of tropical medicine at the turn of the last century may to be seen in this light. It may be argued that tropical medicine itself was a cultural construct, 'the scientific step child of colonial domination and control'.[30] In now burgeoning literature, terms like tropical medicine, imperial medicine, and colonial medicine have often been used interchangeably. But they have specific connotations. Tropical medicine and imperial medicine emphasize the tropics and the empire as units of analysis while colonial medicine stresses the colony. Each may attract different sets of questions. In tropical medicine what ought to be the determining factor—climate, race, geography, or all taken together? What was carried over from the old medicine of tropical civilizations into the new tropical medicine? What attempts were made outside Europe to reconcile the older discourse of body humors and environmental miasmas with the new language of microbes and germs? Interestingly enough, a medical historian described colonialism as 'literally a health hazard'.[31] But to dismiss the colonial doctors reductively as the handmaidens of colonialism or capitalism would also be to ignore a more complex, and more interesting, reality.[32] The doctors had to assume multiple roles. They had little choice. Still one can ask, what role did the 'peripherals' play? Could a synergetic relationship between the core and the periphery develop? These questions assume special significance when viewed against the four centuries of European's struggles in the 'torrid zones' and their transition from early explorers, travellers, and traders to conquerors and ultimate arbiters of the trampled tropics. Earlier, the 'tropical discourse' was viewed through its pioneers; now issues and dichotomies have been given primacy. However, these still abound in metropolitan theorizations and do not include the study of indigenous (non-settler) societies through their own literature and practitioners.

From the Indian point of view, the mid-19th century was a period of looking for fresh opportunities and acquiring new knowledge. Syncretism, not revivalism, was the agenda. Even among the British officials there were some who wanted the government to attempt a fusion of 'both exotic principles and local practices, European theory, and Indian experience', and thereby 'revive, invigorate, enlighten, and liberalize the native medical profession in the mofussil'. Similar views were echoed by the emerging Indian intelligentsia in ample measure. To illustrate, we cite three relatively less known (though important) Indians from the three presidency areas—Raja Serfoji (1798–1832, Tanjore), B. G. Jambhekar (1802–46, Bombay) and S. C. G. Chuckerbutty (1826–74, Calcutta).

Raja Serfoji, the last Maratha ruler of Tanjore, having surrendered real power to the British Resident, spent his time in the pursuit of knowledge. Father Schwartz, a German missionary, was his friend, philosopher, and guide. Fascinated by the different medical system, he had opened an institution for research in medical science and called it the Dhanvantri Mahal (abode of Lord Dhanvantri, the God of medicine). He assembled leading physicians there from the Ayurvedic, Yunani, Siddha, and Western systems. As a result of their interactions and investigations, the best among the tried and effective remedies were collected in a series of works named *Sarabendra Vaidya Muraiga*.[33] These were composed by the court poet in Tamil verse to facilitate easy memorizing and popularization. With the help of Father Schwartz and the British Resident, Serfoji procured hundreds of European medical books and even surgical instruments. He already had a large collection of Tamil and Sanskrit manuscripts. Some of them dealt with diseases of animals and even birds. Ahead of his time, Serfoji also organized a hand-painted herbarium of medicinal plants in natural colours.[34] In the eye wing of his Dhanvantri Mahal, he maintained a set of ophthalmic case sheets in an album, with authentic pictures of the eye and its defects for research purposes. This is perhaps a very early example of 'methodical clinical research' under 'native' patronage, and must have induced the traditional physicians to take cognizance of the new therapies and methods.

Serforji was not an intellectual. He was a man of resources with a genuine interest in medicine, perhaps a self-taught doctor; he is said to have learnt the art of cataract removal. In contrast, Bal Gangadhar Jambhekar was the first Indian to teach mathematics at the Elphinstone College in Bombay. He was also perhaps the first Indian to start a journal for popularizing science (*Bombay Durpan* in 1831) and established the Native Education Society, which later did a commendable job of translating some European works into Marathi and Sanskrit works (like the nosology of Madhav and the anatomy of Susrut) into English. He wanted the native practitioners to improve by studying 'anatomy from the natural subject', even though touching a dead body was taboo at the time.[35] In 1837, his opinion was sought by the Bombay government on the desirability of a medical school in Bombay and the nature of medical education to be given to the natives. In a written reply, Jambhekar asked for (*a*) the education of a limited number of natives in all branches of the science, and (*b*) the dissemination of the elements of medical knowledge among the vaidyas, hakims, and the community of the interior in general through the means of local languages.[36] This dissemination was to be achieved through translations or writing synthetic books specifically for the purpose. Ordinary vaidyas and hakims, he felt, would respond better than the more 'learned' native practitioners, as the latter were quite convinced of their own superiority and were unlikely to compromise their status. Jambhekar wanted the government to go slowly, without ruffling feelings, and be 'as little offensive as possible'. He argued that the repugnance of the Brahmans at dissection, and so on, could be overcome 'by a little perseverance'.[37] How right he was!

S. C. Chuckerbutty came from a Brahman family. He graduated from Calcutta Medical College and was one of the first four Indian medical graduates sent to England for higher studies, in 1945. He was so much charmed by Western values and people that he even embraced Christianity before leaving for England, and put his teacher's name before his surname (he became Soorjo Coomar Goodeve Chuckerbutty). Later, he pronounced 'a day in London' of more value than 'a month in Calcutta'.[38] True to his training, he lambasted indigenous practitioners—'Every Boydo (vaidya) was a born Koberaj (physician)... To suppose that a Boydo could not be a physician unless he passed an examination was to question the ruling of Manu (an ancient law-giver)'.[39] He was not in favour of medical education through Sanskrit or Arabic. He called it 'oriental mania'. But Chuckerbutty's perceptions later changed. He came to support the vernacular medium fully and criticized Calcutta University for representing 'only European opinion and interests' and ignoring 'the national element'.[40]

We have thus seen the views of a native chief, a cultural interlocutor, and a 'modern' doctor. The first was action-oriented, the second persuasive, and the third served the colonial state without being servile.[41] The emerging educated class showed great aptitude for change and new knowledge. But, not the traditional vaidyas. When Madhusudan Gupta dissected a dead body in 1835, a vaidya of high repute, Gangadhar Ray, is said to have left Calcutta in disgust.[42] The traditionalists were convinced that an alien government would not help them.[43] Earlier, the government had abolished medical classes at the Calcutta Madarsa and the Sanskrit College. Several thousand signatures were collected in protest.[44] But nothing could stop, or even dilute, the Anglicists' victory.

In average public esteem, however, the indigenous practitioners continued to hold sway. In Calcutta, Gangaprasad Sen and Neelamber Sen were extremely popular.[45] They introduced fixed consultation fees, priced medicine, the publication of sacred texts, and publicity through advertisements. Gangaprasad started the first Ayurvedic journal in Bengali, *Ayurveda Sanjivani*, and even exported Ayurvedic medicines to Europe and America.[46] These were the indications that certain European practices could be internalized and turned to the advantage of practitioners of indigenous medicine. Even at the conceptual level, the then reigning miasmatic theories and the humoral pathology (of the vaidyas and hakims) were not very incompatible. What the Westerners were averse to was the oriental 'process', not its substance. Almost all of them did recognize the importance of and later emphasized the use of indigenous drugs.[47] But diagnostic procedures and, of course, surgery were to remain major areas of difference for a long time to come.

The Ayurvedic texts written during the early 20th century show a large number of Sanskrit equivalents for terms borrowed from Western medicine, for example, *jivanu* (micro-organism), *samkranti* (transmission of contagious diseases), *svasyantra* (the respiratory tract), and so on. In his *Siddhantanidana*, Gananath Sen (1877–1945) refers to new types of fevers such as *antrikajvara* (enteric or typhoid fever), *granthikajvar* (plague or bubonic fever), *slesmakjvara* (influenza), *kalajvara* (kalazar, a disease).[48] Similar impact can be seen in P. S. Varier's *Astangsarira* which discusses modern anatomy and physiology in 2,045 Sanskrit verses.[49]

DEBATES ON PUBLIC HEALTH

Right from the late 19th century, questions relating to public health engaged both the official and public mind in India and the debates gradually became more intense in the wake of major cholera and plague epidemics. It ranged from assertions of imperial altruism to allegations of colonial callousness. The questions asked were—What was the nature of colonial medical intervention? Was it merely enclavist or could it transcend certain geo-cultural boundaries? How effective it was and what more could have been done? In the end, it left several questions unanswered and several quarters dissatisfied.

A recent work claims that 'supposedly colonial concepts like "public health" had indigenous sub-continental origin... the pre-colonial "scientific" notion of medicine, which was divorced from Persianate civility and which reached out to larger society, became in fact the base of the early British idea of public health'. It also argues that 'local medical patrons (hakims), along with Urdu print culture, played a critical role in sketching out the public welfare concerns of the British in nineteenth century India; indeed they helped crate a public health manifesto... this India-specific manifesto was exported to England to handle the cholera epidemic of the 1830s'.[50]

It is true that local practitioners of all hues saw health as part of public cleanliness and personal hygiene. Next to divine will, diseases were attributed to atmospheric pollutants. The medical reports and works by Ainslie, Moorcroft, Jameson, Corbyn, and so on, were no doubt significant as they did not ignore the 'native' medical opinion. But to claim that there appeared a 'public-health manifesto' is little romantic. India produced no Chadwick. It is good to look beyond the binaries of colonial and national histories. But such flights are very often lean on sources and strong on imagination!

Public health usually refers to organized efforts made under the direction of medical experts for preventing disease and improving the health of the people. Decades before public health moved public opinion, socio-medical activities had called for strong sanitary measures, even a sanitary despotism.[51] This gave birth to the concept of 'sanitary engineering' which gradually developed to denote 'environmental health' rather than the limited original concept of 'plumbing'.[52] Environmental health included not only water, sewage, refuge, and so on, but also equally important subjects like ventilations, lighting, safety, housing, town-planning, and rural sanitation. The concept of public health had thus become virtually all-embracing. To quote an important Rockefeller functionary in India, J. B. Grant—

> Public Health is the science and art of social utilisation of scientific knowledge for medical protection by maintaining health, preventing disease, and curing disease through organised community efforts for (a) the hygiene of the environment, (b) the control of the community infections, (c) the education of the individual in principles of personal hygiene, (d) the organisation of medical and nursing service for the early diagnosis and preventive treatment of disease, and (e) the development of social machinery which will ensure to every individual in the community a standard of living adequate for the maintenance of health. As such public health becomes social medicine and is primarily a field of social activity, applying practically every basic science directed towards a comprehensive programme of community service.[53]

Contemporary medical opinion, however, had different perceptions. Some thought excessive reliance on medical intervention as 'one-sided' and 'dangerous'. For example, J. D. Megaw, who in the early 1930s was the Director General of the Indian Medical Service (IMS) argued—

> Suppose for a moment that the public health services of India were to achieve complete success in stamping out malaria, cholera, small-pox, tuberculosis, and all other great killing diseases of India, and suppose that nothing was done to increase the production of food or to restrict

the growth of population, the inevitable result would be the replacement of the tragedy of death from disease by the greater tragedy of death from starvation.[54]

Medical intervention was thus clearly no panacea. But at the same time, many thought that the control of disease would promptly raise the standards of life and would gradually induce decline in fertility. Yet in the final analysis the situation in India was always found too dismal to warrant such optimism. So the standard official argument would be that public health does not depend only on the control of preventable disease but also on the state of nutrition and general economic conditions. To quote Megaw again, 'a public health policy must be worked out in terms of agricultural and industrial production; it must look ahead and take into account the maintenance of a proper relation between the number of the people and the available supply of the necessities of life'.[55] This indeed was a tall order. The colonial government had neither the intention nor the wherewithal. To the growing demands for greater indigenization of the services, the government responded with a retrenchment policy (vide Inchape Committee Report, 1923). To this were later added severe economy measures in the wake of the Great Depression. Agriculture and public health were obviously the early casualties.

There was a genuine hope that with the spread of education, sanitary consciousness would grow which would gradually force the local bodies and provincial governments to act. But this did not happen. As an American doctor reporting on cholera in India in 1890 wrote, 'youth who will recite Shakespeare and Milton and quote Bentham and J. S. Mill, are ignorant of the first principles of their existence, viz. that pure air and pure water are essential to the maintenance of life'.[56] Well, this tradition (of blaming the other) continued well beyond Katherine Mayo![57] A highly influential IMS regretted, 'the people multiply like rabbits and die like flies'.[58] Many sincerely believed that the European sanitary standards were 'simply above the comprehension of the majority of the natives, whether high or low born'.[59] The problem was no doubt real. Other than evil spirits and goddesses, strange explanations were given. An Indian publicist attributed cholera to the 'alternate blowing of the east and west wind' and smallpox to the 'hailstorm'![60] Many, including the erudite ones, expressed helplessness.[61] Granted that even the high caste and educated Indians lacked 'sanitary conscience',[62] did the Government have it?

SOME LESSONS

Public health has been on the agenda for long. It called for radical changes which no alien government could have risked. In early years, it meant health of the Europeans only and was confined to their housing, ventilation, and so on.[63] Later, public health remained limited to compilation of rather inaccurate vital statistics, vaccination, segregation, and the like. Even these were so wired in government machinery and 'so hopelessly tied in bureaucratic knots' that, as one foreign observer wrote, 'one doubts whether untangling can ever occur and the only hope is for a completely new system'.[64] Not even independence could meet this hope! So why blame the British? It would probably be as wrong as they blaming the poor Indians for all ills. Gandhi was one of the few to provide self-criticism. 'Poverty is no bar to sanitation', he said, while acknowledging that 'chronic poverty and chronic breach of the laws of sanitation are equally to blame for diseases'.[65] As a recent critique notes, 'the solutions offered by Gandhi are deceptively simple in their statement, impeccable in their logic, yet frustratingly difficult to implement'.[66] Still Gandhi was persuasive. On the other hand, the British were tongue-tied, if not aloof or hostile. The real onslaught came from an American publicist, Miss Mayo. She 'meant well'[67] but lacked empathy and cut deep—

> If the celler is full of sewage, if its water supply is poisonous, if the residents are magazines of infection, and if their common habits or domestic relations scandalize me, I am but little affected by whatever virtues may offset these points, or whatever beauty the façade may show. .
>
> My belief is that the wide-spread, the less sparing, the most direct the criticism is, throughout out west, the better it will be for the people of India. They *care* what we *think*. They wince under our disapprobation. The hope is that power will be lashing enough to drive them to act.[68]

Possibilities for improvement were enormous. Examples and suggestions poured but where was the will? Pilgrims to Mecca from Egypt and Indonesia were compulsorily vaccinated against smallpox and cholera. This was held impossible in India.[69] Rogers' suggestion to inoculate the pilgrims going to Prayag Kumbh was considered by the Pilgrim Committee as 'impracticable, inexpedient, and even dangerous'.[70] Enlightened native states like Baroda, Mysore, and Travancore were more open to new ideas and fared better. Mysore was probably the first state in the world to open in 1930 a birth control clinic.[71] In 1935, a

Society for a Study and Promotion of Family Hygiene was formed in Bombay. Later, the National Planning Committee of the Indian National Congress included in its programme separate studies on population and health.[72] Social workers and nationalist leaders knew the enormity of the task.

Notwithstanding the enormous difficulties, medicine did emerge as a nationalist issue in India. Even at the height of colonial power, voices against the dominant medical discourse were heard. The indigenous practitioners vehemently denied that their system was unscientific or irrational, yet they did not see anything wrong in learning and benefiting from the new knowledge. Their emphasis was on reforming the system by adopting 'scientific' method and not on changing the fundamentals of the system. A 'critical anti-colonial spirit', as argued by Neshat Quaiser, permeated the indigenous response. To quote a verse from a hakeem in 1910—

Kuch-ilaj Aya na Kuch Charagiri Ayee:
Tibb-e-Unan Ke Munh Doctory Ayee:
Band Sheeshe Mein Vilayat se Pari Ayee:
Lal-Peeli Hui, Gusse mein Bhari Ayee:
Chaman-e-Tibb se Guldasta Uda Kar Layee:
Nayee Tarkeeb se Bandish Saja Kar Layee.

(Knows no method of treatment, but Doctors dared to challenge Unani. In a closed bottle a fairy has come full of anger from foreign lands. The bouquet stolen from the garden of Unani Tibb has been rearranged in a new fashion).[73]

There were several areas in which the Western and indigenous systems could collaborate but did not. The former put emphasis on the cause of the disease, the latter on *nidana* (treatment). Microbes and microscopes constituted the new medical spectacle.[74] But the vaidyas put emphasis on the power of resistance in the human body. The Westerners were forced to take cognizance of indigenous drugs and the vaidyas took to anatomy, ready delivery of medicine, quick relief, and so forth (as in case with P. S. Varier, 1869–1958 and Hakim Ajmal Khan, 1868–1927). But the comparison ends there. As a recent critique argues, 'they were inclined to borrow but could not create a dialogue between the two epistemics'.[75] Borrowed knowledge seldom develops into organic knowledge.

NOTES

1. Anderson (2002:643–58).
2. Wujastyk (1998:1–38).
3. Majumdar (1935–6:633–54).
4. Meulenbeld (1995:1–10).
5. C. K. Sampath in Subramanian and Madhavan (eds) (1983:1–20).
6. Fascination with alchemy, for example, most probably arose out of early contacts with China where Taoist speculative alchemical tradition had been developing since the second century AD (White 2004:53).
7. Wujastyk (2003:21).
8. Meulenbeld (1999–2000:278).
9. Ibid., p. 286.
10. White, *op. cit.*, 167, Note 6.
11. Wujastyk (2004:6–7).
12. Ibid.
13. The manuscript was first printed by Nawal Kishore Press, Lucknow, in 1877.
14. So is Krishnarama's *Siddhabhesajamanimala* of the 19th century. Meulenbeld, *op. cit.*, 1–9, Note 4.
15. Askari (1957:7–21).
16. Subba Reddy (1957:102–5).
17. Rahman (1982:57).
18. R. L. Verma and N. H. Keswani in Keswani (ed.) (1974: 127–42).
19. Hameed (1986:41).
20. Rahman, *op.cit.*, 129, 165, Note 17.
21. Hameed, *op.cit.*, Note 19.
22. Elgood (1970:88).
23. A European traveller, Edward Ives (1755–7) thus writes of the Indian belief that 'man was divided into two or three hundred thousand part; ten thousand of which were made up of veins, ten thousand of nerves; seventeen thousand of blood, and a certain number of bones, choler, lymph, etc. and all this was laid down without form or order, either of history, disease or treatment'. Quoted in Kaul (1979:299).
24. For details see de Figueredo (1984:225–35).
25. Neelmeghan (1962:12–21).
26. J.Z.Holwell, 1767, *An account of the manner of inoculating for the small pox in the East Indies*, London, p. 24.
27. Pearson (1995:141–70).
28. Cooper and Stoler (eds) (1997).
29. See, Deepak Kumar (1995:180–2); also, Cunningham and Andrews (eds) (1997:172–88).

30. Manderson (1996:10–14).

31. Denoon (1989:52).

32. Bell (1999:10).

33. Rao (1977:I–IV). Numerous books, instruments, and medical case sheets survive as the Modi Raj Records at Saraswati Mahal Library, Thanjavur.

34. R. Venkatraman, 'The impact of modern science on a Tamil traditional system in the eighteenth and nineteenth centuries'. Paper sent to Seminar on Science and Empire, New Delhi, January 1985.

35. *The Bombay Durpan*, 9 January (1835:119–20).

36. Home, Public, No. 18, K.W. Pt. A, 18 July 1838, preserved at National Archive of India (NAI).

37. Ibid.

38. S.C.G. Chuckerbutty, 1870, *Popular Lectures of Subjects of Indian Interest*, Calcutta, p. 56.

39. 'Lecture on the present state of the medical profession in India', dated 2 February 1864. Ibid., p. 138.

40. Lecture on the necessity of forming a Medical Association in Bengal', dated 27 May 1863. Ibid., p. 135.

41. Chuckerbutty may have been uncomfortable with the government. Later, his professorship of *materia medica* was lumped with medical storekeeping and his salary was temporarily stopped. General, Medical, No. 30, June 1867, West Bengal State Archive.

42. B. Gupta in Leslie (ed.) (1977:371).

43. Mukhopadhyay (1923:18).

44. Home, Public, No. 9, 13 March 1835, and Nos. 44–5, 8 April 1835 (NAI).

45. Chuckerbutty records that one of his serious patients asked for Neelamber Sen. When the vaidya arrived people lined up to see him. The patient could not be saved but the day and hour of death foretold by the vaidya proved to be correct. Chuckerbutty, *Popular Lectures*: 139.

46. Gupta, 'Indigenous medicine' *op. cit.*, 372–3, Note 42.

47. W. B. O'Shaughnessy (Professor of Chemistry, Calcutta Medical College, 1835–49) compiled a *Bengal Pharmacopoeia* to facilitate greater use of locally available drug materials and reduce expensive imports from Europe. Later, Dr. Waring published the *Pharmacopoeia of India* in 1868.

48. Meulenbeld, *A History of Indian Medical Literature*, op.cit., 402–04, Note 8.

49. Ibid., p. 377.

50. Alavi (2007:7–8).

51. Cunningham (1888:241–65).

52. J. B. Grant, Director, AIIHPH, to DG, IMS, dt. 26 September 1939, Rockefeller Archive Centre (RAC), IHB, 1.1, 464, B. 6 F. 40.

53. General Address by J. B. Grant on 6 January 1940 at the Indian Science Congress, Madras, printed in *Science and Culture*, 1940, VI(8): 480–6.

54. D. J. Megaw in E. Blunt (ed.) (1938:186).

55. Ibid.

56. E.O.Shakespeare, 1890, *Report on Cholea in Europe and India*, Govt. Press, Washington, p. 391.

57. Katherine Mayo, *Mother India*, Jonathan Cape, London, 1927. This book created a storm and had seven reprints in the very first year of its publication. For an equally sharp rejoinder, see Ranga Iyer (1927).

58. J. D. Megaw to W. S. Carter, 29 October 1928, IHD, 1.1, 464, Box 5, f. 34, RAC.

59. As an example, 'The old bearer who was told to boil the drinking water did so religiously everyday but added a similar quantity of dirty water to it so that it would be sooner ready for the memsahib to drink!' J. C. Hume Papers, GEN 2004, file H-20, Edinburgh University Library.

60. Lall, 1896:III–V. This author was no doctor but President of Kurmi Sadar Sabha, a caste organization.

61. 'I can not imagine how people can keep going at all in such difficult and wretched conditions. In every household people are plagued by rheumatism; their legs swell up; they catch colds and fevers; sick children howl and wail incessantly – nothing can save them, and one by one they die'. Rabindranath Tagore to Indira Devi, 20 September 1894, *Chinnapatrabali* no. 153, in *Selected Short Stories*, tr. W. Radice, Penguin, New Delhi, 1991, 286.

62. J. Kendrick to W. Rose, 14 June 1921, IHB, 5/1.2/Corres/Box 123, f. 1633–34, RAC.

63. Butler (1829:121–56).

64. Diary of J. B. Grant, March 1940, R.G. 12.1 RAC.

65. *Harijan*, 8 February 1947, quoted in Amit Mishra in Kumar (ed.) (2001:249–64).

66. Ibid.

67. Mirza (1954:152).

68. Miss Mayo to Miss E. Rathbone, n.d. (perhaps Nov. 1927), Cornelia Sorabjee Papers, MSS. Eur. F. 165/161, India Office Records, London.

69. J. D. Graham, Health Commissioner to Govt. of India, to L. Rogers, 3 March 1927, Rogers Papers, PP/ROG. C10/69, Wellcome Institute, London.

70. Ibid., C.10/3–4.

71. Family Planning Association Papers, FPA, Box 419, A21/10–11, Wellcome Institute, London.

72. J. N. Sinha in Kumar (ed.) (1991:161–81).

73. Jogi Dakani, quoted in Quaiser (2000:29–42).

74. Anderson (1992:506–29).

75. Panikkar (1992:283–307).

2 Anatomical Knowledge and East-West Exchange

Brothers, there is where our power lies...the real arbiters of the great body politic of society. And think of the social power we even now wield...The people will demand this and the law will give it; we have only to stay awake and be aggressive...Could we ask for firmer standing ground or a longer lever with which to move the world?[1]

> Edgar J. Sprtling, 1902. [Read before the Medical Association of Georgia at its Fifty-third Annual Meeting, Savannah, April, 1902.]

The quoted remark perhaps epitomizes the authority prerogative and social power a professionalized medical practice exerts over society. Its journey unfolds a long tortuous path before us. We would try to understand the contours of its interactions with other medical traditions like Āyurveda. Our primary concern is how exchange of anatomical knowledge between India and Europe occurred and at what levels, during colonial medical encounters.

In European context, Charles V's illness is closely linked with many European countries. He is known to have suffered from 'attacks of gout'. His doctors put him on a severe diet and prescribed purgatives, bed rest for five days, and application of warmth to his legs. After another severe injury, he had to swallow his food in large quantities of Rhine wine and beer. 'Surely, this cannot have been beneficial for the gout attacks!' Authors comment, 'With our modern knowledge of medicine and rheumatology, in particular, we can only speculate on some possible diagnoses...'[2]

Another study of the same case has confirmed the 'probable' case of gout to be the real one. In this study, the only specimen researchers found was the final phalanx of the fifth finger of one of the hands (laterality unknown). A radiographic study was performed. The chemical constitution of the deposits and histologic analyses were analysed by most modern techniques. Researchers assert, 'In addition to biologic confirmation of the *clinical* suspicion of gout, our study also demonstrates the extreme severity of arthritic disease...and how paleopathological studies can provide important information leading to an increased understanding of *history*'.[3] While the former account reveals the history of the Emperor's illness, the later scrutinizes it in the light of modern techniques—it rewrites the history of illness from 'clinical suspicion' to organ localization and diagnosis of the disease. In the first account, it was 'illness narratives' or symptoms revealed to the doctors and making the diagnosis possible. Spatialization of disease was two-dimensional—**symptoms > diagnosis**. The appearance—the symptoms and the signs or verbal testimonies— were sufficient to unravel and differentiate diseases completely; be it aetiologically, epidemiologically, or therapeutically.[4]

In the second, the body is three-dimensional—**symptom > illness > sign**. Disease is located inside the body—in its phalanges, tissues, and bones. They are the signs (the third dimension of the body) to be extracted by doctor. During the 18th–19th centuries, gross anatomy held an intellectual centrality to Western medical science, surpassing anything it enjoyed before or since. Science meant empiricism, epitomized by systematic empirical correlation of symptoms observed at the bedside with lesions found at autopsy. Robert Aronowitz wryly comments, 'This description of progress is not only debatable on its own merits but is also a tautology – molecular research leads to molecular insights than nonmolecular research...and suggest that our formal systems of medical discourse systematically exclude certain categories of knowledge and speculation'.[5]

British people's own biomedical identity was conceptualized within a global context, as part of their own response to the experience of colonial disease. Medical encounters between the two different world views were informed by a dialogue between cultures rather than only imposed by the British or hailed by the 'colonized'. It occurred in an asymmetrically overdetermined space inscribed by unequal and asymmetric translations of meaning. These inequalities were retained in the hybrid interaction of conceptions of the body produced within modern Western medicine and Āyurveda. Arguably, 'the search for cultural legitimacy that characterized Indian science in the nineteenth and early twentieth centuries was displaced by an increasingly dominant discourse of scientific industrialism'.[6] Elsewhere, scholars find that technologies of the body are among the most expansive and intimate of technologies, and they lie, in the modern extra-European world, at a critical intersection between different cultural systems. Moreover, 'there is, after all, no more intimate site of identity than the body. What was the "European" body, and how was it produced and managed – particularly in relation to the "non-European" body?'[7]

To understand how Western knowledge and imagination became victorious 'presupposes a comprehension more deeply grounded in social and epistemological facts than we now possess of how Indian knowledge and imagination lost...'[8]

PREMISE OF EXCHANGE

Metcalf observes, 'The Victorians set out...to order and classify India's "difference" in accordance with scientific systems of "knowing"'.[9] For this purpose, the Raj set out to the production of empirically verifiable knowledge of unknown Indian territories (or space) as part of a larger positivist enterprise. Though, after the revolt of 1857, throughout the later 19th century, 'as they constructed their "India", the British had always to negotiate between a disjuncture: between an acknowledgement of similarity, and an insistence upon difference'.[10] It was, as if, imagined places, they served only, to reflect Europe's gaze back upon itself. The taxonomies of natural history, by constructing secularized and hierarchical notions of the 'modern', and the 'civilized', inevitably emphasized at once the difference, and the inferiority, of non-European societies. The very notions of modernity and civilization were redefined and reconstituted within the metaphor of science. Again, Bengal has its special importance because of the fact 'in climate, as in so much else, what the British called "India" was in fact shaped by their experience in Bengal, the area they knew best'.[11]

Deepak Kumar asks, 'Could a synergetic relationship develop between the core and the periphery?' In his opinion, 'In the scenario of complete homogenization, the possibilities of inter-cultural interactions were rather limited'.[12] How does one adhere to one's local identity while living in a dislocating colonial milieu? In the effort to moor oneself within one's local identity and cultural context, there were convergence, syncretization, and contestation. The reliability of knowledge 'constructed beyond the closed walls of learned societies—especially knowledge constructed out-side Europe—was acutely difficult to establish...'[13]

With this perspective, we shall now proceed to the question of medi-cine and anatomical knowledge in colonial India. 'The colonial discourse on medicine was mediated not only by consideration of political economy but also by several other factors. Polity, biology, ecology, the circum-stances of material life and new knowledge interacted and produced this discourse'.[14] Additionally, colonial scientists like Ronald Ross was more concerned with the financial rather than the humanitarian aspect of na-tional and imperial health.[15]

More on Exchange

Ideas *suit* purposes not because of any logical relationship, 'but because they are naturally suited to particular kinds of use within an existing system of beliefs and norms'.[16] Did encounters between knowledge systems of different origins, valences, hegemonic aspirations (for example, 'Western' medical technologies and non-European 'alternative medicine') produce different bodies? Scholars find that some of these local technologies have even found their way back to Europe, as aspects of the 'alternative medicine' movement show.[17]

To Qaisar, 'at estimating the response of one culture to another perhaps inevitably entails a study of the degree and pattern of contact between members of the concerned culture-groups'.[18] In Indian context, there were distinctly different responses to European technology and knowledge from heterogeneous Indian society.

John Fryer, the 17th century British physician, found '*Bengal* Jug-glers' to show magic 'by Suction or drawing of his Breath, so contracted his lower Belly...as by the most accurate Dissection could be made ap-parent'. He continued, 'The Aetiology whereof I think to be this; that while all the contents of the Belly are moved upwards, all Respiration is expelled, only the voluntary Motion of the Animal Spirits act upon the Nerves (the Mind or Soul commanding them) while the Vital or Natural are compelled to the contrary'.[19] Fryer used specific technical-scientific terms like 'suction', 'accurate dissection', or 'voluntary motion'. He also noted, 'In esteem among them are principally Magick and judicial As-trology...nor are they quite ignorant of Medicks, though Anatomy is not approved, wherein they lean too much on Tradition, being able to give a very slender account of the Rational Part thereof'.[20] In this observation, 'anatomy' confronts 'tradition' and near-absence of 'rational part'. Contrarily, extra-scientific puzzle, according to Fryer, pervaded Indian observation.

Seventeenth century saw the birth, among others, of scientific chemistry, the microscope, and the idea that disease might produce specific changes in the blood which could be detected and would be helpful in the management of the patient. In other words, clinical chemistry and pathological anatomy began to make long strides.[21] With the introduction of stethoscope by Laennec in 1816, medicine became more entrenched to organ-pathology and Linnean identification of 'disease', the two developments which became major contributions of the 19th century to Medicine.[22] Informed by these technological advancements and a different system of knowledge, the British came to conquer geographical territories as well as knowledge world of India.[23]

Indian attitude to European skill in medicine was different for different sections of people. While Indian physicians did not believe or admit that European doctors were properly acquainted with medicine, the masses held a different opinion. In an account of 1634—

> For those Barbarians hold that wherever a Portuguese goes good fortune and skill attend him. Indeed so general is this opinion in those regions, that as soon as any Frangui arrives at a place and it becomes known, they at once bring up their sick, all kinds of diseased persons coming to consult them and beg remedies and drugs for their ailments...[24]

It would perhaps be enough to mention that around 1800 one began to follow Bichat's (1770–1801) maxim 'open up a few corpses', as Foucault laconically remarks.[25] Illness and disease became not a matter of the whole body, but were located in body parts and their pathologies. Bichat taught, 'You may take notes for twenty years from morning to night at the bedside of the sick, and all will be to you only a confusion of symptoms...a train of incoherent phenomena. (But start cutting bodies open and, hey presto), this obscurity will soon disappear'.[26]

When two culture groups confront vis-à-vis, they face the barrier of language. It hinders a deep and meaningful process of mutual appreciation and cultural exchange. 'The British mode of living in India provided cultural blocks to their acquisition of knowledge beyond their problem with language'.[27] To surmount the problem, there was a deluge of translation of Indian texts. Resultantly, 'Seen as a corpus, these texts signal the invasion of an epistemological space occupied by a great number of diverse Indian scholars'.[28]

It may be summarized as—

(a) At the interface of two cultures exchanges occur at various levels with different responses.

(b) More powerful culture (with its political and economic background), operates through—(i) *interaction* (or, knowing the object), (ii) *assimilation* and *experimentation* (ontologically, knowing the nature of the object), (iii) *transformation* (reconstituting the object in a different environment), and (iv) *dissemination* (exporting it to its root—original cultural context—an epistemological question).

(c) In tandem, dislocation occurs at idioms of expression and understanding in both the cultures.[29] For example, while exploring Tropical medical space (including India) 'germ theory' was dislocated by the rise of parasitology, and, finally, giving rise to Tropical Medicine. Simultaneously, there was reconstruction of Āyurvedic knowledge of anatomy and it began to be read and interpreted in the light of modern medical or anatomical knowledge.

DISSECTION, HOSPITAL, AND COLONIAL MEDICINE

Arnold succinctly points to 'the role of physicians as colonial, rather than simply medical, experts and observers, to long-term attitudes to indigenous societies and cultures…'[30] Health of the British soldiers and colonial administrators was of primary importance to the colonizers. For this purpose, they were in utter need of knowing the foreign topography and diseases in India, and to know how these factors came to affect the body.

Against this background, Dr Wade noticed the action of miasma, or marsh alluvia. He put a curb on the emancipation from restraint, giving rise to unlimited indulgence of the soldiers' passions with women, and every possible excess in the gratification of their desire for strong liquors, the neglect of personal cleanliness. Moreover, he stressed on the daily use of the cold bath and frequent intestinal evacuation. Curiously enough, he also related some types of fevers with the 'lunar influence', particularly when they were accompanied by local complaints.[31] Since those very early days, comparative studies were made on differences of treatment patterns between Europe and India. Though applied in Europe, 'Venesection…never to be employed previous to the operation of purgatives, even in the most inflammatory fevers'.[32] As an aside, neologisms like 'marsh fever' were also coined.[33]

Since the 18th century, post-mortem dissection was mandatory, at least, in case of the British patients to establish relationship between symptoms and final diagnosis of disease. 'The clinical "observations" and "illustrations" of Annesley, Morehead, Parkes, and other writers of the period derived their claims to scientific objectivity and authority largely from their studies of morbid anatomy and their attempts to relate the state of diseased internal organs examined after death to the symptoms manifested externally during life'.[34] In case of hepatitis, 'suppurations have been found, on dissection, when there have been no reasons to suspect inflammation or any other disease of this organ'.[35] However, it must be said, sometimes 'Dissections throw no light into the proximate cause of the disease, as they only show its effects'.[36]

Saunders found that 'in India, the fever and dysentery, which are considered as the endemic of the country, have been found on dissection to be accompanied with diseases of the liver'.[37] Moreover, the measures that appeared applicable to European climate were different in Indian practice. He found, 'in Europe, where indeed it is comparatively rare; but in the East Indies, where it is frequent as to be the endemic of that country to European constitutions, a different practice is required'.[38] He also noted, 'by far the greater number of diseases which affect Europeans in India, are connected with, and depend on morbid state of the liver and other biliary organs'.[39] He emphasized the fact that 'the East India hepatitis is not merely a disorder of a tropical climate, but it appears to be almost entirely confined to the Indian continent'.[40] Not only in cases of hepatitis, in dysentery too was autopsy used to examine and understand the nature of pathological changes. Twining noticed, 'The most remarkable circumstances connected with the dysentery of Bengal, are the extensive local inflammation of the mucous membrane of the great intestines, coeval with the commencement of the disease'.[41] Elsewhere, he noted, 'The morbid appearances in the ulterior stages of febrile cholera, very much resemble those seen in the dissection of subjects who have died during the remote stages of remittent fever'.[42]

More precisely, 'The patient dies. The body is permitted to be opened, and this it is supposed to explain every thing'.[43] Curtis concluded, 'Much experience indeed does it require; and many dissections of similar cases, to enable us to judge and distinguish accurately between the causes and effects of disease; and even between the effects of disease, and effects of death'.[44]

Importantly, this new paradigm of organ localization of disease, which was a definite disjuncture from the earlier humoral pathology, was still carrying the traces of humoralism. Dr Paisley commented, 'in a climate where all the capital disorders arise from *putrid bile*, or obstructions, nothing must be shut up'.[45] Another account states, 'The bile however must be excepted, which is considerably increased in quantity, and as some think rendered more acrimonious in quality'.[46]

Treatment followed suit 'by evacuations, relaxing antiphlogistic medicines, and mercury'.[47] A 'Surgeon in India' provided a rueful narrative. 'They bled me while a drop would flow, and blistered me from *top to toe*; from that day I remained perfectly delirious for nearly three weeks... my head was blistered seven times, and my chest four times; I had three bleedings from the arm until I fainted each time'.[48] Twining, like his colleagues, prescribed treatment with 'twelve leeches to the liver', 'copious bleedings', or mercurials. In the year 1776, Charles Maclean did one of the first clinical trials 'concerning the action of mercury upon the living body' in the 'worst ward, in the Calcutta General Hospital, in all India, and probably in the whole world'.[49]

We may now ask what the consequences of these practices were. Some tentative answers may be provided.

First, the practice of dissection provided concrete ground for organ localization of disease—the body was not merely a bodily frame through which saps, humours, and fluids flow, it became a three-dimensional material reality, which can be explored for various investigative purposes. The Indian body image was demystified—no more a 'divine' body—and experiential knowledge was rendered redundant.

Second, although, until the middle of the 19th century, dissection in practice was cohabiting with humoral theory of disease, precise anatomical knowledge yielded excellent surgical results. Symptom or disease to pathology or organ localization was a linear journey, fully complying with *cause-effect* relationship in a positivist-utilitarian social milieu. Twining tersely commented, 'it often happens that the pathological views and the therapeutic methods undergo, in the course of twenty-five or thirty years, a gradual but very complete revolution'.[50]

Third, it had its great social significance too. Radhakanta Deb, an orthodox Hindu, expressed, 'I shall introduce and recommend your advice and medicine both here and in the interior, and the human lives which will thereby be saved will, I trust, be an ample reward for the trouble you have taken...'[51] Rammohan Roy sent a set of 10 Hindu skulls for phrenological examinations to Dr Patterson of Edinburgh. Rammohan wrote to Dr John Patterson—

> Dear Sir, - ...I now have the pleasure of sending you the ten accompanying skulls; and if you find them calculated to answer your purpose, I will, with equal pleasure, send you as many as you may think sufficient for your present researches. If you wish me to procure skulls of different descriptions, you will have the goodness to particularize them, that I may seek an opportunity of meeting your wishes.[52]

Fourth, all the Indian experiences related to medicine, surgery, pathology, and pharmacology found their applications back in Britain and other colonies. European and Indian cases of the tumour of the jaws differed with respect to (*a*) size of the tumour, (*b*) progress of the disease, and (*c*) surgical practices. The mode of 'making the incisions' differed from that 'usually adopted in our country, and appears to have the recommendation of leaving a smaller cicatrix'.[53] Maclean wrote, 'In 1778, during a voyage to India, I discovered the rudiments of a peculiar method of cure in intermittent fevers. In 1790, this plan of treatment was successfully extended, by analogy, to the yellow fever of the West Indies'.[54] Harrison makes it clear that the 'great opportunities presented by the medical work in India were not lost on the Company's surgeons and those of the British armed forces, who were noted during the eighteenth and nineteenth centuries for their innovative and empirical approach to medicine'.[55] Saunders found that it 'becomes of considerable importance to shew also from experience, how far it is safe to transplant the India [*sic*] practice into Europe' and 'to guard against the abuse of a remedy'.[56] In *Indian Hospital Reports* by Hunter, there was early mention of the use of stethoscope for diagnosis. 'The stethoscopic signs, &c, indicated obstruction to the free air into the lungs, and the expectorations, though scanty, was that of bronchitis...'[57]

Duncan Stewart realized, 'nothing more desirable, than that, where the opportunity exists, (as at any of the great Indian hospitals, where liver affections are so common,) an accurate series of *observations should be made, and recorded*, of the real or apparent effects of bile'. Moreover, following this train of logic, 'from which some general law, or theory of its operation in particular circumstances might be derived'.[58] We must note here the importance of Hospital medicine, which was historically a paradigmatic shift from Bedside medicine in Europe. The rise of Hospital medicine 'was the closing hour of medical medievalism'.[59]

An English man complained about Medical College & Hospitals (The Calcutta Medical College) to the editor of *The Statesman*—

> Enter and you will find East Indians and West Indians, Bengalees and Madrasees...These creatures wear the same clothes, and lie on, and use, the same beds and beddings as the Europeans; and as soon as they don the clothes they are *yclept* sahibs! They are of all classes; and (as all patients are distinguished not by *name*, but by *numbers*), were one to ask for 'Now Number Sahib'...[60]

Besides social hierarchy, it is interesting to note how patients became numbers. *Person* of the patient was transformed into *pathology* inside the body in the hospital setting. It reminds us of clinical *objectification* in modern medicine as well as of careful separation among the White and 'black' bodies.

It was also observed that 'many medical men obtain very considerable eminence in their as physician in Calcutta...and no small number turn the experience which they have acquired in India, to good account at home...'[61]

At a much later period, Lambert reported about his trial 'with emetine and bismuth iodide' on Indian patients, 'As this was the first opportunity I had of taking a trial of emetine and bismuth iodide in a series of cases of amoebic dysentery...the following points were considered worthy of investigation'.[62]

Another example comes from Dr Benjamin Guy Babington. He was the 28th president of the Royal Medical and Chirurgical Society of London. He was also the first president of the Epidemiological Society—'a position for which his study of the history of epidemics and the large knowledge of Cholera which he had acquired in India eminently fitted him'.[63]

ANATOMY AND INDIAN SOCIETY[64]

Medicine produces metaphors. On its turn, metaphors go on multiplying new metaphors. However, problems may arise when a metaphor expands in a sphere where it is not challenged or complemented by other equally powerful metaphors which are also expanding. In that case, the metaphor in question may go on expanding its application almost indefinitely. If health is 'a way of tackling existence' in which 'one is not only possessor or bearer but also, if necessary, creator of value, establisher of vital norms', then what constitutes health in one person may well, as Nietzsche said, 'look like the opposite of health in another person'.[65] Medical metaphors fill in the vacuum, especially, when religious or cultural metaphors become marginalized in contestation with the new emerging normative regime of medicine.

In a desperate attempt to become 'modern', even anatomical knowledge of bony ossification was applied to justify the age of marriage of the Hindu girls.[66]

Soorjo Coomar Goodeve Chuckerbutty was a bright student of Medical College. He was possibly the first Indian doctor to extensively use his knowledge of morbid anatomy in diagnosing *typhus* fever in 12 cases in 1864. He used his knowledge in post-mortem examinations to find changes in internal organs in 63 fatal cases of cholera.[67] Such a correlation between manifestation of disease and its anatomical pathology increasingly made indigenous knowledge of 'speculative pathology' and healing marginal.

Another notable example may be the lithotomy operations done by Ram Narin Doss. He was a teacher of surgery in the military class of the Bengal Medical College. He is reported to have performed that operation more than two hundred times with good success.[68] Other important Indian lithotomy surgeons were Dr Bhawoo Dajee and Dr Sadashew Hemraj of Grant Medical College, Bombay. Morehead mentioned of Premanad Sett of Medical College, Calcutta, for successful surgical repair of elephantiasis.[69] Without proliferating examples, it may be safely said that anatomical training in the medical colleges of India did produce perfectly visible surgical results, which had hitherto been unknown to the Indians. One jocose account of 'evacuation' of big hydrocele of a native patient tells us, 'The patient went on his way rejoicing at the resoration to usefulness of an organ which he had not caught sight of for some time and spread about the fame of the hospital where a radical (?) cure had been effected so speedily'.[70]

Dr N. Pan, in the article 'Some Observation on the Gastro-Intestinal Tract of the Hindus', wrote—

The nature of the diet in Indians differs considerably from that of Europeans. In an Indian diet we find a bulky carbohydrate food with a very small proportion of the other proximate principles. This led me to expect that the anatomy of the gastro-intestinal tract in Indians would differ from that of Europeans to a considerable degree...The observations were made on 65 subjects, a very small number, and the conclusions drawn from these cases must be accepted with caution.[71]

Even a cursory reading of the statement makes it clear that the anatomical study undertaken by Dr Pan (or Dr Chuckerbutty) was purely a comparative study (examples of William Hunter, Bichat, William Harvey, or Richard Lower are comparable in this regard). The focus of colonial medical education was to produce 'capable practitioners', not 'capable enquirers and practitioners'. However, the issue that is more interesting is the next part of his observation—

The subjects available for dissection in the Calcutta Medical College are the unclaimed bodies from the Campbell Medical School and Hospital where the majority of the patients come from the poor classes. 'Mahamedans' take a fair proportion of meat in their diet, but no Mahamedan subjects are available for observation. So most of the subjects observed are adult Hindus including Bengalis, Beharis and Uriyas, who subsist on bulky carbohydrate food.[72]

Evidently, the bodies for dissection 'come from the poor classes' and, to add, these must be unclaimed bodies. Consequently, in a populous country like India, there was no need of an Anatomy Act (1832) of England. To note, no 'Mahammedan' subject was available for dissection. Possibly, it was loathsome to them to hand over their bodies to a person of different religion.

In another instance, Charles R. Francis, in 'A Course of Lectures...at the Medical College of Bengal' informed the new students of the Medical College, Calcutta, about a 'moribund pauper' and 'poor wretched skeleton figure', whom 'The police have brought...to great haven of refuge, the Medical College Hospital of Bengal'.[73] Dr Francis' statement points to the fact of abundance of pauper and poor people's bodies ready for dissection.

Anatomical metaphors became the call of the day following colonial medical encounters. Terms and images plucked from the colonial language of medicine and disease began to infiltrate the phraseology of Indian self-expression (or, put otherwise, Indian subjectivity), to become part of the ideological formulation of a new nationalist order.[74] These terms and images, self evidently, were primarily moored on superiority of anatomical knowledge, excellence of surgical practices and, at a later period, diagnostic and therapeutic marvels. Medicine, during colonial period, was intricately related with metaphors of higher civilization,[75] and invasion. Terms like 'microbe hunter', 'disease killers' were usual choice for microbiologists and physicians of the day.[76]

As we have discussed earlier, different sections of the Indian society responded in different ways to Western medicine. The present example would help us to get at the point. A peasant of Birbhum region of Bengal wrote to a person (to whom he owed some money)—'Wreaking evils on you, I went to town. Hence, I have contacted an alien disease. You must know it...And, on getting cured, I must fully repay the debt whatever I owe to you'.[77] This is an account of the 'social body' with its own logic, rules, metaphors, and ethical demands. It is also an account of the subaltern. Dwijendranath, the eldest brother of Rabindranath Tagore, provides another differing contemporaneous 'elite' account, 'Treatment by any means is a wild goose chase! Hence, better not to say anything about *kaviraji chikitsa* (Āyurvedic treatment), even the shimmering rays of the nineteenth century knowledge has failed to penetrate its windows'.[78] He continues, 'Modern medicine starts with *dissecting a corpse*, Āyurveda starts with elaborating on the relationship between *body and mind*. Inspired by 'modernity', he innovatively uses the Āyurvedic categories like *vayu, pitta, ślesmā* (wind, bile, and phlegm) to interpret superiority of Western intellect. In his opinion, persons like Danton belong to the category of pitta or bile and represent 'social dynamics'. Finally, he concludes, 'By the raging light and scorching heat of English education, orthodoxies are being increasingly banished from metropolis to the fringes of villages'. We can see the emergence of the 'medical or anatomical body' as distinct from the 'social body' of the former account. Here remains a subtle difference in the conceptualization of the body *as diseased* in modern medicine, and the body *in disease* in popular or Āyurvedic perception that finally transforms into the 'diseased body' (a hybrid) in metropolitan Bengali perception. While in the former, the body is embedded in its environs, in the latter, it is the disengaged circumscribed biological body.[79]

There occurred an insidious dislocation, evacuation, and reconstruction of the core of indigenous categories and conceptual cosmos. 'The primitive meaning which can be restored does not indicate quite surely the derivative meanings in which the words have been used in the texts'.[80] Semiotics may help us to understand this mechanism in a better way.

An index is a sign that is contiguous with and determined by its object. An idea (symbol) is brought into reality *indexically*, and once it emerges socially in material reality, where its use might spawn a rethinking of the symbol, a new idea—an idea that might change other ideas—change habits, and hence change 'actual behaviour in the outer world' in a continuous dialectical process.[81] Symbols take their meaning not from contiguity with particular objects in particular contexts, but rather from shared understandings that are *independent* of any particular context, that are 'context free'.[82] The indexical relation between anatomical dissection in modern medicine and Āyurveda, can best be described as a metonymic relation, a substantial relation of part to whole and 'habit will have power to influence actual behavior in the outer world'.[83] However, the outer world—the material objective world where signs come into being in use and experience—has a greater effect on the inner world of habit.

Through such mechanisms, the Sankritik connotations of the terms described in Āyurveda were evacuated of their meanings and the vacuum was filled with modern anatomical meanings. Therefore, context-free, universal logic of modern medicine metonymically refigured context-sensitive character of Āyurveda. This metamorphosis was enhanced by excellent surgical results and diagnostic aids like stethoscope, microscope, clinical charts, temperature recording, x-ray, and so on.

Zimmermann brilliantly addresses the problem—

> A more essential example of such changes, the word *pañcakarman*, 'the Five Treatments', can no longer be considered as a generic name for evacuant therapies. *Pañcakarman* might have been originally synonymous with *śodhana*, 'the Purificatory (or Evacuant) Treatments', as both categories encompassed emetics, purgatives, drastic enemas, and errhines. However, since bloodletting (the fifth of the evacuant therapies) has fallen into disuse, it was removed from the set of *pañcakarman*, and replaced by oily enemas. These technical changes, and shifts of meaning, involved a more fundamental change in medical philosophy, *from operative medicine to more gentle methods*.[84]

Interestingly, in his book *Āyurveda Parichay* (Introduction to Āyurveda), Gananath Sen regarded 1830 as the period of Āyurvedic renaissance. Remembering with veneration Madhusudan Gupta as the first dissector of India, he asserted, 'He (Gupta) was the first to chant the *mantra* of Āyurvedic revival'.[85] Meulenbeld comments, 'The renaissance of āyurveda since about the middle of the nineteenth century — historically a fascinating phenomenon...The ancient terms for physiological and pathophysiological processes, nosological entities etc., were diligently reinterpreted to bring them into line with terms derived from Western medicine'.[86]

ANATOMICAL KNOWLEDGE: 1794—COLONIAL INDIA

Although, the British had been exposed to India for a long time, they did not have any knowledge of Indian surgical craft. Contrarily, they used to scoff at the Indian practitioners for their rueful knowledge of anatomy. I would argue that witnessing a case of successful rhinoplasty might have been a befitting answer to their derision about Indian surgical knowledge and drawn their avid interest in ancient Indian medical and surgical practices. B(arak) L(ongmate) wrote to the editor of *Gentleman's Magazine*, 'A friend has transmitted to me, from the East Indies, the following very curious, and, in Europe, I believe, unknown chirurgical operation, which has long been practiced in India with success: namely, affixing a new nose on a man's face'.[87] A *maharatta* (Marathi language as pronounced by Britishers) by the name of Cowasjee (though, he seems to be a Parsee) was a bullock cart driver in the employment of the English Army during the Mysore War of 1793. He was captured by Tipu Sultan's soldiers, who cut off his nose and one of his hands, for his treachery. Cowasjee joined the Bombay Army near Srirangapatnam with a cut nose. His nose was reconstructed by 'a man of the Brickmaker caste' of Satara near Poona. 'Two of the medical gentlemen, Mr. Thomas Cruso and Mr. James Trindlay, of the Bombay presidency, have seen it performed...'

Suśruta's version has the skin flap being taken from the cheek; Cowasjee's was taken from the forehead. Subsequently, the details and an engraving from the painting were reproduced in the October 1794 issue of the *Gentleman's Magazine* of London.[88] 'Barak Longmate's letter appears to have fired the imagination of the English surgeon Joseph Constantine (not John) Carpue (1764–1846) who initially practiced the Indian method of rhinoplasty on cadavers, and waited until a suitable patient presented himself'.[89] Carpue performed his first two rhinoplasties in 1814 and 1815. In 1816, Carpue published the results of these attempts in his landmark work—'*An account of two successful operations for restoring a lost nose from the integuments of the forehead*'.

George Mason noted—

The operation was known and practiced at a very early period of surgery in India by the Brahmans...From India the Sicilian surgeons in all probability received their ideas on the art of restoring noses, and the earliest record we possess on this subject is the report of a Neapolitan bishop in 1442, on an operation of rhinoplasty, performed by Branca.[90]

John Davis informed, 'This is known as the *Indian Method*... They used a secret cement for the adhesion, to which was ascribed special healing power. This is called the *Ancient Indian Method*'.[91] Albrecht Weber too noticed, 'in this department European surgeons might perhaps even at the present day still learn something from them, as indeed they have already learned from them the operation of *rhinoplsty*'.[92]

Manucci was possibly the first traveller to describe Indian rhinoplasty. 'The surgeons belonging to the country cut the skin of the forehead above the eyebrows, and made it fall down over the wounds on the nose...I saw many persons with such noses, and they were not so disfigured as they would have been without any nose at all...'[93]

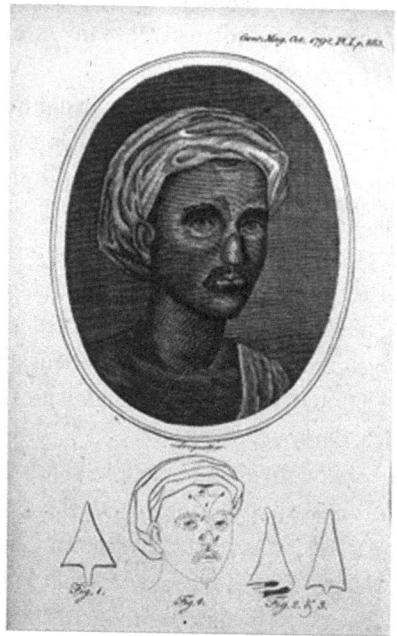

Fig. 2.1: Cowasjee's portrait with the reconstructed nose.

Source: Wellcome Library, London. L0017597 Indian method of the restoration of the nose by plastic surgery, from article by B.L. to Mr Urban, concerning Cowasjee, a man who had his nose reconstructed with the aid of plastic surgery. Line engraving 1794 By: Longmate From: *Gentleman's Magazine* By: B.L. Published: 9 October 1794, Volume 64, part 2, facing page 883.

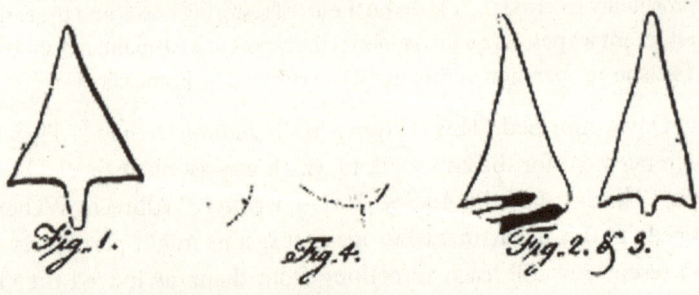

Fig. 2.2: Drawings of the skin flaps used in the operation.
Source: Gentleman's Magazine 1794.

More important, all the major works on Indian medicine were published after 1794. One of the earliest medical works about Indian pharmacopoeia was Ainslie's *Materia Medica of Hindoostan*. He tried to find 'a correct list of what particular articles of of the British Materia Medica could be procured in the Bazars of Hindoostan…or any arranged account of the Materia Mediac of the Native Indians…'[94] Many more books on Indian pharmacopoeia were published thereafter.

In the European context, Urdang made an insightful study. 'It was for the sake of uniformity in the preparation of drugs and the adaptation of the formulas concerned to the special needs and resources of the political units involved that the official pharmacopoeias came into existence… An own pharmacopoeia became gradually a matter of national ambition, a part and a proof of national sovereignty and unity'.[95] In the Indian context, producing new pharmacopoeia was related with bringing about homogeneity amongst numerous synonyms of Sanskrit names and their regional variations. Though Ainslie noted, 'medicine in India is still sunk in a state of empirical darkness'.[96]

Royle found in *Hindoo* medicine 'much fanciful Anatomy, imaginative Physiology, and absurd attention to numbers'.[97] Indigenous surgeons, hakeems and *baids*, were being scrutinized for their absolute lack of anatomical knowledge—'the Hukeem was totally ignorant of anatomy, having no rational idea of the parts to be divided'[98] or 'He had never seen the dissection of the eye of any animal, nor does he believe that any of his family had'.[99] Efforts to bring indigenous surgeries (practiced as family craft) into the mainstream medicine, and thereby relativizing and, finally, marginalizing them, could not erase its survival among low-caste people of India.

Charles Trevelyan emphasized, 'We shall be perfectly content if native students should be found to think as justly, and write as beautifully, in English, as Buchanan, Bacon, and various others did in Latin; or, to come nearer our own times, and in a professional walk, as Harvey, Sydenham, Boerhaave, Haller, Heberden, and Gregory did, in the same language'.[100] Hunter spiritedly observed that modern English education had created a new nexus for the active intellectual elements in the population. It was a nexus interwoven of three strong cords, a common language, common political aims, and a sense of the power of action in common—the products of a common system of education.[101]

The making of new pharmacopoeias coupled with improvement of deplorable state of anatomical knowledge of Āyurveda through modern medical and anatomical education ushered into the germinating new era of nation state. It was perhaps epitomized in the statement—'Under British rule, however, they (*Hakeems* and *Bāeds*) have disappeared altogether from political life, and socially have little or no standing in European society, where they are virtually ignored'.[102] Surpassing all these asymmetric exchanges between East and West, indigenous medicine 'in the enunciatory act of splitting'[103] emerged like the Phoenix amongst Indian population, beyond the reach of metropolitan psyche.

NOTES

1. Spratling (1902:1688–89).
2. Boonen and van der Sj (2005:538).
3. Ordi *et al.* (2006:516–20 [Emphasis added]).
4. Fredriksen (2002:71–3).
5. Aronowitz (1998:1, 3).
6. Harrison (2005:56–63).
7. David Arnold and Gabrielle Hecht, 'Colonialism, Decolonization and Development: Analytic Themes, Research Programmatics, and Collaborative Projects', Internet paper. http://www.histech.nl/tensions/Projecten/CC/Budapest/CD/Budapest/papers/themeworksh/CDAtheme.htm, accessed 28 June 2005.
8. Pollock (2004:24, 19–21).
9. Metcalf (1998:67).
10. Ibid., p. 66.
11. Ibid., p. 171.
12. Deepak Kumar, in Kumar (ed.) (2001:xvix).
13. Raj (2006:24).

14. Deepak Kumar, 2003, 'History of Medicine in South Asia: Some Concerns, Some Questions' [Keynote Address at the first Conference of the Asian Society for the History of Medicine. Institute of History and Philology, Academia Sinica, Taipei, 4–8 November].

15. Fremantle (1911:347).

16. Barnes, Barry in Ian Inkster and Jack Morell (eds) (1983:11–54). [Emphasis in original].

17. Arnold and Hecht (2005).

18. Qaisar (1998:5).

19. Fryer (1912:105).

20. Ibid., p. 103.

21. Foster (1959:173–87).

22. Newman (1960:322–29).

23. Cohn, Bernard S. in Ranajit Guha (ed.) (1999:276–329).

24. Qaisar (1998:16).

25. Foucault (1994:124).

26. Porter (1999:307).

27. Cohn (1997:19).

28. Ibid., p. 21.

29. Hatcher (2000).

30. Arnold (1996:1–19).

31. Wade (1793).

32. Duncan (1794:205).

33. Clarke (1775:126).

34. Arnold (1993:53).

35. Clarke (1775:268).

36. Ibid., p. 134.

37. Saunders (1809:251).

38. Ibid., p. 1.

39. Ibid., p. 15.

40. Ibid., p. 12.

41. Twining (1832:1).

42. Twining (1833:51).

43. Curtis (1807:178).

44. Ibid., p. 179.

45. Saunders (1809:52).

46. William Falconer, 1781, *Remarks on the Influence of Climate, Situation, Nature of Country, Population, Nature of Food, and Way of Life, on the Disposition and Temper, Manners and Behaviour, Intellects, Laws and Customs, Form of Government, and Religion, of Mankind*, C. Dilly, London. Quoted in Smollett,

Tobias George (ed.), 1781, *The Critical Review: or, Annals of Literature*, London, A. Hamilton, p. 100.

47. Saunders (1809:56).

48. 'Indian Treatment of Fever', in *London Medical Gazette* (1828:176–77).

49. Charles Maclean, 1817,. *Results of an Investigation, respecting Epidemic and Pestilential Diseases; including Researches in the Levant, concerning the Plague*, London: Thomas and George Underwood, Vol. II, p. 502. Also, see, U. Trohler and I. MacLean Chalmers, 1818, Comparing Like with Like and Recognizing Ethical Double Standards in Therapeutic Experimentation, URL : http://www. jameslindlibrary.org/trial_records/19th_Century/maclean/maclean_commentary. html

50. 'Mr. Twining on Diseases of Bengal', in *Edinburgh Medical and Surgical Journal* (1835:133).

51. 'Native Medical Institution of Bengal', in *Oriental Herald and Journal of General Literature* (1826:17–25 (21)).

52. *Transactions of the Phrenological Society* (1824 : 434–35).

53. O'Sahughnessy (1845:45).

54. Maclean (1817:56).

55. Pati, Biswamoy and Harrison, Mark (ed.) (2009:176).

56 Saunders (1809:8).

57. Hunter (1836:382–84).

58. Stewart (1835:363–88). [Emphasis added].

59. For the pioneering work on this topic, see, Ackernecht (1967:33).

60. *The Statesman*, Wednesday, 23 June 1880, Calcutta. Quoted in Ray Chaudhuri (1987:4). [Emphasis added]

61. Roberts (1838:245–52).

62. Lambert (1918:116–118).

63. *The Royal Medical and Chirurgical Society of London* (1905:275–76).

64. For recent accounts on anatomical knowledge and Indian society, see, Harrison, Mark in Pati, Biswamoy and Harrison, Mark (ed.) (2009). Bhattacharya (2009:1–51). Wujastyk (2009:189–228).

65. Boyd (2000: 9–17).

66. Sanyal (1888:5–13).

67. Sengupta (1970:183–91).

68. Morehead (1860:506).

69. Ibid., p. 701.

70. Anonymous in *Centenary Volume*, Medical College, Calcutta (158–9). This was originally published in *Indian Medical Gazette*, LX (1925:127–29).

71. N.Pan, 1919, '*Some Observation on the Gastro-Intestinal Tract of the Hindus, Journal of Anatomy* 53(2–3):259–65.

72. Ibid., p. 259.

73. Francis (1868:97–9).

74. Arnold (1993:241).

75. Prakash (2000).

76. Otis (1999).

77. Mandal (1953: 80)

78. Dwijendranath Tagore read this essay at the 8th session of Kambuliatola Learning Society (কম্বুলিয়াটোলা পাঠ সমিতি), Calcutta. The date of publication in the Bengal Library Catalogue is 24 August, 1891, p. 82. (Visva Bharati archives)

79. Bhattacharya, Jayanta in Kalitzkas, Vera and Twohig Peter L. (ed.) (2004:31–54). [Emphasis added]

80. Filliozat (1964:144). Wujastyk expresses similar concern in his *The Roots of Ayurveda* (1998:29–38).

81. Charles S.Peirce, 1955 *Philosophical Writings* (edited by Justus Buchler), New York, Dover Publications, pp.98–119. Also, see, Burnum (1993:939–43).

82. Mines (1997:33–44).

83. Peirce (1955:284). Also, see, Culler (2001:51–87).

84. Francis Zimmermann in Paul Unschuld (ed.) (1989:141–51).

85. Sen (1943:31).

86. Meulenbeld (1999–2000).

87. Longmate (1794:891–92).

88. Joseph (1987:217–221).

89. Van De Graaf (2009:226).

90. Mason (1873:138–39).

91. John Staige Davis, 1919, *Plastic Surgery: Its Principles and Practices*, P. Blackistone's Son & Co., p. 1.

92. Weber (1882:270).

93. Manucci (1907:301).

94. Ainslie (1813:i).

95. Urdang (1946:46–70).

96. Ainslie (1826:v).

97. Royle (1837:48).

98. Lindsay (1829:440–2).

99. Scott (1817:156–62).

100. Trvelyan (1838:215).

101. Hunter (1891:1).

102. Anonymous in *Indian Medical Gazette* (1868:87–9).

103. Bhabha (1994:128).

3 From Bazaar Medicine to Hospital Medicine

Calomel, India, and the British Empire, c.1750–c.1800

MARK HARRISON

A s is well known, the colonies provided access to a range of drugs
that were not commonly available in Europe, most of which were
botanical remedies, famously cinchona and ipecacaunha. However,
British India was also the source of a major revolution in therapeutics
based on the use of calomel, or mercurous chloride. Calomel was one
of the number of chemical remedies pioneered in the hospitals of the
East India Company in the 18th century and early 19th centuries, which
had an important impact on medicine in Britain, and elsewhere in its
empire. As I shall suggest below, the use of mercurial drugs to treat non-
venereal complaints, while not totally unprecedented, was to say the
least, unusual in European medicine. Thus, their employment in a wide
range of diseases in India, from the 1750s, marked a radical departure
from established practice. In taking a different view of the uses of
mercury, the Company's surgeons were demonstrating the view that
tropical diseases were distinctive and their practices shed further light
on what historians have seen as the development of a distinct branch of
Western medicine—the medicine of hot or warm climates. And yet, this
episode also demonstrates that tropical practice could make an impact
on medicine back 'at home'; a fact all the more remarkable because the
treatment may have originated in Indian medical practices. Hence the
title of this chapter— 'from bazaar medicine to hospital medicine'.

The remainder of the chapter traces the development of mercurial therapy, beginning in southern India, with later excursions to the West Indies and to Britain. My main aim in doing so is to demonstrate the importance of colonial hospitals as sites of medical innovation. India and other British settlements provided a context which was highly conducive to innovation. There, Western practitioners, of course, had ready access to a wide range of exotic remedies. But this was not the only, nor the most important reason, why new practices emerged. More important, was the degree of licence afforded to practitioners in the settings just described and the opportunities presented there for systematic clinical observation and trials. No less significant was the fact that the imperatives of medical practice differed radically from those in Britain. The medicine of warm climates developed substantially within the medical services of the armed forces and its overriding imperative was to find cheap and effective mass remedies, rather than the more individualized requirements typical of civilian practice. Equally, the fact that some tropical diseases proceeded rapidly towards an often fatal termination meant that drastic intervention was generally thought necessary. The no-nonsense, practical ethos of the military and naval services was in any case disposed towards such treatment, and in this respect, the professional identity of their surgeons was not unlike the practitioners described by Warner in his study of American therapeutics.[1] Like their counterparts in early 19th century America, colonial practitioners considered themselves men of action and therapeutic intervention—often drastic—was their *raison d'être*. There was a good deal of similarity between the likes of Bejamin Rush of Philadelphia, for example, and prominent colonial practitioners; indeed, they often contributed to the same journals, belonged to the same societies, and possessed similar outlooks on matters of politics. Many of the remedies which they used and advocated were the same and their therapeutic practices were determined largely by the perceived centrality of climate and locality in disease.

The increasing use of chemical remedies in mid-18th century India was based on the putrid theory of fevers which held sway in both the East and West Indies, and particularly a variant which attributed most diseases suffered by Europeans to 'superabundant and acrimonious bile'. It was widely held that the liver was very sensitive to hot climates and generally liable to become 'deranged' and inflamed. Moreover, it was held that hot climates stimulated the production of more bile than could be absorbed in the normal process of digestion, causing the excess bile to become corrupt, giving rise to putrefactive diseases, including fevers and dysentery.

The rise of mercurial remedies was closely linked to the biliary theory of fevers, which came to dominate Anglo-Indian and then West-Indian medicine in the last decades of the 18th century. Mercury served as a powerful purgative that would rapidly cleanse the intestines of redundant and corrupted bile.

But the growing reputation of mercury as a treatment for a wide range of tropical ailments placed tropical practitioners at odds with most practitioners in Britain. In the mid-18th century, mercurial remedies were largely confined to the treatment of syphilis and, partly because of their Paracelsian connotations, were still regarded by some physicians with a deal of suspicion. Although Boerhaave had recommended mercurial drugs in the treatment of flux, for example, but such remedies do not appear to have used as a matter of course.[2] The widespread and liberal use of mercury in the tropics was therefore a wholly new development in British medicine, and one which was to prove highly controversial. Yet, by the end of the 18th century, variants of the practices developed in India were being employed not only in other tropical colonies but also in Britain itself. Mercurial therapy for non-venereal complaints, thus represents a clear case of a therapy making the transition from the colonies to affect British medicine as a whole.

In the middle of the 18th century, Company surgeons began to administer mercury in the form of calomel pills to patients suffering from inflammatory diseases of the liver. In these pills, calomel was generally mixed with gum arabic and ipecacaunha, which was already an established medicine for dysentery. These were generally given every three to four hours, until the patient's urine turned pale,[3] or sometimes in sufficient quantities to make the patient salivate. This practice began in the Company's hospital in Madras in the 1750s, under the direction of two surgeons, John Wilson and Gilbert Pasley.[4] An acute form of hepatitis had been affecting European troops on the Coromandel Coast in large numbers and it had assumed epidemic proportions. Finding that traditional antiphlogistic treatments made no impact on the disease, the two men turned to calomel as their primary remedy, but the exact reasons for this are unclear. It may well be the case that Wilson and Pasley knew that Beorhaave had endorsed its use, but calomel does not appear to have been used in Europe in the relief of liver complaints. A more likely source was the nearby bazaar, in which Indian practitioners sold mercurial remedies. Mercurial remedies entered *Ayurvedic* medicine in the 14th century, partly through the influence of tantrism and partly through *unani-tibb*. In south India, the local medical tradition, *siddha*, which was more directly influenced by tantrism, made extensive use of chemical remedies including mercury, and we know that itinerant salesmen-practitioners move from bazaar to bazaar selling and using mercurial remedies.[5] In view of the fact that the latter were likely to be practicing medicine without much reference to classic texts, we cannot be sure of the ways in which they employed mercury. But in siddha medicine, it was common to use mineral remedies including mercury (*rasam*) to relieve 'obstructions' of the humours and cure fevers, which is similar to the manner in which calomel was employed by Pasley and Wilson. Both men had a contract to supply their hospital with bazaar medicines and would have been familiar with local practices;[6] they would have also regularly purchased mercury, which was already extensively used to treat venereal complaints. Indeed, the Madras hospital had separate rooms in which patients were given mercury to the point of salivation.[7] The hospital also possessed a laboratory, which had been established at the initiative of Pasley and Wilson, so as to enable them to manufacture remedies from local ingredients; Indian practitioners were engaged to work in the laboratory as compounders.[8]

In the coming decade, the fame of Wilson and Pasley spread throughout India and practitioners in other stations appear to have corresponded with them, as we shall see below. Patients in need of treatment for liver diseases also travelled to Madras to seek their assistance, while by the early 1770s, mercurial remedies were being taken by those who wished to relieve themselves of tropical ailments. In 1771, for example, Gustavus Ducarel, who appears to have been an officer in the Bengal Army, requested his uncle to send him Kyser's Pills, not 'for a certain Disorder' (syphilis) but because 'they will always be of great value either for myself or my Friends, as the mild preparation of the Mercury renders them the fittest Medicine for this Country'.[9] But as news of mercurial treatment filtered back to Britain, it was greeted with scepticism and dismay by some eminent physicians. One London physician, Dr Silvester, wrote to Sir George Colebrooke, at the Court of Directors, claiming that 'Your People have not always the best Physical Assistance' and suggesting that castor oil might be used instead of calomel to treat liver diseases. Pasley wrote the Court of Directors a long letter ridiculing the suggestion. 'There are Bilious Disorders in India which sometimes end in general obstruction of the Viscera' he explained, 'where the Liver and every other glandular part contained in the Belly enlarge considerably and form together a production of the Bowels, which becomes a Chronick Case of difficult Cure. Castor Oil under such Circumstances would be trifling with the health of the Patient'.[10]

Pasley seems to have received support from both the Governor of Madras in Council and from the Court of Directors, and the practice of using mercury continued at the hospital in Madras and, indeed, quickly spread elsewhere in India. The fact that the Company was prepared to protect its surgeons against interference from physicians at home is highly significant because it demonstrates that the opinions of the former carried great weight. Claims made by Company surgeons about the peculiar dangers of the Indian disease environment, and of the need for remedies more powerful than those used in Britain, seem to have been accepted. Indeed, in the same decade, some Company surgeons were committing their observations to print with the sanction of the Company. The first to do so appears to have been the Company Marine surgeon John Clark, who had spent several years in Madras. Like Pasley and Wilson, Clark recommended calomel in cases of inflamed and obstructed liver—

> In cold climates, the cure, as in all other inflammations, depends on plentiful bleeding, antiphlogistic purges, and the application of a blister to the part affected. But in the East Indies, this method being found unsuccessful, and the disorder in general proving soon fatal, the most experienced practitioners in that part of the world prescribe mercury as a specific. They apply it externally upon the part, and give it internally in such doses as excite a general salivation.[11]

However, Clark was at that time uncertain about the efficacy of mercurial preparations in cases of fever. Indeed, he warned that the profuse sweating caused by large doses of mercury could actually prove injurious in the putrid fevers of hot climates.[12]

But it was not long before calomel and other mercurial remedies came to be recommended for a much wider range of diseases. As the efficacy of mercury lay in its effects on the liver and on its ability to clear large quantities of peccant matter rapidly, it seemed logical to use

it in complaints which were also supposed to arise from excessive bile.
By the 1780s, this included most of the principal ailments common
among Europeans in India, including nearly all fevers and fluxes. The
first British-Indian writer to recommend mercury for the treatment of
fevers was the Calcutta-based physician Dr Francis Balfour.[13] It will be
recalled that Balfour was one of the number of practitioners in British
India who wrote on sol-lunar influences on fever and he attempted to
devise a therapeutic regimen in accord with the lunar cycle.[14] He appears
to have placed increasing reliance on mercury throughout his career.
His first monograph—his *Treatise on the Influence of the Moon in Fevers*
(1784)—advocated a mixture of treatments, in which mercurial therapies did not figure largely.[15] But mercury was far more in evidence in
his later *Treatise on Putrid Intestinal Remitting Fevers* (1790), in which
Balfour's favoured method of treatment was to expel putrid matter with
a mixture of emetics and purgatives. Of the latter, he believed calomel to
be especially valuable.[16]

By the late 1780s, mercury in the form of calomel pills had come to
dominate British medical practice in India, where it was used in high
doses to treat many common ailments, including dysentery and fevers.
In Britain, by contrast, mercury was still used predominantly for venereal
complaints and most physicians regarded its liberal use in cases of hepatitis and fevers as dangerous and unsophisticated, preferring less drastic
and more individualized remedies.[17] But the Company's surgeons paid
little heed to criticism from doctors in Britain. Like their counterparts in
the Army and Navy, the vast majority did not possess medical degrees,
but had attended a course of lectures at one of the Scottish universities—
usually Edinburgh—or one of the new surgical schools established in
London. The ethos of these institutions was empirical and experimen-
tal, and was compatible with the robust practicalities of military life.
Although physicians were perhaps more inclined to experiment than
we have been led to believe, the Company's surgeons saw the medical
elite of London—the Oxbridge-educated MDs of the Royal College of
Physicians—as effete and irrelevant. Until the end of the 18th century,
there was a good deal of suspicion and ill feeling on both sides. Thus, Sir
Paul Jodrell (1746–1803), who had been recommended to the Nawab of
Arcot by Sir George Baker, President of the Royal College of Physicians,
reckoned that 'it is not the custom here to practice Physic as we do in
England, the Company's Servants being all Surgeons'.[18]

Mercury was now 'lord paramount' of all the remedies administered in the hospitals of British India, as one later critic was to put it,[19]
its dominance being clearly indicated in the writings of the prominent
surgeon and orientalist, John Wade. Wade wrote at length on its use in
the treatment of fevers in an essay on the 'Nature and Effects of Emetics,
Purgatives, Mercurials, and Low Diet, in Disorders of Bengal and similar
Latitudes' (1792) and in his 'Paper on the Prevention and Treatment of
the Disorders of Seamen and Soldiers in Bengal' (1793). In common with
many other British practitioners in India, he believed that vitiated bile
was the cause of intermittent fevers and many other 'tropical conditions'.
This seemed to be confirmed by Wade's post-mortem examinations of
patients who had died of fever and which usually showed that the liver
was more damaged than other organs.[20] Since it was now normal to treat
hepatic disorders with mercurial preparations, he argued, it seemed reasonable to apply them in all cases of fevers linked to some derangement
of the liver. In his first publication, which was addressed to his brother
Charles Wade, a physician in Lisbon, he claimed that calomel generally
worked where the bark did not, such as in the deadly 'pukka' and jungle
fevers of Bengal.[21] Indeed, Wade had found on many occasions that 'the
medicines chiefly in use in Europe' had been used in vain and that calomel was often the only remedy that was effective.[22]

Wade had been converted to the biliary theory of fever by Pasley, who
recommended an initial purge with castor oil, followed by the gradual administration of mercury pills.[23] In a letter to a young surgeon on the Bengal
establishment—which was probably Wade—Pasley had declared that—

> Mercury, in judicious hands, is a safe and tractable medicine, and it is the
> only safe and powerful deobstruant in glandular obstructions, it is of
> consequence the only medicine to be depended upon in those latent de-
> fects of the system, which entail diseases or impede recovery; however, it
> often requires assistance from other medicines, from exercise, from spas,
> or from medicated aqueous medicines.[24]

Wade was convinced of the efficacy of Pasley's remedies and believed that
his knowledge of liver complaints was second to none. The successful
treatment of liver disorders, he claimed, 'has long been understood in
the honourable company's settlements in the East Indies, and perhaps
there only'.[25] Indeed, Wade thought that the use of calomel and other
purgatives to treat fevers amounted to a 'therapeutic revolution'.

Certainly, from the 1780s to the 1820s, scarcely anyone in India doubted the 'absolute necessity of mercurializing every patient affected with fever, dysentery or hepatic affections'.[26]

The sovereignty of mercury in British India was due in large part to widely held assumptions about the climate and its effects on the human body, but its dominance was also due to the robust way in which its advocates dealt with contrary viewpoints. Although most advocates of mercury were wary of excessive salivation, and seldom relied on mercury alone, they took pains to denounce rival systems of treatment. Wade argued that hitherto common therapies, such as treatment with Peruvian bark, were of little use in India. He could accept that bark was 'a medicine occasionally applicable to the various modifications of fever ... as they occur in Europe' but maintained that such occasions were 'very infrequent in warm climates', even in the case of intermittent fevers which were generally thought to respond well to this treatment.[27] Stimulants such as wine were also of little use in the tropics, he claimed, and in some cases, they had been positively detrimental because they had been given in enormous quantities. Those who advocated such practices, he argued, had usually little experience of fevers in India.[28] Indeed, Wade insisted that surgeons arriving in India dispense with any 'prejudices acquired at the university or at the shop',[29] and warned that 'the diseases of warmer latitudes differ very materially from such as afflict the inhabitants of cold climates, and the methods of treating them should consequently vary'.

The denunciation of rival practices shows that a new orthodoxy had emerged in British-Indian medical practice—grounded in the biliary theory of fevers, and manifest in the overriding emphasis on mercury as a therapy. Although the military context provided many of the conditions necessary for innovation in medical practice, and though military surgeons prided themselves on their empiricism, it also enabled senior medical officers to impose their views upon juniors. This could be done to some extent through the exercise of patronage, without which the aspiring surgeon had no chance of appointment to the Company or the armed forces medical services, or of advancement through the ranks. Once in the service, surgeons or physicians in charge of hospitals were in complete control of the purchase of medicines and were in a position to regulate their use. Above these surgeons came the inspectors and deputy inspector-generals of hospitals and the Medical Boards (in India there was one for each presidency) that had the power to enforce certain practices on pain of disciplinary action. Some medical offices viewed the powers wielded by these individuals as tyrannical,[30] and there is one well documented case of a medical officer falling foul of the Indian medical authorities for pursuing practices at variance with the official line—that of the British Army surgeon Thomas Clark.

Clark's *Observations on the Nature and Cure of Fevers, and of Diseases of the West and East Indies* (1801) is unusual in that it was written not so much to communicate new ideas, as to vindicate its author, who had recently been accused of malpractice in the military hospital at Colombo. Clark joined the Army as an assistant surgeon at the end of 1790 and was sent immediately to Canada. In August 1793, he was dispatched to Barbados and served there, and on several islands in the West Indies, before purchasing a surgeoncy with the 113th Regiment in Ireland. In October of that year, the regiment embarked for India and Clark arrived in Madras in November 1796. Shortly afterwards, he was ordered to Ceylon to take charge of the military hospital at Colombo. When Clark arrived in the East Indies, he was a very experienced surgeon and had learnt much about the diseases of warm climates; his approach was flexible and empirical, in the best tradition of British military medicine. While at Colombo, however, he fell foul of the Medical Board in Madras and, in particular, of Dr Ewart, the Inspector-General of Hospitals. Ewart, a British Army physician, appears to have had authority over both Crown and Company hospitals, and issued general orders that applied to both.[31]

One such order was that all surgeons working in hospitals had to fill in case-books describing the patient's symptoms and the treatment given; a rule that was generally flouted owing to competing claims on surgeons' time. Clark was one of the few who carried out these orders and, though ill himself, ordered his assistants to complete the forms. They did this for one month and, towards the end of 1798, Clark dispatched the form to the Inspector-General as requested.[32] Shortly afterwards, Ewart replied to Clark enclosing 'a long and elaborate dissertation upon his Case-Books, in which he was pleased totally to reprobate the Medical Practice Reported in them'.[33] Ewart even went so far as to accuse Clark of killing one of his patients by using inappropriate treatments. Unfortunately, Clark did not specify which treatments Ewart complained of in his letter, and the latter's 'dissertation' was lost by Clark when returning from India. However, it is clear from Clark's writings, and the subsequent actions of

Ewart, that they disagreed fundamentally about the causation of diseases like fever and dysentery and about their treatment.

Whereas Ewart subscribed to the conventional British-Indian view that fevers and dysentery originated in disorders of the liver, and were most effectively treated with mercury, Clark believed that both fevers and dysentery—while often connected with liver disorders—often developed independently. Clark further believed that the primary cause of all these diseases was the 'sedative' action of tropical climates, which checked perspiration, causing the body to overheat and the heart and arteries to become over excited. Heat also led, he believed, to a marked 'determination' of the blood from the skin towards the thoracic and abdominal organs, causing them to become distended and inflamed; this—rather than superabundant bile—was the cause of fevers, dysentery, and hepatic disorders. In Clark's opinion, all these complaints could be treated effectively by bleeding, as it reduced the quantity of blood and diminished inflammation.[34] Clark's advocacy of bloodletting in these diseases was clearly at odds with British-Indian orthodoxy. As he later pointed out, Ewart was of the opinion that 'fever, and likewise dysentery, were almost always occasioned by the state of the liver',[35] thus their respective approaches to the treatment of these diseases necessarily differed.

However, Clark did not advocate bleeding to the exclusion of all other treatments. In cases of fever, bleeding was followed by the administration of large doses of calomel, or Dr James' antimonial powder.[36] The latter would have been acceptable to Ewart and the Medical Board, but Clark's primary course of bleeding was not; nor was his insistence on ipecacaunha (rather than mercury) as a remedy for dysentery. When Ewart visited the Colombo hospital in November 1798, shortly after having sent his comments to Clark, he took over the running of the hospital and immediately abolished the use of ipecacaunha.[37] Shortly after this, Clark was arrested and threatened with a court-martial for disobeying orders, on the grounds that his assistants were no longer keeping a log of treatments. However, given that most surgeons regarded this as an 'intolerable piece of drudgery'[38] and refused to comply with Ewart's orders, it seems likely that the charge was merely a pretext to exclude Clark from practice. Ultimately, Clark did not face trial but was kept under arrest for around three months, during which his health deteriorated further. After his release, in 1799, he was forced to leave Ceylon and to return to Britain, where he wrote his extraordinary vindication.

Although mercury therapy never became totally dominant in British India, the treatment of fevers came to display a certain amount of rigidity and uniformity. Any tendency to conformity arising from convictions about the uniqueness of the Indian disease environment was compounded by the hierarchical organization of the military medical services and the boards that regulated military and naval hospitals. Heroic treatments such as purgation with mercury also befitted a military service and suggested a worldly, no-nonsense approach to those who had fallen sick. Too many in the army and navy, sickness seemed rather ignoble and was closely associated with poor discipline; indeed, many illnesses were ascribed, in part, to disorder or intemperance. Back in the 17th century, Bontius had written of the need to 'restrain the fury of rioting morbific matter' in cases of cholera,[39] and analogies between putrefaction and social decay abound in the literature on Indian fevers in the 18th century. In view of such anxieties, and the low esteem in which British soldiers were held, it may well have been that vigorous purging had a disciplinary element—a subconscious desire to purge Europeans of any harmful alien elements.

All these factors may help to explain the prevalence of mercury therapy for fevers in late 18th and early 19th century India, but it is likely that the resort to large quantities of mercury was indicative of desperation as much as anything. In one of his first letters home, the Company surgeon Francis Maxwell told his father (who seems to have possessed some knowledge of medicine) that—

> You would be surprised, and, I'll venture to say, so would every Medical man in Glasgow, at the quantity of Mercury we give in Feveres [sic], Fluxes, etc., for diseases here are such that if we do not stop them soon by vigorous remedies, they will save us trouble by killing the patients. As you are a bit of a doctor, you may form some idea of your practice when I inform you I frequently give a man 70 or 80 grains of Calomel in 24 hours, and perhaps continue the same for some days.[40]

However, patients often took some convincing that mercury therapy was in their best interests, as George Cormack, a cornet in the Bengal Army, recalled when recovering from an attack of bilious fever—

> The fatigue I underwent brought on a Bilious Fever and this is the first letter I have written since my recovery. The Fever did not annoy me above five days, but the Doctor, a cabbage headed West Country Medicine Pounder, crammed me with such a quantity of Calomel as salivated me completely for 25 days. I had no use of either gums or teeth.[41]

The unpleasant side effects of mercury and its failure, in many instances, to arrest the progress of disease, later induced many practitioners in India to turn against it. But by the 1790s, mercurial remedies were being employed as a matter of course, not only in India but in the West Indies, too. According to the Jamaican physician, William Wright, he had learned of the method used in the Madras hospital as early as 1860, in a conversation with Lind of Haslar. Four years later he, too, began to use mercury in the treatment of visceral obstructions, and afterwards began to use calomel freely, not only in hepatic disorders, but in all acute diseases he encountered. At about the same time, according to Wright, one Dr Drummond, also of Jamaica, began to use calomel to treat fevers and pleurisies, but at that time the two practitioners had no knowledge of each other. Rather, Wright had learned of Drummond's method from a Dr Smith of Savannah, Georgia, who gave calomel in doses of 20 grains in acute diseases.[42]

However, mercurial treatment for non-venereal complaints does not appear to have been common in the West Indies until the 1790s, when its rising popularity was largely a function of the desperation many felt in the face of the yellow fever epidemic that claimed so many lives on St Domingo. One of its chief advocates was Colin Chisholm, author of *An Essay on the Malignant Pestilential Fever* (1795).[43] More commonly known as yellow fever, this disease was thought to be a putrid bilious fever—like many of the fevers in India—even though the symptoms, most notably yellow staining of the skin, marked it out as different to some degree. The black vomit that was characteristic of the later stages of the disease seemed to suggest that the victim's bile had putrefied; hence the apparent utility of treatment with mercury. The logical of Chisholm's argument appealed to a number of other surgeons working in the West Indies. One such was James Bryce, formerly a surgeon on the East-Indiaman, the *Busbridge*, and his own experience in using calomel in the treatment of yellow fever was such that he was 'most anxious to recommend a more free use of calomel, than has hitherto been common even in warm climates, being fully convinced that the greatest part, if not all the acute diseases of those regions, proceed, either immediately or remotely, from accumulations of offending matter in the bowels'.[44]

The powers of mercury had also caught the imagination of the Army surgeon James Clark, who like many other British surgeons, employed it in the treatment of the disease on St Domingo. Of the different treatments for yellow fever employed on the island, mercury stood out as being by far the most effective. Its main rivals—such as bloodletting, which was used extensively by the French—were considered dangerous by Clark and most other British surgeons.[45] The British method of treatment consisted in moderate purging with jalap followed by six to eight mercurial pills given as quickly as possible, followed by two to three more every hour until they began to take effect. If this course of treatment did not arrest the symptoms, the dose of calomel was increased to 10 grains. Calomel pills continued to be administered throughout the febrile stage and often for several days afterwards, but, according to Clark, this method 'seldom failed to remove the fever in twenty-four or thirty-six hours'. He was aware that some would consider the amount of calomel used too large and even dangerous, but, he explained, in 'this most desperate of all diseases, it is necessary to oppose, very speedily, the most powerful, and seemingly desperate remedies'. Like Bryce and Chisholm, he believed that its beneficial affects lay in expelling and correcting 'a vitiated and superabundant secretion of bile'.[46]

By the 1800s, the treatment of yellow fever with mercury was well established amongst British Army surgeons in the West Indies,[47] and, in 1812, when Robert Jackson took charge of the medical department of the British Army in the West Indies, the practice generally adopted in fever was still to 'saturate the system with mercury'.[48] The same was true of naval outposts in the West Indies, according to Leonard Gillespie. In 1799, he recorded in his journal that the method employed by most surgeons on that station was to bleed, if necessary, on the first attack of fever and then to administer a calomel purge—'about five grains every hour until the mouth became affected'. He added that a concoction of ginger was sometimes necessary to allow such large quantities to remain in the stomach until the point of salivation was reached.[49] Calomel was also used to treat dysentery on naval vessels in the West Indies, one surgeon noting that a combination of calomel and ipecacaunha worked particularly well, notwithstanding the opinion of some British authorities such as Dr Robertson. The same surgeon also noted that he and his naval colleagues in the West Indies had learned of the practice from 'the writings of East India Practitioners'.[50]

Some held that the propensity of mercury to bring forth salivation was greater in tropical climates but the quantities used in the East and West Indies suggest that this belief did little to moderate its use.[51] Salivation, indeed, had become the touch stone of mercurial treatment, being recommended by some of the principal authorities on yellow fever such as Clark and Rush.[52] Practitioners in the West Indies were so confident in this that they thought little of criticism at home. An anonymous correspondent to a London-based surgeon, Mr Chamberlain, claimed that—

> I am astonished to hear that some of the practitioners in England have written to their friends here [Jamaica] of the "madness of our practice". I shall not call them mad; but I think them blameably [sic] presumptive in writing of what they know nothing at all. For, if they are eminent, their opinions may poison the minds of such unfortunate strangers as may be taken ill, so as to make them object to the only treatment that has a chance of saving them from the most fatal of all diseases yet known, scarcely the plague itself excepted.

He added, 'whenever you may have an opportunity of giving advice to adventurers coming this way, never neglect to recommend having the salivary glands slightly affected before they embark, or immediately on their arrival on the spots of infection'.[53]

The extensive employment of mercury in the West Indies was, as we have seen, justified on the grounds that tropical diseases required more drastic treatments than those in Britain. And yet a number of practitioners came to advocate the use of mercury in diseases analogous to those found in the Indies, although in lesser quantities. Practitioners in Britain came to hear of the way in which mercury was used in India as early as the 1760s, with an account given of its use in the treatment of dysentery in the *Medical Museum*.[54] Favourable reports of its use had also been communicated by Lind in his *Essay on the Diseases of Hot Climates*,[55] and it was used with apparent success by John Clark after his return from India to treat hepatitis and stubborn cases fever encountered in his practice at the Newcastle Infirmary.[56] It was also strongly advocated by Daniel Lyssons, of Bath, in the treatment of epidemic fevers.[57] But it was not really until the 1780s that publications on the subject appeared with sufficient frequency to make much of an impact in Britain. One of those who advocated its use then was Dr Robert Hamilton, a physician in the Norfolk town of Lynn Regis (King's Lynn), who had employed mercury in the treatment of inflammatory diseases for some 18 years. He had discussed the treatment with Pringle[58] who had given him encouragement and expressed the hope that it would be given trial in some of the public hospitals. But 'so little was it consonant to common practice', he claimed, 'and so difficult is it to overcome prejudices, that I apprehended it never was tried'.[59] Hamilton had learned of the practice from a 'worthy surgeon of the navy' who had worked at a hospital on the Coromandel Coast for eight years, before his return to England in 1764. It was he who had suggested that the same practice might work in England, particularly in the low-lying country around Lynn, which in several respects resembled India. 'Our diseases are nearly the same with those of similar situations in India', Hamilton wrote, 'particularly the bilious autumnal remittent and intermittent fevers, an allowance being made for their difference in violence and magnitude'. Like the south-east coast of India, the fens also suffered from 'a most dangerous hepatitis'.[60]

A few years later, the former EIC surgeon James Lind, now a royal physician based at Windsor, also extolled the virtues of mercury in the treatment of inflammatory diseases and dysentery. In 1787, he was already able to report that it was used by a number of distinguished practitioners in Britain, although he warned that British physicians ought to be more moderate in the quantity they administered and guard against salivation.[61] By the 1800s, there were quite a number of doctors in Britain itself recommending purgation with mercury. These included fever expert, Sir William Fordyce,[62] liver expert, Dr William Saunders, and a host of other practitioners who believed it useful in everything from hepatitis to the diseases of children.[63] But there were still, of course, many sceptics. The Grenada-based military surgeon, Colin Chisholm, declared that there was a 'powerful prejudice' against the practice in the medical department of the Navy,[64] although, as we have seen, this was by no means true of all naval surgeons. To the extent that it was true, resistance to mercury may be ascribed to the nervous theory of fevers popularized by such influential naval practitioners as Thomas Trotter (1760–1832).[65] However, there were still many practitioners who remained suspicious of calomel on pragmatic grounds, fearing its toxicity and its associations with quackery.

Mercury remained well entrenched in medical practice in Britain and the tropics until the 1820s, at about which time the growing dominance of the nervous theory of disease undermined the old rationale for using powerful purgatives such as mercury. Practitioners moved increasingly towards the use of stimulants and bloodletting—a practice which had formerly been rejected as inappropriate for warm climates. It would require at least another chapter to explain and describe this process fully but the main point is that mercurial remedies were no longer regarded as panaceas in the way they had been formerly. Although mercurial treatment of non-venereal complaints remained common, the drug no longer occupied a central place in therapeutics, either in the colonies or in Britain. However, what the case of calomel shows is that a practice which originated in colonial hospitals was capable of profoundly affecting the development of British medicine more generally. The growing sense of distinctiveness which marked out medical practice in the tropics was not a barrier to the transmission of ideas and practices to the homeland. Tropical practitioners tried to have it both ways—when it suited them, they stressed the uniqueness of tropical practice and their unique expertise; but if they returned to practice in Britain, they stressed the relevance of their experience of fevers to the treatment of fevers there.

NOTES

1. Warner (1997: especially Chapter 1).

2. See, Andreas-Holger Maehle, 1999, *Drugs on Trial*, pp. 15–17; W. F. Bynum in W. F. Bynum and Roy Porter (eds) (1987:5–28); Gunter B.Risse, 1986, *Hospital Life in Enlightenment*, Cambridge: Cambridge University Press, pp. 199–200. Goldwater (1972:239–48).

3. Goodeve (1837:145).

4. Pasley's name is spelt in at least three ways in contemporary sources, *viz.*, 'Pasly', 'Paisley', and 'Pasley'.

5. T. L. Folly, 1798, 'The Preparation or Sublimation of Mercury by the Malabars', *Tranquebar*.

6. No. 192, 3 May 1763, No. 143, 12 April 1763, P/240/21, Madras Public Consultations, OIOC.

7. Letter from Robert Twining and James Wilson detailing repairs and additions needed to make the hospital larger and fit for the purpose. No. 462, 1757, P/240/14, Madras Public Consultations, OIOC.

8. Madras Public Consultations: No. 177, 26 February 1762, P/240/20; No. 155, 9 March 1762, P240/20; No. 491, 18 October 1765, Letter from Mr Gilbert Pasley to Robert Palk, President and Governor Ft. St. George, 14 October 1765, No. 494, P/240/23, OIOC.

9. Gustavus Ducarel, Purnea, to James C. Ducarel, St Germaine, France, 4 January 1771, Records of Ducarel Family, D. 2091, F/7/5, GCRO.

10. Letter from Gilbert Pasley to Governor of Madras in Council, Nos. 167–172, 29 March 1771, P/240/31, Madras Public Consultations, OIOC.

11. Clark (1801:269).

12. Ibid., p. 139.

13. Francis Balfour (d. 1767) obtained an MD at Edinburgh University in 1767 and joined the Company's Bengal service as an assistant-surgeon in 1769; he resigned his combat commission on promotion to surgeon in 1777 and he became head surgeon in 1786. In 1788, Balfour gained a prestigious post as a member of the medical board, on which he sat until 1796; he was re-appointed to the board in 1800 and remained a member until he retired in 1807. In addition to the works cited in this chapter, he was the author of *Dissertatio de Gonorrhea virulenta* (1767), *The Forms of Herkern* (1781), and a lost translation of the *Seir-I-Mutakherin*. Crawford (1930:15).

14. See, Harrison (2000:25–48).

15. Francis Balfour (1784:17–20) believed that the so-called '*Pucca* Fever' of Bengal could not be cured with anything but bark, which checked the process of putrefaction; Balfour was in correspondence with Pringle and was aware of the latter's experiments which appeared to show that bark had an antiseptic quality. However, Balfour allowed that purely bilious fevers could be cured simply through evacuation (Ibid., p. 21).

16. Editorial, *India Journal of Medical Science*, n.s., 2 (1837:306); Balfour (1784:111–12, 129–30).

17. For example, 'J.M.', *The Medical Museum: Or, A Repository of Cases, Experiments, Researches, and Discoveries Collected at Home and Abroad by Gentlemen of the Faculty* (1764:611–12); Gilbert Pasly to Hon. Court of Directors, 29 March 1771, Madras Public Proceedings, P/240/3, OIOC, BL; Gustavus Ducarel to James Ducarel, 4 January 1771, Ducarel Papers, D.2091, Gloucestershire County Record Office; Lind (1787:534); Wade (1793:150–62).

18. Jodrell to Earl of Salisbury, f.4065, undated, Letters from Sir Paul Jodrell, 9/35/177, Wiltshire and Swindon Record Office.

19. Ibid., p. 145.

20. Wade (1793:116–17, 129).

21. John Peter Wade, 1792, *Nature and Effects of Emetics*, 57.

22. Ibid., p. 297.

23. Wade (1793:155).

24. Paisly quoted Ibid., p. 162.

25. Ibid., p. 112.

26. Goodeve (1837:147).

27. Wade (1793:59).

28. Ibid., pp. 62–3.

29. Ibid., p. 48.

30. Maclean (1810:90).

31. Clark (1801:vi).

32. Ibid., pp. vi–vi.

33. Ibid., p. vii.

34. Ibid., pp. 18–19, 30–4, 39.

35. Ibid., p. 234.

36. Ibid., p. 19.

37. Ibid., p. 234.

38. Ibid., p. vii.

39. Bontius (1769:27–8).

40. Maxwell to his father, undated c. August 1798, Letters from Dr Francis Maxwell, MSS. Eur. C.101, OIOC.

41. Letter from George Cormack, 17 November 1804, in Alexander Allan Cormack (ed.), *The Mahratta Wars 1792–1805: Letters from the Front by Three Brothers - Nicholas, George and Thomas Carnegie of Charleton, Montrose*, RAMC 715/6, CMAC.

42. Wright (1797:23–4).

43. Chisholm (1795:163). The treatment was also developed by others simultaneously. For example, Dr Maclarty (1796:328–33).

44. Bryce (1796:52).

45. Clark (1797:24–5).

46. Ibid., pp. 30, 37–8.

47. Mabit (1804:17).

48. M'Cabe (1825:13).

49. Leonard Gillespie, 'Medical Journal of His Majesty's Ship, Arab, from the 27th day of March 1799 to the 27th day of March 1800', ADM 101/85/4, TNA.

50. Alexander Meline, 'A Journal of Physical and Surgical Cases that occurred on Board of His Majesty's Ship L'Aimable between the 5th day of September 1797 and the 4th day of September 1798; during which time the said ship was employed in the West Indies and on her passage for England', pp. 15–23, 36–7, ADM 101/81/4, TNA.

51. Quier (1778:22).

52. (1799:79).

53. Letter to Mr Chamberlain, Kingston, Jamaica, 15 September 1800, 'Miscellaneous Intelligence, Observations and Hints' (1800:568).

54. Samuel J.M. Alberti, 2011, *Morbid Curiosities: Medical Museums in Nineteenth Century Britain*, Oxford: Oxford University Press, p. 611.

55. Lind, *Essay* (1808:104, 107).

56. Falck (1776); Letter from Dr Robert Hamilton to Dr Duncan, giving 'An Account of a successful Method of treating Inflammatory Diseases, by Mercury and Opium', *Medical Commentaries*, 9 (1783–4:191–205, at p. 204).

57. Lyssons, *Effects of Camphire and Calomel*; Bryce (1796:54–5). Bryce refers to the use of calomel by Dr Carmichael Smyth of London, to treat victims of an outbreak of goal fever at Winchester.

58. Dr. John Pringle, Bart of Pall Mall (1707–82), President of the Royal Society. He was the author of the book *Observations on the Diseases of the Army in Camp and Garrison.*

59. Ibid., pp. 191–2.

60. Ibid., p. 194.

61. Lind (1787:43–56, at pp. 43–4).

62. See, Wade (1793:52–3).

63. See, for example: Houlston (1784); Saunders (1809); Letter from 'A Medical Practitioner', Gloucester, 13 November 1801, *The Medical and Physical Journal*, 7 (1807:38–9); Currie (1809).

64. Chisholm (1795:163).

65. For Trotter's views on yellow fever (1797:334–6).

4 Dietetics, Mimesis, and Alterity

Food in Asian Medical Traditions and East-West Exchanges[†]

DAVID ARNOLD[¥]

In the 30 years since the publication of Charles Leslie's landmark volume, *Asian Medical Systems*,[1] the scholarship on medicine in Asia has ranged widely across time and space, revealing many different themes and perspectives. It would be almost impossible to summarize or even to categorize that enormous body of work, but, in the main, it can be said that historical work has focussed considerably more on questions of disease, on morbidity and mortality, than on issues of how health was maintained—or sought to be—in various social and cultural contexts. This prevailing emphasis on disease is perhaps unsurprising. Disease—especially the epidemic diseases in which so much of the earlier history of medicine in Asia (and elsewhere) was grounded— makes for a more dramatic and conveniently episodic story than the continuing, day-to-day history of health. The history of health is often more difficult to document, precisely because it is an everyday history, and it raises complex issues as to what different cultures and classes, different governmental regimes and state agencies, envisage as 'health' in the first place. Our scholarly concerns have mostly been pathological,

† An earlier version of this chapter was presented at the conference on 'Health and Medicine in History: East-West Exchange' held at JNU in November 2006.

¥ I am grateful to the organizers for inviting me to attend the conference and to those participants whose comments and criticisms I have tried to incorporate here. Additional thanks are due to Dominik Wujastyk, Shang-Jen Li, and Projit Mukharji.

and for that reason we may have done an interpretive injustice to the wider field of health, disease, and medicine.

This chapter is one attempt to address that imbalance by focussing on the significance of food and dietetics in different medical traditions, as they relate especially to India. In so doing, the discussion takes a critical view of the idea of 'exchange' as it pertains to relations between indigenous and colonial (Western) medicine in South Asia and, following the lead of Michael Taussig and Jean M. Langford, makes alternative use of concepts of mimesis and alterity.[2]

FOOD AND *AYURVEDA*

The Ayurvedic tradition of South Asia has commonly been regarded (as in Charles Leslie's pioneering collection of essays) as a 'medical system', and on that basis comparable with other Asian medical systems—which Leslie identified principally as the Chinese and the 'Mediterranean' (that is, the Hippocratic, Galenic, and *Unani*) systems. Leaving aside the question of whether we can really call these 'systems' at all (given their enormous internal diversity, diverse agencies, and complex trajectories over time), there is a presumption in this 'systems' approach to comparative medicine that what makes these (and later 'cosmopolitan' or Western medicine) amenable to comparison is that they have in common a corpus of canonical medical texts, specialist medical practitioners, and a set of diagnostic tools and therapeutic functions that aligns them with rationality, science, and secularism rather than with sorcery, magic, and divination. They also belong to literate (or part-literate) societies and, in terms of practitioners and patients, to the elite strata within them (in this sense, at least by implication, alterity lies in the subaltern or folk medical traditions).[3] But defining them as systems of *medicine* alone is clearly insufficient. Thus, it has been widely acknowledged that Ayurveda was—or aspired to be—considerably more than this. It was a 'science of life', a body of knowledge about how to sustain health and prolong human existence.[4]

Certainly, a substantial part of the textual material brought together in the canonical compilations (the *samhitas*) of Charaka and Susruta by the early centuries of the Common Era was concerned with the identification and treatment of specific diseases, with various branches of medical practice, with the proper conduct of the physician, and with the appropriate instruments and techniques to be employed. But this

Indian system of knowledge was directed at maintaining health and
was concerned with preventing as well as curing diseases. Further, as
A. L. Basham remarked in discussing Ayurveda, 'The concept of medicine as a means of preserving health rather than curing disease led to
much emphasis on dietetics'.[5] The 'classic' Ayurvedic texts devoted considerable space to the nature, properties, and uses of various food items,
and to dietetics as the body of rules and principles for regulating health
and controlling disease through diet. They attribute, often in remarkable
detail, the healing, health-sustaining, or disease-inducing properties of
different foods, including many varieties of rice and other grains, pulses,
vegetables, fruits, dairy products, and animal flesh, and the appropriate
forms of cooking or other modes of preparation required to optimise
the therapeutic value of each one.[6] Indeed, the very idea of digestion is
a central explanatory mechanism within Ayurvedic physiology. What is
ingested through eating is transformed into the five fundamental elements (the *mahabhutas*) of which the body is composed and so affects its
overall balance and general state of well-being or disorder.[7] Food feeds
and sustains the bodily system but also has the contrary capacity to con-
found its proper working.

The study of dietetics and the taxonomy of foods were central elements in Ayurvedic diagnosis and preventive medicine. The Caraka
samhita speaks of food, along with sleep and a chaste life, as being one
of the 'three pillars' of health—the abuse of food, as by overindulgence,
is correspondingly seen as a source of disease. The text prescribes eight
rules for appropriate eating and explains the humoral consequences of
abstinence and fasting.[8] The Susruta samhita considers the four different
means by which food is consumed (chewing, drinking, licking, and eating) and the means by which it is converted into nutritive juices (*rasa*)
within the body—from this process come blood, flesh, bone, and semen.
The text further recounts the need to safeguard food and drink from
poisoning—Ayurveda is almost as rich in toxicology as it is in dietetics.[9]
A later author, Vagbhata, in the 6th or 7th century CE discusses seasonal
foods and their 'heating', 'cooling', and other properties, idioms that
reflect the wider cultural evaluation of the properties of specific foodstuffs in South Asia.[10] Subsequent authors and compilers continued to
add to this diet-related medical discourse—Bhavamishra, for instance, in
the 16th century gave a description of lathyrism, a condition caused by
consumption of the vetch, *Lathyrus sativus*.[11]

Food, moreover, provides continuity between the individual and, as Francis Zimmermann so effectively argued in *The Jungle and the Aroma of Meats*,[12] the physical environment he (or she) inhabits. It unites the individual with the cosmos and registers the variations that characterize each season and every environmental zone. Hot, dry places produce certain kinds of foods, animal as well as vegetable, or foods whose distinctive properties might contribute to particular manifestations of disorder or could, conversely, be used to counter or cure a specific ailment. Ayurvedic medicine exists in part as the assemblage and interpretation of this knowledge of how food, and the physical environment in which it is found and eaten, inform the bodily condition. But it is also a kind of secondary resource—the need for a physician can be obviated so long as one eats the right thing in the right place and in the appropriate season. Food, of course, is by no means the only factor invoked to explain disease and healing processes in Ayurvedic texts, but it is one of the most fundamental.

Were the other medical traditions similarly food-fixated? Probably so, but not uniformly. The oft-cited Hippocratic text 'Airs, Waters and Places' gives far more weight to the changing seasons, to winds, waters, and physical location, than to food. Only marginally and rather indeterminately does the author refer to the greater susceptibility to disease of 'heavy drinkers and eaters' or the effects of seasonal changes in relation to diet. In this canonical Hippocratic text, food seems to have no privileged relationship with disease, its aetiology, and symptomatology—this is especially so when its author turns to discuss the all-important question of the causation of epidemics. Only in speaking of the nature of the medical regimen is reference made to suitable and unsuitable foods—but even this, when compared to the elaborate cataloguing of foods and their properties in Charaka, Susruta, and other Ayurvedic texts, appears scant and superficial and to entail little speculation on the effects different foods have on human physiology.[13]

But within the evolving context of humoral thought, food (and drink) became installed as one of the six 'non-naturals' of Galenic medicine,[14] and some works of this tradition do give substantial weight to food as a factor in health and disease, notably Galen's text *On the Power of Foods*, dating from around 180 CE. A concern with diet may well reflect the affluent lifestyles of the upper social strata of Greco-Roman society and hence those who patronized the practitioners of this medical system.

Although the boundary between culinary taste and dietary medicine was far from clear-cut, it has been argued that through the study of dietetics, diet was 'raised from mere eating for the sustenance of the body to a higher philosophical plane that bolstered its importance within medicine as a whole'.[15]

A similar 'medico-culinary-dietetic tradition' flourished in the Islamic world from around the 8th century CE. Again, information concerning dietetics, the proper preparation of foods, and their health preserving or harmful properties, was not a monopoly of physicians alone but 'was shared by other sectors of the cultured urban public'.[16] Dietetics played a prominent part, too, in the Chinese medical tradition and its *materia medica* from at least the Tang dynasty and probably much earlier.[17] The Ayurvedic tradition was, therefore, probably not alone in the importance it attached to dietetics, though the degree to which the properties of individual food substances were identified and classified may, even so, have been exceptional. Arguably, this common ground facilitated the sharing of 'medico-culinary' ideas between different Eurasian elites and their medical traditions; but this commonality may also have generated very different interpretations of how different food substances, especially exotic and unfamiliar ones, might be used and to what bodily effect. 'Exchange' did not necessarily signify agreement as to the powers and utility of the commodity that was being exchanged.[18]

The Unani tradition as it developed in South Asia from the 13th century onwards—in association with Ayurveda and with a physical and cultural environment distinctive from that of the eastern Mediterranean and Middle East in which it originated—developed a similar preoccupation with the disease-preventing and curative properties of specific foodstuffs, and assigned value to particular items of food as tonics, elixirs, and aphrodisiacs. The centuries-long transmission and translation of texts, the dissemination of foods that were once regionally specific, the shared use of therapeutic substances, and the common understanding of the importance of diet to health and disease, should make us cautious about over-privileging the importance of the subsequent 'exchange' between East and West, between South Asia and Europe, from the 15th century onwards.[19] It has, after all, been one of the trends in the recent historiography of medieval and early modern South Asia to stress the subcontinent's interconnectedness with other regions across the Eurasian *ecumene* in the centuries before the coming of European trade and domination. Through the trade in spices and medicinal drugs, through the movement of medical texts and specialists, and the flow of medical ideas and practices, the history of food as medicine deserves a significant place in this wider cultural and commercial history.[20]

It should likewise be noted that Ayurvedic pharmacology, far from being regionally confined, drew upon an extended network of commercial exchanges (of which Indian bazaars were often only the ultimate transactional sites), using medicinal substances drawn not just from the different ecological zones of South Asia but also from across Eurasia— from China to East Africa and even, by the 18th and 19th centuries, from the Americas.[21] New items of food, introduced from the Atlantic world, such as okra (*bhindi*), were incorporated into Ayurvedic and Unani materia medica, often without reference to their exotic origins, and assigned properties compatible with those epistemological traditions.[22] At the same time, though, as Leslie notes, these and other medical systems retained their separate identities and their distinctive ways of thinking about the body, about health, environment, and disease.[23] Even in late Unani texts, many substances continued to be identified as 'Indian medicines', or as drugs known only from their inclusion in Indian medical works, as if to distance them from those more familiar from (and whose use is thereby authenticated in) Arabic and Persian sources.

ENCOUNTERS WITH WESTERN MEDICINE
To what extent did the Ayurvedic concern with dietetics, and hence with the medicinal, life-preserving or life-enhancing properties of specific foods, inform Western medicine in India from the mid-18th century onwards—or form part of an epistemic and therapeutic 'exchange' between East and West? Certainly there was substantial European interest in the late 18th and early 19th centuries, in Indian 'cooling regimes' (including the use of 'cooling' foods) as used in the treatment of particular diseases, such as smallpox and malaria, and in the value, for Europeans residing in the tropics, of avoiding overindulgence and following a 'temperate' diet. For a while, the modest, vegetarian diets of (some) Indians were admired and praised as a model of moderation worthy of European emulation.

Thus, James Johnson, one of the leading medical authorities of the period, remarked—'That vegetable food, generally speaking, is better adapted to a tropical climate than animal, I think we may admit'.[24]

Charles Curtis, similarly, observed that newcomers to India 'cannot too soon adopt the regimen of the Europeans who have resided in the climate, and accustom themselves to what are called the native dishes, which consist for the most part of boiled rice, and fruits, highly seasoned with hot aromatics, along with meat stews, and sauces, with but a small proportion of solid animal matter'. He recommended that newly arrived Europeans follow the example of long-established residents 'in the management of what have been called the Non-naturals' (including diet).[25] Conversely, early 19th century British physicians were often tentative about interfering in dietary practices of the Indian in their charge, if only because they believed that Indian diets were already modest, even abstemious, by European standards. Discussing the treatment of dysentery, the Calcutta surgeon William Twining remarked in 1832—'The natives of Bengal are so scrupulously attentive to propriety in diet, when they are ill, that we have no difficulty in restraining them to as small a quantity of food as may be consistent with the cure of their diseases'. A little sago and rice-water would suffice, he believed, 'for that which would be to Europeans a low diet, is stimulant and injurious to Asiatics, while any degree of acute disease exists'.[26]

But Twining, a surgeon at Calcutta's General Hospital, was somewhat exceptional among Western physicians at the time in the degree of attention he paid to Indian diets and the recommendations of 'native practitioners'.[27] Much of the discussion on disease by East India Company surgeons followed a neo-Hippocratic climatic and 'miasmatic' explanation of disease (especially with respect to those epidemic diseases that were a primary European concern in South Asia), in which diet received scant consideration or was seen as a predisposing or aggravating factor rather than a causative one. Hence, the possibility that the outbreak of cholera in Jessore district in Bengal in 1817 might have been due to some defect in the grain consumed locally was briefly touted by the local magistrate but swiftly rejected as 'wholly untenable'—preference was given to the role of 'atmospheric vicissitudes' and other climatic disturbances.[28] A government enquiry into the cause of an 'epidemic fever' that swept through the southern districts of the Madras Presidency concluded that even though quantities of 'unwholesome grain' had been consumed in the affected districts, it could not be included among the causes of the epidemic. The grain might have induced debility and so rendered the effects of the epidemic more fatal, but, the medical committee concluded,

the 'unnatural state of the atmosphere' and the resultant 'morbific mias-
mata' were a more plausible explanation for the epidemic.[29] The Western
physicians' emphasis on anatomy (and, by contrast, its neglect among
contemporary Indian practitioners), the use of post-mortems in identifying diseases and in establishing their physiological effects, the perceived
need for 'heroic' treatments to stem the rapid and fatal tide of disease in
the tropics—all these further militated against a sustained cross-cultural
discussion of dietetics and fostered divergent views on the importance of
diet to health and healing.

That is not to say, though, that the dietetic element in Indian medical traditions was altogether ignored by Western commentators, especially when discussing Ayurveda. In 1837, in one of the most influential
works of medical Orientalism, the former East India Company surgeon
J. F. Royle, debated at length the antiquity of 'Hindoo medicine' and
noted, in passing, the importance of diet in ancient Indian texts (which
he knew only through English translations). He observed, 'As we might
expect from the mild habits, simple diet, and unexcitable constitutions
of the Hindoos, with attention to regimen, there is a long list of what
are translated [as] assuaging and depuratory medicines'. But, he added,
reverting to the perceived need for more rigorous therapeutics in India's
tropical environment, 'in a country where the accession of disease is as
sudden as is the rapid accumulation of fearfully fatal symptoms', it was
necessary for the physician to adopt measures characterized by 'prompt-
ness of decision, and vigour of practice'—that is by recourse to the use
of leeches, bloodletting and drastic purgatives rather than slow-acting
dietary measures.[30] In his account of what was 'interesting and instruc-
tive' in the 'Hindu system of medicine', T. A. Wise of the Bengal Medical
Service similarly mentioned diet. He noted how, according to Caraka
and Susruta, environment, climate, season, and diet influenced human
health and affected humoral balance; but he, too, tended to regard dietetics as a secondary feature of the 'Hindu system', of significant value only
in treating the first stage of a disease.[31]

By the 1840s, if not earlier, what European physicians looked for in
Ayurveda (and Unani *tibb*) was an 'empirical history of diseases and
remedies', a set of diagnostics and therapeutic practices, combined with
a convenient storehouse of materia medica,[32] that could be selectively
incorporated into Western medical practice. British interest in Indian
diets arose from other sources rather than through any 'exchange' with,

or mediation through, Ayurveda. It came principally through investigations into the nature of the food consumed by the labouring classes and
the need to provide life-sustaining diets for Indian prisoners, especially
once, in the mid-1840s, prisoners were being denied the right to feed
themselves. These enquiries, especially those instituted by provincial
governments in the 1860s, made scant reference to Indian dietetic ideas
and instead related diet to contemporary Western medical and scientific
findings.[33] This divergence—rather than mimesis or exchange—signi-
fied a shift not just away from engagement with the indigenous systems
of medicine but also from the health of individuals and the 'medico-
culinary' concerns of Indian elites. The surveys represented a move,
however imperfectly executed, towards a new spirit of colonial governmentality. The investigation of diet was coming to be seen as a means of
disciplining the poor (most evidently those institutionalized in prisons
or famine camps). It was a means of acquiring effective knowledge about
the food habits of the different classes of the population, especially the
'industrial and labouring classes', and of assessing the work value of the
foodstuffs they consumed.[34]

REINSTATING DIETETICS

When the revival of Ayurveda began in the late 19th century it was,
in the main, self-consciously as an ancient and indigenous system
of *medicine*.[35] It claimed to be comparable to Western medicine in
its ability to diagnose and treat disease, but had the added virtue of
possessing drugs and techniques unknown to the West, of having a
materia medica particularly suited to Indian constitutions and the
diseases and physical environment of South Asia, and the impoverished
economic circumstances of colonial India (the elitist bias in classical
Ayurveda, in which treating the poor was discouraged and serving the
king the highest honour and duty, was patriotically overlooked). Thus,
in an address given at the opening of the Benares Hindu University in
1916, Kaviraj Gananath Sen, one of the leading advocates for Ayurveda,
remarked that 'Western medical men should do well to remember
that fundamentally the principles of treatment recommended in
Ayurveda are almost identical with those of Western Medicine—only
the drugs and indigenous and methods of administration are somewhat
different'.[36] The move to make Ayurvedic remedies widely available to
a mass market, through newspaper advertisements and pre-prepared

ointments and pills sold through the post or over the counter, further militated against close consideration of the patient's individual dietary requirements or the need to prescribe specific foods in order to correct humoral imbalances.

One reads little in the speeches and writings of these Ayurvedic revivalists—or in those of their critics[37]—about the centrality of diet. For instance, in the early 20th century, Kabiraj Nagendra Nath Sen Gupta published a three-volume account in English of *The Ayurvedic System of Medicine* based on the Sanskrit authorities. His work opened with a brief account of health, but the subject of food occupied only two pages of his opening remarks, and these were more about how food should be eaten than on the health-reserving or life-sustaining properties of individual foodstuffs.[38] In the many hundreds of pages that followed, food and dietetics received hardly a mention.[39]

If the question of dietetics did, from time to time, appear in revivalist texts, it was as a secondary voice, as a plea for the reinstatement of something unaccountably lost or as an exemplification of the abiding differences between the Eastern and Western systems of medicine. For instance, in the now celebrated report of the Madras Committee of Enquiry into 'the indigenous systems of medicine' in 1923, there was much discussion of the *tridosha* theory (or the theory of three bodily humours, *vata* or wind, *pitta* or choler and *kapha* or phlegm) and its supposedly scientific basis, but there was almost nothing on dietetics. One has to turn to one of the many appended statements of written and oral evidence, that given by an out-of-town *kaviraj* (physician) Haran Chandra Chakrabarthi, to find the following statement—

As regards our country, the Ayurvedic system of treatment is undoubtedly more efficacious than any other system of medical treatment, in as much as its principles of treatment are based on full consideration of the place, time, diet and customs of our country. In the first place as regards diet, the injunctions of Ayurveda are best suited to our countrymen. The Western system of medicine has hardly discussed the dietetics and customs of our country, while Ayurveda has laid down what is particularly beneficial or detrimental to our health after due consideration of the merits and defects of every one of our food-stuffs in all their different conditions and forms and everyone of our actions. It has further enjoined that in selecting every diet, the physician should closely observe the condition of the place, time, vitality, natural constitution, habits and age of the patient. In the West the

consideration of diets is based on chemical analysis of those ingredients;
but in a majority of cases, such a process hardly yields any useful result.[40]

In a further statement of difference, the kaviraj added that 'without
due consideration are the Western physicians prescribing for us diets
examined in their own lands and this is causing us much harm'. He
claimed that there were no Western medicines for prolonging life and
generative powers—only Ayurveda could offer these.[41]

The significance of dietetics was not, therefore, altogether absent but
in the debates of the time such a strong emphasis, as that given by Haran
Chandra Chakrabarthi on diet, was a minority view. Far more attention
was paid to the validity of Ayurvedic pathology, diagnostics, and especially to the recuperation and deployment of its 'useful' drugs. This raises
interesting questions about the nature and meaning of 'exchanges',[42] but
also of medical mimesis. In some respects, the Ayurvedic revival was
mimetic—it took up from earlier Western Orientalists claims for the antiquity of 'Hindu medicine', for its status as a 'system' and 'science', and
a source of drugs and therapies not available in Western medicine. It also
followed medical Orientalists like Royle and Wise in downplaying the
role of dietetics and in marginalizing the elaborate and detailed discourse
on food, along with its properties and powers, to be found in Susruta and
other canonical texts. It could further be argued that there were elements
of a medical 'exchange' in the late 18th and early 19th centuries, as the
reference in European texts to specific items of Indian materia medica
indicate. But this was not a comprehensive or egalitarian 'exchange' as
between two equally rated systems of medical knowledge. Only a small
and selected part of the Ayurvedic and Unani corpus was taken up for
consideration—and much of that was rejected on grounds of inefficacy,
obscurity, or irrationality. Thus, despite the prominence given to food
and dietetics in the Susruta samhita (even in the early 19th century a
much quoted source), almost none of this passed into Western medical
discourse or, in consequence, the Ayurvedic revival.[43]

One of the difficulties the Ayurvedic revivalists experienced in seeking
to incorporate an ancient system of medicine into present-day praxis was
the nature of the dietary prescriptions laid down by Susruta, in particular. These included the flesh of numerous different animals,[44] whereas
the modern medicine sought to express itself—and the Hinduism it
represented—in essentially vegetarian terms and to play down what
Zimmermann refers to as Ayurveda's 'violent therapeutics' and 'the

equivocal nature of the Ayurvedic doctrine, caught ... between violence and vegetarianism'.[45] Indeed, in a further mimetic instance, Western medical texts had exhibited a similar tendency to see 'Hindu civilization' in vegetarian terms. Perhaps, partly because those texts were compiled by surgeon-botanists like J. F. Royle or W. B. O'Shaughnessy, whose primary interest was in locating and investigating the properties of medicinal plants, they played down or omitted references to meat in Ayurvedic therapeutics and Indian materia medica.[46] Similarly, as already noted, Ayurveda originated as part of an elite tradition and its dietary concerns (like those of many Galenic and Unani texts) were with foods familiar to the wealthier classes. They were not directed at those low-status groups who lived in poverty and had little, if any, choice about the kind of food they consumed. In seeking to make itself, in opposition to Western medicine and the costly British medical establishment in India, a popular and affordable system of medicine, Ayurveda needed to shed this elitism and present itself in ways that would commend it to the Hindu population at large. In part, what was happening here was the bifurcation of an earlier 'medico-culinary' tradition. Just as aphrodisiacs and elixirs were being edited out of mainstream Ayurvedic and Unani texts in order to demonstrate their scientific nature, so matters pertaining to food and diet were being relegated to cookery and the kitchen.

In one sense, the disengagement of Ayurvedic medicine from its own dietetic tradition is ironic, for it occurred at precisely the time that Western medicine was developing its own scientifically articulated concern for diet—but this was expressed in a language of carbohydrates, proteins, calorific values, vitamins, and diet surveys that further distanced it from the humoral pathology of Ayurveda. In the short-term, at least, this new direction in Western thinking about health and illness offered even less likelihood of a mutual 'exchange' with Indian medicine. Between systems, dietetics served to emphasis alterity rather than similitude, highlighting differences that were cultural as much as corporeal. Hence, there was a patriotically inspired as well as empirically grounded sentiment that even though the subject of Indian diets was important, Western observers were ill-qualified to comment on them because they knew so little about them.

As early as 1869, Mahendralal Sircar (who as a homeopath, a former practitioner of Western medicine, and an advocate for the selective revival of Ayurvedic medicine, straddled three different medical traditions) reported with enthusiasm the recent publication of Baron von Liebig's work on the chemistry of food and urged that it be widely read in India, where the subject was 'grossly neglected'. As a medical reformer, he noted that the indigenous practitioners, the *vaidyas* and hakims, had traditionally ascribed a high value to the consumption of suitable foods, but, assuming a scientific stance, he claimed that without the modern knowledge of chemistry and physiology, their supposed knowledge was 'perfectly useless'. On the other hand, he argued, European physicians in India were 'little acquainted with the foods usually consumed by the natives; consequently much value can hardly be placed upon their advice in this matter'.[47] In fact, as we have seen, the nature of Indian diets had already become a matter of colonial enquiry. At the same time, too, the British brought their own prejudices and preconceptions to the evaluation of Indian diets, regarding vegetarian—especially rice-based—diets as a cause of Indians' physical weakness, or as grounds for making a contrast between the healthy and 'masculine' wheat diets of the north and North-West and the enfeebling and effeminizing rice diets of Bengal and Madras.[48]

Partly in response to European diatribes against vegetarian diets, there was, though, an emerging Indian middle-class discourse in which poor or improper diets were cited as a factor in the 'decline' and 'degeneration' of modern Hindus.[49] Thus, in a lecture in 1929, Chunilal Bose, professor of chemistry at the Calcutta Medical College, observed that 'our present Indian diet is defective and ill-balanced and is directly responsible for the progressive deterioration of the physical health of the people, particularly of Bengal, and indirectly affecting their moral and economic well-being'.[50] He went on to discuss dietetics and the modern science of nutrition in relation to Indian food staples, but strikingly he did so without connecting this with Ayurveda, even though he argued that Bengalis' diets and physique had been far better in earlier times. He concluded, 'It is the duty of every true son of Bengal to devise means and adopt measures for the increased supply of milk and fish throughout the province. This will improve the diet of the people and make the country smile once again in health and prosperity'.[51]

One could perhaps argue that the dietary preoccupations of the Ayurvedic tradition resurfaced in other forms than in revivalist discourse. Gandhi, for instance, had no great faith in Ayurveda or in any other medical 'system' that took responsibility for maintaining health and coping with disease away from the individual. But, even so, his recourse to fasting and his ideas of health and diet seem to reflect key elements of Ayurveda (though Gandhi's thinking, as with respect to vegetarianism, also reflected his profound engagement with the West).[52]

It is hard to judge how far the actual practice of Ayurveda changed as a result of its encounter with the West and the consequent playing down in revivalist discourse on the importance of dietetics. Did diet, in fact, remain a powerful diagnostic tool and therapeutic response, despite its relative absence from revivalist speeches, textbooks, and tracts? Perhaps so. It is worth considering in this connection an interesting passage from the *Handbook of Tropical Therapeutics* published by R. N. Chopra of the Indian Medical Service in 1936 and addressed to both an Indian and European readership. Chopra shared something of Mahendralal Sircar's eclecticism—he was a practitioner of Western medicine (which he taught at the Calcutta School of Tropical Medicine) but also a proponent of the scientific investigation of indigenous medicine in India. In 1930–1, he chaired an investigation into indigenous drugs and in 1946–8, presided over the Government of India's committee of enquiry into the indigenous systems of medicine.[53]

Chapter 7 of Chopra's 1936 *Handbook* was devoted to 'Diet and Dietetics in the Tropics'. He began by remarking that—

> The importance that the Indian patient attaches to his diet is not fully appreciated by Western practitioners. The Hakims and Kavirajes lay great stress on the subject of diet. In Sushruta, the well-known book on Hindu medicine, it is said that 'The physician that does not know the principles of dietetics cannot cure disease'. This idea is ingrained in the minds of Indian patients and unless proper attention is paid to this aspect, patients are not convinced about the utility of a particular line of treatment. It is surprising, however, how few physicians practising Western medicine pay any special attention to this important subject.[54]

After discussing the technical aspects of diet, including the role of vitamins and proteins, Chopra turned to 'the Indian dietary', observing—

> The importance that the Indian ryot [peasant] attaches to his diet is hardly realised by Western practitioners. It is not uncommon to find a practitioner writing up prescriptions for medicines without any directions as to the nature of the diet his patient should take. The patients often remain dissatisfied in this respect and may lose faith in the physician.[55]

This suggests that the practical and ideological gap, the divergence, between Western and indigenous medicine, remained considerable.

CONCLUSION

Consideration of dietetics—and its changing cross-cultural fortunes—suggests one possible way among many of focusing on issues of health in Asian medical history. But it also invites a degree of scepticism about the idea of 'East-West exchange'. For one thing, the process of 'exchange' was an ancient one, long preceding the arrival of the European West and was represented, *inter alia*, in the mutual borrowings of (but continuing distinctions between) the Ayurvedic and Unani medical traditions. The idea of 'East-West exchange' is certainly to be welcomed as a way of countering facile assumptions about the simple imposition (or uncontested hegemony) of Western medicine over South Asian societies, and clearly there were some significant 'exchanges' taking place between European medicine and Ayurveda, from the time of the Portuguese arrival,[56] and perhaps especially, at a time of intensified contact, in the late 18th and early 19th centuries. But, as recent debates about 'colonial knowledge' should remind us, in the asymmetrical power relationship that unfolded under British colonialism, these 'exchanges' were often rather limited or skewed to meet the particular needs and perceptions of the colonial rulers.

The British had little sustained or practical interest in Ayurveda's remarkably rich tradition of dietetics and, as a part of a dual process of mimesis and the construction of alterity, Ayurveda remodelled itself in ways that tended to stress its comparability with Western medicine, and so downplayed dietetics. When in the course of the 19th century Western medicine developed its own concern with diet and nutrition, it was not in dialogue with Ayurveda but along lines laid down by scientific enquiry in the West or in the interests of colonial governmentality. But, in a further mimetic turn, hostile Western views of Indian diets, especially rice-base, vegetarian ones, helped to shape reformist and nationalist attitudes and to inspire calls for dietary change. Within Ayurveda itself, the role of diet was marginalized and it was left to sympathetic investigators like R. N. Chopra to argue that dietetics remained indispensable to Ayurvedic doctrine, and an aspect of medical practice that made it distinct from, and irreplaceable by, Western medicine. Overall, then, in the colonial period, dietetics served more to articulate mimesis and alterity between different medical traditions rather than an active process of 'exchange'.

NOTES

1. Leslie (ed.) (1976).
2. Taussig (1993); Langford (2002).
3. Leslie, 'Introduction', in Leslie (ed.) (1976:1–12).
4. Basham. 'The Practice of Medicine in Ancient and Medieval India', in Ibid., p. 22
5. Ibid., p. 22; Leslie in Leslie, Charles, and Allan Young (eds) (1992:197).
6. Ray, Gupta, and Roy (1980:32–7, 110–226).
7. Wujastyk (2001:5, 7).
8. Ibid., pp. 67, 91.
9. Ibid., pp. 157–9, 181.
10. Ibid., pp. 243–6, 266–80.
11. Ibid., p. 15.
12. Zimmermann (1987).
13. Lloyd (1978:136, 148–69, 186–205, 272–6). Cf. the many foods and their properties in Ayurveda: Wujastyk (2001:278–9).
14. Nutton in Bynum, W. F., and Roy Porter (eds) (1993:288).
15. Grant (2000:7).
16. Waines (1999:233).
17. Engelhardt in Hsu, Elizabeth (ed.) (2001:173–91). My thanks to Shang-Jen Li for this reference.
18. Note, for instance, Galen's rather dismissive view of rice (Grant (2000:96)), and the cautious reception given to aubergines, a 'new' vegetable from India, in early Islamic texts (Waines (1999:237)).
19. For the use of animal and vegetable foodstuffs in Unani medicine, including as tonics, febrifuges, and aphrodisiacs, see Gladwin (translator) (1793), and Playfair (translator) (1833).
20. Chaudhuri (1985); Wink (1996–7).
21. Fleming (1810:1685–6); *Report of the Proceedings of the Central Indigenous Drugs Committee of India* (1899:10–19).
22. Playfair (1833:51).
23. Leslie, 'Introduction' (1976:2–3).
24. Johnson (1813:433). On Western views of health and medicine in this period, see, Harrison (1999:48–53, 80–4).
25. Curtis (1807:280, 283).
26. Twining (1832:125).
27. As in the treatment of 'spleen diseases': Ibid., pp. 287–8.
28. Jameson (1820:91, 159).
29. Ainslie, W., A. Smith and M. Christy (1816:77, 92).
30. Royle (1837:52–3).

31. Wise (1860[1845]:95–105) (first published in Calcutta in 1845). For earlier observations on the importance assigned by Susruta to dietary change on the first appearance of a disease, see, Wilson (1825:27–8).

32. Ainslie (1826); O'Shaughnessy (1844); Anon. 'Hindu medicine' (1847:379–433).

33. Hutchinson (1845); Leith (1851–2:114–27); *Report on the Diet of Prisoners and of the Industrial and Labouring Classes in the Bombay Presidency*, Education Society's Press, Bombay, 1865; *Report by Civil Medical Officers on the Nature, Growth and Mode of Preparation of the Various Alimentary Articles Consumed as Food by the Industrial and Laboring Population in the Several Districts of Bengal, North-Western Provinces, Punjab, Oude and British Burmah*, Home Secretariat, Calcutta, 1863. More generally, see, Arnold (1994:1–26).

34. For a Foucauldian view of diet (albeit mediated through Marx and Weber), see, Turner (1992), especially Chapter 6.

35. For the nature and course of the Ayurvedic revival, see, Mukhopadhyaya (1923–6).

36. Sen (1916:20).

37. As in the investigation of indigenous drugs by M. C. Koman in Madras in 1918–21, in V27/850/41, India Office Records [IOR], British Library, London, where questions of cost and efficacy dominate.

38. Sen Gupta (1901:6–8).

39. The relative absence in contemporary Ayurveda of dietary prescriptions, as compared with pharmaceutical ones, is noted by Langford (2002:165). But Ayurveda did not turn its back on diet entirely—for example, Sen Gupta (1901:129), suggests that since indigestion helped cause cholera, the patient should fast and avoid heavy food, especially ghee and fried articles. On fasting as one of the principal tools of Ayurveda, see, Ram Bhishagratna (1909:6).

40. *The Report of the Committee on the Indigenous Systems of Medicine, Madras. Part II: Written and Oral Evidence*, Government Press, Madras, 1923, 21.

41. Ibid.

42. The idea of long-distance and transoceanic 'exchanges' gained authority from Crosby (1972); but some of the limitations of that concept, especially with respect to the role of human agency and the transferability of knowledge systems, have since become apparent—for example, Carney (2001:4–5, 85–9).

43. One has to turn to recent interpretive works, like Zimmermann's *Jungle* (1987), or Ray Priyadaranjan, Hirendranath Gupta, and Mira Roy's synopsis and commentary on the *Susruta Samhita* (1980) to appreciate the full extent and importance of this dietary discourse.

44. Ray Priyadaranjan, Hirendranath Gupta and Mira Roy, *Susruta Samhita*, 32 f. note more than a hundred kinds of flesh for health and medicinal use.

Table I (Ibid., 110 f.) lists the physiological action associated with each of these animal foods.

45. Zimmermann (1987:170–1). 'Herbs and plants' were seen to be the essence of Ayurveda. 'The tropical country, as it [India] is, must rely on the indigenous system only... The seers have studied the effects of these herbs and plants with reference to time and place and this system is therefore most suitable to the country but the other systems are allien [sic] however much excellent they may be in other climates': Ethirajulu Naidu (1918:10).

46. For example, O'Shaughnessy (1842), where animal materia medica occupies only a dozen pages in a work of 700 pages almost entirely devoted to plant products. Note, too, Whitlaw Ainslie's remarks on sending a catalogue of edible vegetables and medicinal plants to the East India Company's Court of Directors on 12 April 1810: 'Having long thought that in a country like this, so great a part of whose inhabitants eat no animal food, it might be interesting (as connected with an important branch of the materia medica) to ascertain, and bring under one head, the numerous vegetable productions which are in consequence used as diets': Board's Collections, F/4/379: 9495, IOR.

47. *Calcutta Journal of Medicine* (1869:191).

48. Twining (1835:418). For a more technical evaluation that reaches similar conclusions, see, Church (1886).

49. On the defects of 'Hindu' diets, see, Dey (1866:9). Echoing European strictures, Dey attributed the Bengalis' 'diminutive stature' and their 'want of vitality and energy' to eating too many sweets and living largely on rice by contrast with the wheat-diets of the North-West which produced 'a more robust and healthy race of men'. For the internalization of these dietary views by Bankim Chandra Chattopadhyay and other nationalists, see, Chowdhury (1998:22–3, 35–6). The decline of Indian health under colonialism and the consequent need for Indian remedies is discussed in Langford (2002:20,63–84).

50. Bose (1930:2–3,).

51. Ibid. p. 94.

52. Alter (2000:Chapter 1); Gandhi (1949).

53. On the Chopra Report, see Langford (2002:112–116). In this report, dietetics were again seen as a distinctive feature of indigenous medicine and contrasted with the Western emphasis on 'microbes' and other factors affecting the body from outside: *Report of the Committee on Indigenous Systems of Medicine.* (1948:79–80).

54. Chopra (1936:146).

55. Ibid., p. 159.

56. Pearson (1995:141–70); *idem*, 'First contacts between Indian and European medical systems: Goa in the sixteenth century', in Arnold, David (ed.) (1996:20–41).

5 Health and Sovereignty in the New Asia

The Decline and Rise of the Tropics

SUNIL AMRITH

> Already in Tokyo, house-fronts are dirty and Asian, but Hong Kong in the East, just as Cairo in the West, is the first true symbol, of clothes drying on projecting iron rods, or tattered gunny bags making do as screens, of ill-fed and diseased children, of fouled humanity sprawling on the road-sides...this Asia of teeming millions, of dirty and impotent millions. All Asia is prostrate with the common disease of poverty...[1]
>
> Ram Manohar Lohia (1952)

This declaration by Ram Manohar Lohia to a conference of fellow Asian socialists in Rangoon, in 1952, captures some crucial features of the imagination of development in post-colonial Asia, shared by colonial and post-colonial, socialist and conservative commentators—the notion of common sights, smells, and dispositions across 'Asia'; the focus on the thickness of population, the 'teeming millions'; the biologization of poverty ('a disease'). In Lohia's vision, there is more than an echo of a long tradition of discourse that David Arnold has called 'tropicality'—Asia as an area of heat and humidity which possessed distinctive vegetation, flora and fauna, a distinctive epidemiology, and produced distinctive (distinctively undesirable) human and social characteristics.[2] This was a vision of tropical Asia dominated by the power of nature, and 'naturally' poor. Yet, Lohia departed from many of his colonial forebears in his optimism that radical economic and social reform—that is to say, policy—could overcome the sloth and despair induced by geography. 'This is no time for laissez-faire', Lohia concluded, 'at least in Asia'.[3]

This chapter examines the shifting role of nature—and particularly of disease—in shaping visions of Asian development. The basic narrative of the chapter lies in the gradual shift from optimism to pessimism about the possibility of conquering tropical nature, and I argue that this shift was shaped by the particularly complex bio-political terrain of Asia's borderlands, on the one hand, and growing cities on the other. The starting point of the chapter is the argument that David Arnold has made for the pervasive importance of 'the tropics' in shaping colonial visions of Asia's past, present, and future. A number of Asian nationalists and social reformers, I suggest, drew on aspects of colonial discourses about tropical Asia, but took a more optimistic view, that the tropics could be 'conquered' in the name of national development. From the early 20th century, the belief grew that technology, discipline, and social reform could conquer the tropics, thus transforming not only the natural environment, but social structures, and even embodied behaviours. Within that vision—shared by a diverse group of scientists, officials, and political activists—there were contrasting emphases—a dominant view, which placed technology front and centre, and an increasingly marginal view that emphasized redistribution and social transformation.

Given its easy availability, its widespread political acceptability, and the sense of enthusiasm it was able to evoke, the techno-centric approach to conquering the tropics prevailed. The global malaria eradication campaign of the 1950s, which focused intensively on Asia, epitomized the faith in this approach, and represented the apogee of late-colonial-into-post-colonial optimism. However, the malaria eradication programme encountered several difficulties, and experience began to suggest that 'nature' would not be so easily subdued. Two questions in particular troubled governments and observers: the first was that the space of malarial distribution did not correspond to the increasingly well-defined spaces of national economies—the anopheles mosquito was no respecter of sovereignty, and at times, cast doubt on the ability of states to master 'their' territory. The second area where the narrative of epidemiological transition broke down was in Asia's growing cities, increasingly central to the problematic of development.

By the 1960s, nature re-emerged as an explanation for poverty, for the inaction of states, and as the primordial condition of Asia. Frustrated states turned, more or less gradually, towards two kinds of policies which would characterize Asian approaches to development in the following generation, even as the paths of Asian nation-states diverged—an obsessive focus on population control, and an increasingly coercive urban policy of 'slum clearance' and 'beautification'.

CONQUERING THE TROPICS

By the 1930s, a more optimistic narrative emerged to challenge the determinism of tropical medicine, out of the conjunction of nationalist thought and international professional networks. On this view, technology, knowledge, and education could overcome the diseases of the tropics, and also the habits and bodily dispositions of tropical peoples. The historian of medicine, Warwick Anderson, has characterized this shift as the moment where 'biomedical science ceases to be an environmental discourse in the Asian Tropics and becomes primarily a discourse on social citizenship'.[4] An increasing number of observers—from colonial medical officials to Asian social reformers— felt that education might lead to the 'modification' of the human characteristics produced by tropical conditions.[5]

The new knowledge of nutrition played a central role in this transformation, by suggesting a materialist critique of the notion of tropical medicine. The global economic depression of the 1930s served as a catalyst for the wider circulation of new knowledge of human nutrition, with the League of Nations playing a central role in its transmission. Beginning with an investigation of the impact of unemployment on the nutritional status of workers in a number of European countries, the League swiftly moved to an authoritative declaration on minimum standards of human nutrition. Notably, the League's seminal report suggested that their findings were as significant in tropical countries as in temperate, industrial lands. Developments in the scientific knowledge of vitamins provided a language that could draw together Europe and the colonies, 'core' and 'periphery', economics, geopolitics, and the government of the individual human body.

The explicitly comparative framework of nutritional discourse was open to application to colonial problems. Indeed, a significant amount of the 'new knowledge of nutrition' emerged from colonial laboratories. Perhaps, the best known of the new nutritional studies were John Boyd Orr's contrast of the diets and health of the Maasai and Kikuyu, and

Robert McCarrison's experiments contrasting the health and vigour of rats fed with Punjabi diets with the malnutrition experienced by their counterparts fed on the rice-based diet of the 'Bengalis and Tamils'.[6] W. R. Aykroyd, director of the Coonoor Nutrition Research Laboratories, undertook the most wide-ranging research on questions of nutrition in south India. His pioneering research with Indian colleagues had shown that the preponderance of highly milled rice in the south Indian diet led to a range of nutritional deficiencies, as a result of the lack of proteins and of 'protective foods', and a particular lack of leafy vegetables and proteins. Significantly, Aykroyd and others suggested that nutritional deficiencies, more than the 'tropics' or particular cultural failings, explained the acute susceptibility of the Indian poor to infectious disease.

The implication was that education, and even a 'nutritional policy', might improve public health. A range of Asian nationalists took up the nutritional critique, their visions of the future sought to transcend the pessimism of colonial discourse on the tropics. Foremost amongst them was Gandhi. Gandhi's writings on nutrition are full of references to the latest research on the subject. He gave pride of place—because of its authority and its universality—to the League of Nations Health Committee's seminal findings on the Physiological Bases of Human Nutrition in 1936. A summary of the report immediately appeared in the pages of *Harijan*.[7]

In Gandhi's view, harnessing this international scientific knowledge could go towards increasing national vigour and vitality. Underlying Gandhi's experiments with food and hygiene was a critique of the economic impact of colonial rule on rural India. Not only did polished rice weaken the vitality of the Indian 'race', it was an example of the (economic and moral) impoverishment of India's villages through mechanisation—

> If rice can be pounded in the villages after the old fashion the wages will fill the pockets of the rice pounding sisters and the rice eating millions will get some sustenance from the unpolished rice instead of pure starch which the polished rice provides. Human greed, which takes no count of the health or the wealth of the people who come under its heels, is responsible for the hideous rice-mills one sees in all the rice-producing tracts.[8]

In an article simply entitled 'Green Leaves', Gandhi declared that 'since the economic reorganization of the villages has been commenced with food reform, it is necessary to find out the simplest and cheapest foods that would enable villagers to regain lost health'.[9] Gandhi's critique culminated in the redefinition of his Constructive Programme in 1940—'it is impossible for unhealthy people to win *swaraj*', Gandhi declared, 'therefore we should no longer be guilty of the neglect of the health of our people'.[10]

Interestingly, a regional imagination continued to shape the discussion of health in Asia, but now in a more complex way. An undifferentiated discussion of the epidemiology of 'the tropics' gave way, in nutritional analysis, to a consideration of the problems of the 'rice-eaters' of Asia. Aykroyd suggested, for example, that the illnesses common to a large part of the South, South-East, and Eastern Asia came not from the determining influence of the environment, or even the ecology of rice cultivation, but from the interconnected regional economy. Malnutrition, he suggested, was a consequence of the regional economy, involving the import of rice by the densely-settled parts of eastern India (and southern China) in exchange for the export of labour and skills to the frontier lands of Burma, Malaya, and Ceylon.[11] During the Depression, the price of rice fell more sharply even than that of other commodities, and cheap, poor quality imported rice continued to flood south India.[12]

Alongside nutritional knowledge, new technologies of birth control, new insecticides, innovations in housing, and in technologies of latrine construction, allowed for the emergence of a more optimistic view of the possibility of transcending the tropics. As Warwick Anderson has put it, by the 1930s, 'it is the irresistible technical force of modern colonialism—better cooling, refrigeration, "physiological" housing, railways, the telegraph—that stuns the new generation of scientists, exciting wonder and trepidation', where once it had been sublime tropical nature that had fulfilled this role.[13] Often with the support of the Rockefeller Foundation, keen to spread the gospel of 'scientific' social organization, demonstration areas and model health centres sprouted up across Asia in the 1930s—from northern China to Ceylon and South India. One of the most ambitious, and most publicized, was the Dutch colonial government's Poekwerto Health centre in Java, run by the Rockefeller official, Dr J. L. Hydrick, whose faith in rural public health as a panacea for all ills is oddly touching. The League of Nations' conference on Rural Hygiene in the Far East, held in Bandung in 1937, provided a forum for the exchange of ideas and enthusiasm, bringing British, French, and Dutch colonial officials together with Chinese, Japanese, and Siamese public health experts. The optimism was infectious. In their plans for the health services of post-independence India, the Congress Party's National Planning Committee declared that India's young health workers needed to be imbued with 'missionary spirit'. 'By example and persuasion', these workers would 'spread the gospel of healthy living, communal and personal, and thus take other villagers a step or two away from their age-long prejudices and superstition on the road to better living'.[14]

As Asian nationalists began to 'see like a state', public health assumed a central place in their visions of national development, because it promised a way of overcoming natural conditions. That is to say, precisely those conditions which colonial officials had long used to explain Asia's poverty and excuse themselves from responsibility—the tropical environment, and its production of lassitude, inertia, and sloth, and sensual excess. Perhaps, the example par excellence of this transformation in nationalist thought—characterized by Partha Chatterjee as the 'moment of arrival' of Indian nationalism[15]—is the National Planning Committee of the Indian National Congress, in which Jawaharlal Nehru and Subhas Chandra Bose were the driving forces. In a series of reports on public health, population, and on 'women's place in the planned economy', the Planning Committee gave voice to a vision of the future where science, technology, and personal and national discipline would conquer tropical poverty.

The Planning Committee decried the vicious circle of poverty and under-nutrition leaving the Indian poor with 'inadequate safeguards against the rigours of nature or ravages of disease to resist which they are very poorly equipped'.[16] In the eyes of the Planning Committee, the qualitative issues of individual nutrition linked closely with the question of the quantity and 'quality' of the population as a whole. Increasing food production, as much as redistributing its consumption, was at the heart of the Planning Committee's vision. The Planning Committee declared that—'all social customs, religious taboos and injunctions which now stand in the way of the husbandry of soil resources and efficient utilisation of available food resources have now to be abjured to mitigate the effects of chronic food shortage and poverty'.[17] The health of the population became a reason of state. An unhealthy population would pose an obstacle to the State's plans for industrialization and social transformation.

This was but a first step. The Planning Committee declared itself interested in the 'possibilities inherent in careful scientific breeding of the human race'; in creating a new, improved race of Indian bodies that, healthy and vigorous, would allow for the country's 'development'.[18] The health of the population becomes, here, an instrument, a tool for government in the service of greater aims—planned industrial development, and socio-cultural modernization. In the words of Mohan Rao's recent study, the Planning Committee's vision was one of 'harnessing bodies not just for the economy, but for a sublime, and sublimating, nation state'.[19]

The techno-scientific breakthroughs of the Second World War—the insecticide DDT, anti-biotic drugs, and X-ray technology—cemented the optimistic, transformative narrative of health and development. Converted bombers taking flight to blanket swathes of land with DDT transformed the bounds of the possible, suggesting the real possibility of disease control. This technology, married with the winning of sovereignty and state power by a newly mobilized and confident cohort of Asian nationalist leaders, made the post-tropical future look bright. Many were confident that, once the tropics were conquered by technology, history—human, secular history—would prevail over geography.

POST-COLONIAL VISIONS OF DEVELOPMENT

What emerged at the end of the Second World War, in fact, was a layered, regional, imagination of development. Two overlapping narratives tied together questions of health, ecology, and economic transformation in Asia. The first was the older, tropical, narrative, that is, the vision of what Pierre Gourou called 'hot, wet Asia', sharing fundamental, biological, and political characteristics.[20] The second was a historical discourse on poverty—an explanation of Asia's poverty in terms of a shared history of colonial exploitation and underdevelopment, the solution to which would lie in the assertion of national economic sovereignty, perhaps within the framework of some sort of broader, regional cooperation.

Thus, a number of discussions immediately after the war revolved around the idea that Asia posed a particular, and unified, set of problems with respect to the government of welfare; a set of commonalities and regularities in the sphere of political economy, governed by climate, resources, population and—as a residual category—'culture'. Implicit in these discussions was a quest to define the scope of action open to post-colonial Asian states. Asian governments and the new international organizations alike saw a set of deeper regularities governing the conditions of life and health across Asia.

The conception of 'Asia' as an administrative category for the government of life and welfare drew on a range of disciplines, many of them colonial disciplines. The first was tropical geography and tropical medicine. 'Asia' found its unity, on this view, in patterns of climate and disease ecology. In the words of a World Health Organization (WHO) expert, writing in 1947—

> The Central and South-Eastern parts of Asia, together with Indonesia, i.e. the 'Monsoon Asia' of geographers, should be considered as one epidemi-ological area. It would include the endemic foci of cholera and territories most readily infectible [sic.] by that disease ... it is free from yellow fever but is severely affected by malaria, by flea-borne and mite-borne rickett-sioses and by the ubiquitous smallpox. Most of the area suffers from the food deficiencies of the rice eaters, from a high tuberculosis morbidity and mortality in its cities and the extension of the prevalence of that disease in the rural districts.[21]

The leaders and administrators of post-colonial states reinforced this view of 'Asia', as possessing a certain unity, but their focus was less on the disease environment and more on the ontological fact of Asia's poverty. Indeed, a focus on Asia's poverty undermined the power of tropical nature as an explanation for the region's disease patterns. Jawaharlal Nehru suggested, at the anti-colonial Asian Relations Conference of 1947, that 'backwardness' was the essential problem that united Asia; across the region, he said, 'standards of life are appallingly low'.[22] There was an unfortunate commonality in that 'most of the Asian countries suffered from extreme backwardness in respect of health'. A committee at the Asian Relations Conference explained the persistently high mortality and morbidity across Asia in terms of material deprivation—'the reason for infant mortality and lower vitality', they argued, 'is also largely economic. It was stated that in Ceylon two-fifths of the population did not obtain sufficient energy from their diet'.[23]

The Social Welfare Committee of the Asian Relations Conference discussed the continent's problems in singular terms. The high levels of mortality and morbidity in 'Asia' were due to a veritable catalogue of ills—'an extreme inadequacy of existing health services'; 'unhygienic en-vironmental conditions'; a 'lack of education and certain social practices which have had an adverse impact on the physical and mental health of the people'. Above all, illness was due to poverty.[24]

There were clear implications of this definition of the problem of pub-lic health as part of a broader nexus of poverty and under-development had clear implications. The new international organizations and post-colonial Asian governments held the view that concerted policies of public health might form part of a broader series of interventions to bring about agrarian transformation and industrial development. A number of modernizing colonial administrators, and some British and American doctors, concurred.[25]

The relationship between health and development remained ambiguous. On the one hand, public health policies would constitute an effort to liberate Asia from the deadening hand of 'nature'. Yet, there was also, in the immediate post-war period, a counter-argument, which held that liberation from the tropics would come not through technology, but with social justice, and the redress of historical inequalities. The tropics continued to exert an influence on how development was imagined, but now in dialogue with a more transformative, social, rather than environmentalist, discourse.

THE LIMITS OF PLANNING

The 1950s and early 1960s saw the height of techno-optimism in the imagination of healthy development. The orthodoxy in international public health, by the early 1950s, was that radical new technologies would allow for the control, or even eradication, of 'tropical' diseases, as a precondition for development. Deploying an agricultural metaphor, a UN report declared that there was 'the tangle, the jungle undergrowth, of disease which has to be cleared before a country has a fair chance of development'.[26] Most prominent amidst this 'jungle undergrowth' was malaria, widely accepted as the number one international health priority—not least because of the availability of DDT, and its seemingly miraculous results during and immediately after the Second World War. David Arnold has shown that 'the identification of malaria with tropical backwardness and torpor became a recurring theme', particularly in the writings of Pierre Gourou.[27]

The notion that malaria was one of the most important factors underlying the prospects of development was widely held. Jawaharlal Nehru, addressing an Asian Malaria Conference in Delhi, put the challenge in universal terms—'In this, as in other matters which affect us underdeveloped countries', he declared, 'the pace, the speed of advance, become all the more important. ... If you don't go fast enough, the others will'. 'The others', in this case, referred to all manner of natural forces, from evolving anopheles mosquitoes to the 'iron laws' of human population growth. And Nehru himself suggested that non-human actors might shape the outcome of events—'In many of these regions of Asia, maybe elsewhere, malaria has been a more powerful determinant in the course of human history than people imagine'; the implication was that it might still prove to be so.[28]

Nothing better symbolized the narrative linking biology with development than public representations of the malaria control programme, from the mid-1950s. In 1954, the Indian government issued a postage stamp to mark the intensification of anti-malarial efforts under the Five Year Plan, funded and orchestrated by the WHO and the American Economic Cooperation Administration.[29] Within a year, the Indian initiatives formed part of a now-global campaign to eradicate malaria altogether.

The dominant narrative throughout the malaria eradication programme was a developmentalist one. Wrote *The Hindu*—'In India anti-malarial campaigns, undertaken with WHO assistance, have been successful. There has been an increase in the population of the Terai region and the area under cultivation has gone up 40 thousand acres. Equally striking successes are claimed in the eradication of malaria in some of the most deadly hotbeds of the disease in Burma'.[30]

Spraying with DDT was a means of making land cultivable and releasing labour for the modern industrial economy. Indeed, malaria eradication would cement the space of the 'national economy' itself, making the space of production congruent with the space of state sovereignty, removing 'natural' obstacles to cultivation. The invocation of the Terai region signifies an escape from the tropics, for it had been notorious in the colonial imagination as representing the lethality of the Indian environment. The Terai, David Arnold has shown, was once 'almost defined by death. This tract was considered so deadly as to be impassable for Indians and Europeans a like through a large part of the year'.[31] The key was to be able to show that malaria eradication would allow for an increase in food production, at a time when, from East and West, alarm grew about the global 'population explosion'.

It was not long, however, before the language of 'natural forces' re-emerged strongly, with increasing reports of natural resistance to DDT, of obstacles and shortcomings standing in the way of the smooth workings of the malaria eradication machine. Already in 1955, exhorting the world's governments to support an intensification of the malaria control programme, American malariologist Paul Russell posed the problem as an acute struggle between nature and development—

Already four or five of the fifty-odd major malaria-carrying anopheline species had developed different kinds of resistance to DDT in certain areas ... Since there was not at present any satisfactory substitute method of attacking malaria, it was very important to eradicate the disease before the vector anophelines became resistant to the insecticide. It was not known exactly how many years the insects would remain sufficiently susceptible to DDT to allow of malaria eradication; the minimum appeared to be six or seven years and the maximum ten.[32]

Perhaps as significant as 'natural' resistance was the fact that national sovereignty was always vulnerable to the influence of transnational movement. The international health campaigns of the 1950s were organized on a territorial basis, each centred on a pilot project or a training centre—the most important of them staffed by international consultants. The boundaries of these regions were assumed fixed, usually according to geographical or epidemiological features (Burma's hill zones, Ceylon's 'dry', 'intermediate', and 'wet' zones), or, as in India, according to the lines of provincial boundaries.[33]

Yet the population of South and South-East Asia, in the 1950s, was anything but stable. If the borders between nation states were increasingly rigid, the boundaries of regions were constantly in flux.[34] The 1950s saw a significant and continuing movement of population across the borders of India's partition. Civil and political conflict spurred the frequent movement of population in Burma and Indonesia, to say nothing of the tens of thousands of Asian Muslims who made the pilgrimage to Mecca each year.[35]

Not only were the pathogenic targets of the international health campaigns constantly slipping out of control, so, too, were human victims, or 'vectors', of infection. The plans for disease eradication assumed populations to reside within static regions, densely or sparsely populated, hypo- or hyper-endemic with malaria. They assumed, furthermore, that the space of claimed sovereignty would also constitute the space of national disease control programmes. Yet, as Agnese Lockwood, an American political scientist, observed in Burma at the time—

The whole programme...is seriously jeopardized by the inaccessibility of insurgent-held regions. To be effective, a programme must cover the infested areas and their population 100 per cent. Not only do mosquitoes fly from one place to another but, even more serious, they gradually develop resistance to insecticides. At the present time, a race is developing in Burma between the vector resistance and the government's ability to make the entire country accessible to malaria spray teams.[36]

There was a constant 'threat of infection across borders with India, Pakistan, China, Laos, Thailand'.[37]

Although the malaria control programme was conceived as a transnational initiative, the WHO planners ultimately assumed a series of 'homogeneous' national spaces that did not exist. Where the reach of state sovereignty was weakest, so the threat of infections crossing borders was greater. At the end of the 1950s, Edmund Leach concluded that the Burmese state's 'claims regarding territorial suzerainty were optimistic in the extreme'. Leach argued that 'the authority exercised by the central government over the Independent Sovereign State of Burma over its outlying regions in the year 1959' was in some senses 'a fiction'. Nor did the sharp dichotomy between the densely populated Valleys of Burma and the 'isolated' Highland societies prove an adequate representation of Burmese society.[38] Even anecdotal evidence from the time suggests that people, including sick people, were very mobile, presenting a picture of 'population' very different from the one established in the documents on malaria and tuberculosis control in Burma. Ludu U Hla, a Burmese journalist and folklorist, collected, in the 1950s, a series of life histories, narratives of his fellow prisoners in Rangoon central jail—each was a story of movement, from the Karen lands to lower Burma, from Rangoon to the Tamil Nadu countryside and back again; and, almost universally, from the country to the city.[39] Borderlands have always posed a particular problem for the planners of development in post-colonial Asia.

THE CHALLENGE OF THE TROPICAL CITY

Development was, to adapt Raymond Williams, imagined as a journey from the country to the city. In the realm of economic theory, this found expression in W. Arthur Lewis's vision of the 'dual economy' and the transfer of labour from the 'economic darkness' of the 'traditional' sector to the 'fructification' of the modern capitalist economy.[40] The journey from country to the city formed an almost ubiquitous cultural narrative in the post-colonial world—in cinema, in literature, both high-brow and low-brow, and in the popular imagination. With his genius for synthesis and comparison, Mike Davis has recently shown that the 1950s and 1960s marked the 'takeoff' of the mega-cities of the South, and, with it, the growth of urban slums.[41] The 'housing problem' remained one of the most pressing challenges of development, and one of the most neglected.

It was in the alleyways of Asia's growing urban slums that the dreams of disease eradication were lost; the lanes through which, quite literally, pathogens and the 'carriers' of disease could not be traced. The city was where the narrative of epidemiological transition crumbled. Whereas medical science and modernization theory, put together, suggested that the transition from the country to the city would signify a transition from epidemic to chronic disease, the true picture was more complicated, and less predictable; a recent account suggests that—'The urban poor are the interface between underdevelopment and industrialization, and their disease patterns reflect the problems of both. From the first they carry a heavy burden of infectious diseases and malnutrition, while from the second they suffer from the typical spectrum of chronic and social diseases'.[42]

Early optimism that the revolution in pharmaceutical technology might circumvent the problems of poor housing and overcrowding, for example, in the treatment of tuberculosis, proved ill-founded. Instead, Indian medical researchers in the early 1960s found that the urban environment posed formidable obstacles to the penetration of the medical gaze. The very chaos of the urban landscape and the fluidity of population rendered any hope of tight control over patients taking drugs at home very difficult. Investigators at the National Tuberculosis Institute of Bangalore pointed out that they could not find, let alone supervise, the tuberculosis patients whose courses of drug treatment they were overseeing—...in many cities in India, and presumably in several other countries, an address is not necessarily adequately described in terms of a street and a number. One needs description in terms of landmarks, distances and directions from these, perhaps in terms of names of inhabitants of neighbouring houses, for example, those of shop owners.

While there seemed to be scope for 'improvement in address-taking', the researchers concluded that 'it would seem unlikely that this problem can be solved until the whole street-naming and house-numbering system has been improved'.[43] That is to say, a degree of control over tuberculosis patients taking chemotherapy could not be achieved until the map of South India's cities had been rendered more 'legible' to bureaucrats and medical policymakers.[44] These problems were, in a sense, a symptom of the social change and massive urban influx of the 1950s and 1960s.[45]

The lanes through which the WHO and its local partners had to pursue recalcitrant patients were difficult to navigate, if they were marked on the map at all. As one of the early social surveys of Bangalore made clear, 'the area between Commercial Street and Russel Market are mostly congested. In the above areas, there are no sufficient open places between houses. The streets with the houses on both the sides are very narrow. Dust and dirt surround these houses. Sanitation is very poor in these localities'.[46]

The fundamental problem was an almost complete absence of the kinds of diffuse medical surveillance which Michel Foucault, David Armstrong, and others have highlighted in their writings on public health in modern European history.[47] Michel Foucault observed, in the case of 18th century Europe, that for a process of outpatient treatment (the shift towards a 'domestic form of hospitalization') to work, there needed to be a 'medical corps dispersed throughout the social body, and able to offer treatment for free or as cheaply as possible'.[48] In Asia's growing metropolises, it was precisely this level of dispersion of medical care within society that was missing.

Thus, even as international organizations armed with wonder drugs aimed to 'universalize' the Third World city as a site for technological intervention against disease, another kind of universalism threatened to re-assert itself: the 'universal' colonial—and now post-colonial—city: unchanging; filthy; pathogenic, and capable of subverting even the wonder-drugs of the age.[49] The problems of environmental sanitation which a 1949 Government of India report had highlighted remained intractable.[50]

What emerges, strongly, in many accounts of the urban environment is an almost miasmic theory of disease; contagion comes from the filth of the environment, which is the ultimate 'menace to public health'. 'The sewage and sullage tend to settle down', one Madras census commissioner declared in 1965, 'causing a perpetual stench that pervades the entire neighbourhood, pollutes nearby wells in houses and constitutes a menace to public health and the aesthetic susceptibilities of the people'.[51] One of the striking features of his despairing, yet almost lyrical, report on Madras City, is its timeless nature. The descriptions of pathogenic urban squalor move rapidly across time and space—contemporary accounts from the early 1960s are juxtaposed with extracts from colonial reports of the early 20th century, suggesting that nothing much had changed.[52] The census commissioner's description of Madras's housing problem is substantiated by a description of the Greater Bombay Housing Scheme Committee in 1946—

overcrowding in rooms or tenements, close construction, bad lighting and ventilation, dirty and dilapidated appearance owing to total neglect of maintenance, filthy surroundings, insufficient and substandard sanitary arrangements and amenities and on the whole a sub-human sickening look and atmosphere about the place, often reeking with the smell of rotting food or garbage thrown round about, sluch, overflowing sewage owing to chokes and filthy soil pans, with most of the pull chains missing and flushing tanks out of order.[53]

The reach of this environmentalist discourse on ill-health was broad.

I suggested earlier that 'Asia' was imagined as a single category for the administration of public health policies. Observers in the international organizations, and many of their counterparts in national governments, saw Asia in terms of a set of shared problems and shared conditions, all of them amenable to technological intervention. However, an older discourse on 'Asia', focusing on the almost insurmountable problems of 'filth' and the tropical environment, had not disappeared.[54]

The teeming tropical city became a frequently used trope in support of arguments for a shifting approach to development—away from welfare and social transformation and towards a narrow focus on population control. It appeared that the cities of the South, and particularly of Asia, held the power to evoke almost physical revulsion on the part of outsiders. This was present, most infamously, in the opening lines of Paul Ehrlich's crude Malthusian tract, *The Population Bomb*, describing a 'stinking hot night' in Delhi—'As we crawled through the city, we entered a crowded slum area.... the streets seemed alive with people. People eating, people washing, people sleeping. People visiting, arguing, and screaming. People thrusting their hands through the taxi window, begging. People defecating and urinating.... People, people, people, people'.[55]

This, Ehrlich declared, was 'the *feel* of overpopulation'.[56] More thoughtful observers, like Claude Levi-Strauss, were no more immune to this vision of the teeming urban tropics. Arriving in Calcutta, Levi-Strauss described 'the herding together of individuals whose only reason for living is to herd together in millions, whatever the conditions of life may be. Filth, chaos, promiscuity, congestion; ruins, huts, mud, dirt; dung, urine, pus, humous, secretions and running sores...'.[57] Views such as these, increasingly widely expressed, backed a rising crescendo of calls for population control, using coercion if need be. The problem of development was not poverty but overpopulation; poverty was a direct result of overpopulation. As Vijay Prashad has shown, by the early 1960s, the 'housing problem' in Delhi was, once again, the problem of how to keep the urban poor out of the city, a path that would lead to the grotesque excesses of 'slum clearance' and 'beautification'.[58]

It was not outsiders alone who produced this discourse on the pathogenic urban tropics, silencing issues that had, for a time, featured in discussions of development—land ownership, and power relations. It was, equally, a discourse generated by Asians, in Asia. This focus upon the pathogenic dangers of the urban environment spanned from India to Singapore, from Kuala Lumpur to Rangoon. Colonial and post-colonial, national and international medical discourses amalgamated in a way that challenged the optimistic narrative of progress in international public health.[59]

What we see, then, is the re-emergence of what David Arnold has called 'tropicality', but in a specifically urban, pathogenic form. A specifically 'tropical' form of social medicine was taking root. One of the foremost centres for the revival of this tropical medicine within Asia was the Department of Social Medicine at the University of Singapore Medical School in the 1950s—attracting students from throughout the region.

In this environmentalist discourse on health, the late-colonial (and post-colonial) metropolis remains defiantly mired in filth.[60] Within this environment, the threat of infection was everywhere. Mobile food hawkers were viewed with particular suspicion by public health authorities across South and South-East Asia; they were the ultimate 'vectors' of disease.[61] In the words of a Burmese student of public health, writing a thesis on post-colonial Rangoon whilst at the University of Malaya in the mid-1950s—'the itinerant hawker is a very difficult person to locate when the authorities suspect him to be the cause of ill-health in consumers…some do not have a fixed place nor travel the same streets'.[62] It was deemed that 'as carriers of communicable diseases the sherbet (prepared cold drink) seller, and the ice cream vendor [are] the most dangerous'. Ignorance, of course, was at the root of the problem. The author of the thesis lamented that 'society sees no evil in consuming food from a hawker or a road side stall. Many people do not have the basic knowledge of hygiene. Plainly, they do not know the consequences of eating dirtily. Or even if they do, as some do vaguely, they do not care'.[63]

This provides an illuminating illustration of the complex relationship between medical discourse and the narrative of development. A narrative of progress, enlightenment, and prosperity was always juxtaposed with a nihilistic picture of insurmountable environmental obstacles. The language of WHO reports and technical assistance publications, of techno-science triumphing over nature, was never unchallenged; always, there remained a language of 'natural forces', of overcrowding and over-population in a tropical environment which needed 'ceaseless disinfection'.[64]

Yet, if it could be employed to raise the spectre of breeding masses in the Third World, the persistence of poverty and risky environments could also be used by those in the Third World, to mock the promises of governments and international organizations; to question what it really meant to speak of a 'right to health'. Such was the case of an Indonesian account of disease and death, which is mocking, even contemptuous, of the possibility of liberation through the international 'gospel of hygiene', or by modern medical care. The work in question is a short story entitled 'My Kampung', published in 1952 by Pramoedya Ananta Toer.

The story appears in a collection of tales and sketches set in the Djakarta of the late 1940s and early 1950s, its characters are Djakarta's labouring poor. The subtitle to the collection, 'Caricatures of Circumstances and Their Human Beings', is strongly suggestive of the tone of the stories, with their atmosphere of futility and acquiescence.[65] 'My Kampung' begins, then, with a caricatured image of filth and pestilence, so characteristic of the colonial discourse on the tropical environment. Pramoedya evokes the grotesque and the corporeal, even as his tone alternates between resignation and sarcasm. The story begins—'Friend, you've heard the name of my Kampung, haven't you? Kebun Djahe Kober, five hundred metres in a straight line from the palace. And you also know, don't you? Its gutters are covered in shit of the *kampung* residents' (p. 77). The proximity of the kampung to the Palace is an irony that runs through the story.

The narrator declares that not even a 'small guerrilla squad'—writing, here, in the aftermath of Indonesia's bloody war of independence—would suffer the mortality of this kampung, 'with its stink and condition', where 'people die one after another' (p. 78). There follows a sordid catalogue of the many residents of the narrator's alley, one of seven in the kampung, who had suffered 'cheap' deaths. There is the case of the man who dies from 'chronic venereal disease'; the mother who kills her favourite child with an overdose of worm medicine; the print setter who dies of lead poisoning, and the Chinese shop owner who flees on a ship to 'die in [his] own country', leaving his wife to die in the kampung. And then there are the countless victims of tuberculosis—'T.B. did not surprise anyone in my kampung anymore; it was something routine' (p. 83). In keeping with the tone of tragedy, bordering on farce, the narrator makes no attempt to pass judgement on the situation. Instead, he implicitly mocks the discourse of hygiene and public health—'If killing with weapons is punished by the government, killing because of ignorance and poverty is not prohibited in my *kampung*, even if the killing is of one's own child. It is a routine situation and perhaps quite understandable' (p. 82).

If this portrait of the kampung Kebun Djahe Kober appears to mock the promises of positive health, hygiene, and development, which were so prevalent in the early 1950s, the effect was entirely intentional. It is the conclusion of 'My Kampung' that makes it such an explicit, and interesting, commentary on the global discourse of public health. 'You too, friend, can come to my *kampung* sometime', the narrator says, 'finding it is not hard at all' (p. 84). The kampung, after all, is a stone's throw from the Palace—'five hundred metres in a straight line towards the southwest, there my *kampung* stands in all its glory, defying the doctors and the technical professionals' (p. 84). And then this striking point is repeated once more—'the *kampung*'s located so near the palace where everyone's health, and every little detail is guaranteed' (p. 84).

CONCLUSION

David Arnold traces a direct line between colonial discourses of 'tropicality' and later, post-colonial visions of development—'The image of the tropics as a world set apart by nature, a world characterized by poverty, disease and backwardness thus acquired a new scientific authority and specificity: the foundations had been laid for a reconceptualizaton of the "backward" tropics as the Third World'.[66]

Undoubtedly, works by the likes of Pierre Gourou provide a direct line of continuity between 19th century colonial views, and the notion of 'tropical development'. However, I would argue that the specific form taken by discourses about tropical 'nature' in Asia by the 1960s owed much to debates within Asia, and between Asian scientists, politicians, and writers—often conducted within the new international organizations. In particular, the 'return of nature' to explanations of Asia's poverty stemmed from the frustrations encountered by post-colonial visions of an escape from nature through technology, social reform, and nationalist revolution, directed by sovereign states.

Above all, I would suggest that the notion of Asia as hostage to natural forces—the laws of human reproduction as much as the spread of pathogens—emerged out of the 'ungovernable spaces' frustrating attempts at planned transformation.[67] Modern power, Foucault argued, involved the development of governmental technologies to understand and control the 'mass effects characteristic of a population', a technology which 'tries to predict the probability of these events'—the birth rate, the death rate, rates of disease, life expectancies—and control for them.[68] This chapter has suggested that in two realms, in particular, it seemed by the 1960s that such regularities all-too-often slipped beyond the grasp of governmental power—at the borders between states, and in the growing urban centres.

Although subsequent decades have seen very different histories of development across Asia—some states, this one in particular, are more 'governmentalized' than others—it would seem fair to suggest that borderlands and urban centres are still those spaces least amenable to government and development.

NOTES

1. Ram Manohar Lohia, 1963, 'An Asian Policy' in *Marx, Gandhi, and Socialism*, Hyderabad: Navahind.

2. Arnold (2000:6–19).

3. Lohia (1963:292).

4. Anderson in P. Greenough and A. Lowenhaupt-Tsing (eds) (2003).

5. Ibid., pp. 40–1.

6. J. Boyd Orr and J. L. Gilks, 1931, *Studies in Nutrition*, London.

7. Findings of the International Commission of Experts appointed by the Health Committee of the League of Nations', *Harijan*, 25 April 1936. The original report was: League of Nations, *Report on the Physiological Bases of Nutrition*, League of Nations Document A.12 (a), 1936.

8. Gandhi (1949:44–6).

9. Ibid., p. 51.

10. *Collected Works of Mahatma Gandhi*, 1994, CW.72 July 6, 1937 to February 20, 1938, p. 380, Delhi: Publications Division, Ministry of Information and Broadcasting.

11. Baker (1981:325–39).

12. Ibid.

13. Anderson (2003:42).

14. National Planning Committee (1947:43–4).

15. Chatterjee (1986).

16. National Planning Committee (1948:8). See also National Planning Committee (1948). Although the proceedings of the Planning Committee were published in edited form after the war, the discussions took place between 1938 and 1940.

17. NPC, *Population* (1948:127).

18. Ominously, the Planning Committee included Nazi Germany on its list of countries where 'successful' experiments on eugenic lines had been conducted.

19. Rao (2004: 20).

20. Gourou and Ladorbe (1953).

21. World Health Organization Archives, Geneva. First Generation Files 452-1-5. 'Delimitation of Regional Health Areas on an Epidemiological Basis', Third Session of the Interim Commission of the WHO, 31 March 1947.

22. *Asian Relations: Report of the Proceedings and Documentation of the First Asian Relations Conference, New Delhi, March-April 1947* (1948).

23. 'Report on Social Services', in *Asian Relations* (1948:183–5).

24. K.C.K.E. Raja, *Health Problems of India*, Pamphlet from the Asian Relations Conference (Indian Council of World Affairs, 1947) [Nehru Memorial Library collection].

25. On British colonial views on post-war development in their African territories, see, Cooper (1996); Lewis (2000).

26. UN, *Preliminary Report on the World Social Situation* (1952:25).

27. Arnold (1999:15). See, Gourou (1966).

28. *Report on the Third Asian Malaria Conference*, New Delhi, 19–21 March 1959, WHO Print Archives, WHO Library, Geneva. WHO. SEA/Mal/16, Annex 3, Opening Address by Jawaharlal Nehru.

29. On the intensified National Malaria Control Programme in India, see, D.K.Viswanathan, 1958, *The Conquest of Malaria in India*, Bombay; Government of India, Directorate General of Health Services, *Annual Reports*, various years; Jeffery (1988).

30. *The Hindu*, 9 April 1955.

31. Arnold (2005:49).

32. WHO, Committee on Programme and Budget, Sixth Session, *OR*, 63 (1955:198).

33. WHO. SEA/Mal/5 (1956); WHO. SEA/Mal.7 (1957); WHO. SEA/Mal/6 (1956).

34. See the essays in P. Kratoska, R. Raben and H. Schulte Nordholt (eds) (2005).

35. A report on the implications of the Haj for malaria eradication exposed another challenge posed by population movement, this time of an inter-regional kind: M. A. Farid, 'The Pilgrimage and its Implications in a Regional Malaria Eradication Programme', 9 April 1956, WHO/Mal/168.

36. Agnese Lockwood, *The Burma Road to Pyidawtha*, Carnegie Endowment for International Peace, *International Conciliation*, No. 518, May 1958, p. 433.

37. Ibid., p. 433.

38. Leach (1960:49–86).

39. Hla (1986).

40. Williams (1960).

41. Davis (2006).

42. Werna, Blue and Harpham, cited in Davis (2006:147).

43. The 1961 census of Madras, too, talks of 'a number of dwellings ... [which] offer no surface on which a number could be painted, not even a substantial door post or indeed a door at all': Government of India, *Census of India, 1961*, Volume 9, Part 11 C, 'Slums of Madras City', (1965:96).

44. This is James C. Scott's term. Scott, 1998, *Seeing Like a State*, New Haven and London.

45. A social survey of Bangalore noted that: 'The rapid growth of industries and trade attracted many outsiders to settle and work in some factory or other in the city ... Government service, domestic services, general labour, factory labour, cart driving, brick laying and mason work, trade and money lending businesses have attracted outsiders'. K.Venkatarayappa, 1957, *Bangalore: A Socio-Ecological Study*, p. 32.

46. Ibid., p. 41.

47. M. Foucault, 1984, 'The Politics of Health in the Eighteenth Century', in P. Rainbow(ed.), *The Foucault Reader*, London; Armstrong (1983).

48. Foucault (1984:285).

49. On this tradition of colonial medical discourse, see, W. Anderson, 'Excremental Colonialism', and D. Chakrabarty (1991:15–31).

50. Government of India, Ministry of Health, *Report of the Environmental Hygiene Committee*, October 1949 (1956).

51. Government of India, *Census of India, 1961*, Volume XI: Madras. Part I—A (i): General Report, P. K. Nambiar, Superintendent of Census Operations (1966:225–6).

52. The report, for example, quotes from the 1908 Imperial Gazeteer of Madras: *Census of India 1961*, Volume XI: Madras (44).

53. Government of India, *Census of India*, 1961, Volume XI, Part 11 C: Slums of Madras City (1965:6).

54. Cf. Anderson, 'The Third World Body'.

55. Ehrlich (1971).

56. Ibid., pp. 15–16.

57. Ibid.

58. Ehrlich and Ornstein (2010).

59. On earlier colonial discourses on sanitation and the urban environment in Singapore, see, Yeoh (1996).

60. See also, Lim (1956).

61. The 'hawker' problem absorbed much energy within the colonial government of Singapore in the 1950s. See, for example, National Archives of Singapore [NAS], Ministry of Health Subject Files (MH/630), DMS 4068/60, 'Ad Hoc Committee on Hawkers', and the voluminous correspondence therein. For an early post-independence statement on the 'hawker problem' in Indian cities, see, Government of India, Ministry of Health, *Report of the Environmental Hygiene Committee* [October 1949], (Delhi, 1956).

62. Tin Maung Maung, 1958, 'Hawkers and Roadside Foodstalls in Rangoon', DPH Thesis, Singapore: University of Malaya.

63. Ibid.

64. The phrase is from Warwick Anderson, 'Excremental Colonialism'.

65. P.A.Toer, 2000, 'My Kapung', *Tales from Djakarta* (tr. by Sumit Mandal), Jakarta and Singapore: Equinox Publishing, pp. 75–86.

66. Arnold, 'Representations of the Tropical World' (1999:16).

67. Watts (2004:6–34). Watts argues that 'the Foucauldian project from which governmentality is derived is often chided for its panoptical sense of closure and overwhelming aura of domination, but …[the case of Nigeria] reveals ragged, unstable, perhaps ungovernable, spaces and analytics of government that hardly correspond to the well-oiled machine of disciplinary biopower'.

68. Foucault (2003:249).

II

The Differing Perceptions

6 Cholera, Heroic Therapies, and Rise of Homoeopathy in 19th Century India†

DHRUB KUMAR SINGH

This chapter examines the debates pertaining to the treatment of cholera in two distinct pathies, and alludes to a particular context in which schism in Western medical thought found expression in the choleraic colony of 19th century India. Attempts by medical men of the age to come up with a successful prophylactic breakthrough in the treatment of cholera revealed the limitations of dominant 'heroic' therapies of Western medicine. However, as will be seen, cholera not only challenged the limits of heroic and rational medicine, but actually became the contextualizing disease which contributed to the emergence, proliferation, and entrenchment of a new alternative pathy in colonial Bengal.

THERAPIES, THERAPISTS, AND THERAPEUTICS

The entire 19th century was mediated by several outbreaks of 'Asiatic Cholera' the world over.[1] India was construed as the primary seat and site of this scourge with Bengal regarded as its cradle and 'habitual domain'. In 1817, it travelled from here and reached Europe. Indeed from 1817, 'when cholera first burst out of Bengal to start its international career, it had never been absent from some or the other region of the Indian peninsula. In 1847 it entered European Russia again, as it had done in

---

† Earlier versions of this chapter have been published but with different emphasis and slant.

1829 and reached Britain again by way of the Baltic, in 1848'.[2] Earlier in 1831–2, in Britain and France, it had fueled unfounded rumours among the laity and accentuated 'divided opinions' and medical controversies among doctors. Cholera 'created panic' and 'posed puzzles' both in the colony and metropole as it occasioned exchange of medical ideas from India to Europe and vice versa.

While alluding to the various therapies and therapeutics that were employed by medical men to combat cholera in 19th century India and re-emphasizing the relationship between cholera and broader contours of colonialism which circumscribed it, this chapter's concern is more about how cholera mutated some aspects of medical thought and ideas, and how the career of cholera challenged and changed the career of a doctor in the colony.

In the case of cholera, the prophylactic employment of various therapies and therapeutics is intimately linked to the understanding of the etiological and epidemiological parameters of the disease and their impact on the diseased population. Both these parameters regarding cholera remained controversial all along the 19th century. Amidst these controversies about the nature and cause of the disease, its symptoms and their variations at various stages of the disease were recorded consistently and meticulously. The 'empirics' of the disease was established but the 'rationale' behind those controversies still eluded medicine. The divided opinions about the nature of this disease and the mode by which it was transmitted[3] remained the marked feature of the medical literature on cholera in the 19th century.

It is a well-documented and well-established fact of medical history that medicine for the larger period of the post-Enlightenment era was crude and heroic. Heavily influenced by the Cartesian mechanistic model of science, medicine was continuously streamlining and nuancing its understanding of human anatomy and physiology and the alteration caused by diseases to them. Both nosology and pathology were poised to acquire their distinct shape by the middle of the 19th century. However, at the prophylactic and curative levels, medicine was crude and heroic and, by today's standards, even barbaric. The pharmacopeia of this heroic age was slim, the barber's blade was sharp, and there was no anaesthesia[4] to soothe the pain. How did medical men grapple with cholera in this broader context of 19th-century medicine will be the focus. In what manner did the context of heroic therapy allow for the emergence of an alternative pathy—homoeopathy—within Western medicine and how this strand was picked up by some colonial medical men will be our concern. Cholera will serve as the contextualizing disease for the early conversion of some of the allopaths in the colony. This account will be anchored on one of the most famous and early converts to homoeopathy—Dr Mahendra Lal Sarkar[5]—for understanding the interlinked context of cholera and the rise of homoeopathy. The hostile reaction meted out to Sarkar by his allopathic peers and the medical establishment will shed light on the working of colonialism as well as highlight the tensions within a particular paradigm of medical knowledge and its attempted contextual resolution.

In the choleraic context, the claims of therapeutic efficacy and its superiority can be assessed if one allows the voices from some of the 'rival traditions' to speak out, and here, Sarkar's voice as a physician allows us to do so. This is important because, as one flips through the voluminous treatises on cholera written during the course of the 19th century, one is struck by the paucity of accounts on therapies and therapeutics related to its treatment. One is compelled to conclude that, for much of the cholera history in the 19th century, the number of 'curative' measures/entities within the *materia medica*, were indeed few. Moreover, the drugs used to manage the patient were not administered on fixed principles and much depended on the exigencies of circumstances and on the personal conviction of individual doctors. The anxiety fostered by the baffling disease often compelled them to adopt vigorous medical treatments like bleeding and paraboiling, which increased the risk of iatrogenic damage. Pessimism was manifest in the articulations of many medical men who encountered the disease. More often than not, medical men, frankly but cynically, admitted that in the virtual absence of effective drugs, simply helping nature to take its own course would, in many cases, have promised as good if not better results. Advocates of vigorous medical styles like Sir Thomas Watson,[6] who belonged to the dominant pathy, in the context of cholera epidemics conceded that—'[t]o many patients, no doubt, this busy interference made all the difference between life and death. But if the balance could be fairly struck, and the exact truth ascertained, I question whether we should find that the aggregate mortality *was in any way disturbed by our craft'.*[7]

For Lebert, another commentator on medicine, 'cholera in its well-pronounced, typical, and perfectly developed form slays the half of all persons attacked,' and that 'internal medicines, according to all experience hitherto, have proved useless during the attack'.[8] In India, the first well-documented major cholera epidemic occurred from 1817 to 1821.[9] In the absence of vital statistics in India, until the mid-1860s, it was impossible to arrive at an accurate figure of cholera deaths. 'From such statistics as are available, it would appear that at least twenty-three million people died of the disease in British India between 1865 and 1947. It is likely that a further ten to fifteen million deaths occurred during the previous fifty years'.[10] Bengal, the cradle of cholera, as per J. Jameson's report of 1820, shows mortality exceeding 10,000 for many districts including Jessore, where more than 10,000 perished in two months of 1817 alone.[11]

This high mortality rate and the dismal record of dominant medicine pertaining to cholera for the larger part of the 19th century challenged Sarkar to tread a path different from what his professional brethren had adopted. That heroic therapy had not much to recommend against cholera was Sarkar's despair. 'Beyond the recommendations of the vaguest generalities, as quarantine, cleanliness, and disinfectants the old school is entirely silent on the subject',[12] he lamented. He looked towards new drug provings with hope—'it is to the new school that the credit of suggesting prophylactic remedies is due'.[13] He was prepared to give it a fair trial on this basis. But before we come to Sarkar's inheritance of the 'schism' in Western medical thought and his expatiation of cholera according to the 'new school' of medicine in the 1870s, let us recount the sufferings of the 1817 epidemic and revisit the early therapeutic encounters of medical men with cholera in India.[14]

EARLY CHOLERAIC ERUPTIONS AND ENCOUNTERS

When after 1817, cholera reports were authored, the ardent urge and pursuit for a clue in therapeutics led many medical men to scan Ayurvedic sources with the help of *vaidyan*s or indigenous medical practitioners. *The Cholera Report of the Madras Presidency* compiled by William Scot, the Surgeon and Secretary to the Medical Board in 1824, cited the *Chintamani*, authored, as per the Report, by the mythological sage Dhanwantri, as an important indigenous medical source. This text, according to the Report, had references to a disease resembling cholera, and it was 'classed under the generic term *Sannipata*, which includes all paralytic and spasmodic affections. The species of Sannipata, supposed to be spasmodic or epidemic cholera, [was] called *Sitanga*[15] which was characterized by the 'chillness like coldness of the moon over the whole body, vomiting, thirst, fainting, great looseness of bowels, and trembling of the limbs'.[16] Another name for spasmodic and epidemic cholera was *Vidhumar Vishuchi*, described as 'most rapid in its effects; its symptoms were dimness of sight in both eyes, perspiration, sudden swooning, loss of understanding, derangement of the external and internal senses, pains in the knees and calves of the legs, griping pains in the belly, extreme thirst, lowness of bilious and windy pulses and coldness in the hands, feet and the whole body'.[17]

One finds the reconciliation[18] of the symptoms of Sitanga and Vishuchi in the term *Bisuchika* that became synonymous with cholera; one was considered to be the virulent form of the other. For the afflicted, death offered the final reconciliation in both. The kin of the afflicted were advised beforehand to prepare for the cremation of their sick relatives or neighbours under the spell of Bisuchika, as the diseased 'may [have to be] taken out to be burnt as he will not recover'.[19] Cholera was considered the cause and context for the last journey—an inevitable fate. The blame of pessimism was attributed by Western medical men to Ayurveda and *Unani*, and to the vaidyans and hakims who practiced them. It was perceived to be ingrained in Ayurveda and this precluded the possibilities of using indigenous cures for Bisuchika as prescribed by Ayurvedic texts.[20] These possibilities became dimmer as the oriental romance of the earlier encounter ebbed away and derision towards indigenous systems of medicine gradually crept in. 'The first cholera epidemics coincided with the beginning of the western assault on Indian medicine. Initially a patron of Ayurveda, in the 1830s the East India Company reversed its attitude and, as part of the triumph of "Anglicists" over "Orientalists", identified itself exclusively with western medicine'.[21]

Nevertheless, in the phase of the 'orientalist commitment' with its implicit 'enumerative modalities', many lists and compendiums of native materia medicas and bazaar medicines were prepared by European medical men. It was emphatically claimed that 'nearly all the articles of real efficacy used by the natives are found in our pharmacopeia,'[22] and, as articles such as 'gamboge, impure calomel, pure corrosive sublimate, arsenious acid, senna, cassia fistula, sulphur, mercury, opium, musk, castor, croton-tiglium, rhubarb, turbeth root, jalap, impure potash and soda, the impure mineral acids and several others'[23] were already present in their (that is, European) pharmacopoeia, there was no need to look towards the ridiculous prescriptions of the vaidyans which, was construed by various parallelisms and analogies, to be based on the 'Paraselcian adage'. The Europeans painted the 'native practice of physic' as an inferior science bordering on quackery.

During the cholera eruptions of November 1818, in Travancore, Staff Surgeon Hay's confidence in the efficacy of Western medicine was to be the sole guarantor of life and property and any expectancy of gaining knowledge from traditional medicine was undermined when he saw the *vythian*s (that is, the vaidyans) unscrupulously fleeing in the wake of *veshoo-u-geka*[24] eruptions.[25] This cowardice on the part of the vythians, for Hay, underscored the message that Ayurveda had no succour to offer to their dying brethren and also revealed the weakness of Ayurveda. With a heightened sense of responsibility, Hay recounted in his evidence before the Madras Medical Board how he recruited, reinstated, and recasted native medical men in their professional roles as vythians, by arming them with ample instructions and medicines. In a self-congratulatory exercise, Hay delighted in his efforts towards co-opting the vythians as carriers of Western medicine in the hinterland. Still, Hay feared high mortality owing to the 'general inattentive habits' of native physicians and was apprehensive that, in spite of his instructions, the vythians may flee in panic on the day of the epidemic visitation and trial, leaving the sick unattended and unassisted.[26]

In contrast to Hay, the Judge and Magistrate of Zillah Jessore, C. Chapman, was more impartial in his account of the fleeing population while reporting about the cholera epidemic of 1817, refraining from airing such a triumphalist account of the medicines employed. Chapman understood that the fleeing away of the population was not due to cowardice, but was to be attributed more to the 'impossibility of affording any effectual medical aid from the suddenness of attack,'[27] which he thought was enough to undermine the 'spirits of [even] the stoutest heart'.[28] He rationalized his own orders to close the court and sought the 'approbation' of this step from the government, as a preventive step taken 'with the object of decreasing, as much as possible, the number of inhabitants in the town'.[29] Though Chapman appreciated the 'active exertions' of the attending Assistant Surgeon Dr Tytler to administer medicine, he emphasized prudence which demanded that 'every person who could obtain the means of conveyance [be] removed to a distance from [his] place and [his] neighbourhood'.[30] For our present focus and concern, the pertinent question relates to those wonder drugs which Hay and Tytler dispensed. Was it calomel[31] or was it opium?[32] Perhaps, both because, they were regarded as the 'wondrous drugs', used by Tytler liberally during the Jessore epidemic of 1817.

THE RHETORIC AND REALITY OF HEROIC THERAPY

Surgeon Tytler relied on the 'prompt exhibition of the calomel and opium'.[33] 'The consumption of calomel was so great'[34] that within the last 12 days of August 1817, the entire stock in Tytler's possession got expended and, as he had to resort to frequent borrowings, he signaled for immediate and speedy supply of calomel by Dâk from Fort William to save the already thinning population of Zillah Jessore.[35] Such a high consumption by the small population living under the shadow of cholera reveals the heroic doses that were lavishly administered by Tytler. For the Surgeon, '[i]t was gratifying to be acquainted with the fact that no example of failure has occurred, where, before the symptoms were allowed to proceed too far, recourse was had to the remedy prescribed— *the free use of calomel*, in the first instance, and **opium** administered in small doses when the vomiting was excessive and long protracted'.[36] The Medical Board at Fort William 'approv[ed] the practice pursued by Dr Tytler in the treatment of the disease'.[37] The supply of calomel required by the doctor was transmitted to him without delay by Dâk. Tytler who had found the cause of cholera in the use of 'new rice' by the natives, went on to prescribe and administer large doses of calomel. Calomel rapidly established itself as a panacea, 'scruple after scruple of calomel'. Scot's cholera report of 1824 found that calomel was being 'universally administered in cholera [cases] from 15 to 20 generally 20 grains of dry calomel being placed upon the tongue, [which] was washed down by 100 drops of T. Opii (Tincture of opium)'.[38]

Clearly, there was not one Tytler but many. Dr Ayre once gave 580 grains of calomel in three days[39] and recorded no disagreeable effects. 'Heroic doses of calomel' 'which under ordinary circumstances [would] have **salivated** a troop of dragoons, and as much opium powder and tincture as would have **stupefied** a company of infantry,'[40] were witnessed by Dr Moor of Bengal Army, as being prescribed by many doctors as late as 1850. A large variety of liquors, decoctions of spices, and aromatics added extra colour and effect to this heroic therapy of calomel and opium in vogue. Did a malady arising from the consumption of 'new rice' require such heroic doses of these drugs? Nevertheless, the brave doctors had set the stage for the employment of heroic therapy against the humbling symptoms of cholera.

As the spatial expanse and virulence of the 1817 epidemic increased, memorandums pertaining to the symptoms and plan of treatment to be adopted were issued to surgeons and magistrates of the Presidency. Broad guidelines were made in English as well as in Bengali, for the recruitment and guidance of native physician-interlocutors, so that the 'wondrous drugs' supplied could be transmitted far and wide. With the non-availability of doctors and surgeons at every choleraic place, any European officer or gentleman with a 'rational mind' was to be entrusted with the responsibility of supervising native physicians in their administration of 'rational medicine'. 40 to 50 such native physicians were employed at Calcutta alone.[41] It was through them that the efficacy of Western medicine was established among the 'reluctant' and 'sly' natives. In Jessore, Tytler recommended 'small pecuniary' rewards for two such native doctor-interlocutors, Muhammad Zukee and Balram, for their laudable conduct and longstanding loyalty of 13 and 9 years, respectively.[42] 'Their exertions in administering the medicines and explaining the cause contributed, in an eminent degree, to the relief of the sick and removal of the disorder'[43] being attempted by Tytler. Definitely the 'embattled minority' might have recruited many more local native interlocutors, like Zukee and Balram, in their battle against cholera, as also in their battles against native princes and principalities.

As the general symptoms of this 'fell disease' were marked, the Medical Board sought to establish order among the 'diversity of opinion and practice' so that a general principle of conduct could be evolved and put forward. In the plan of treatment adopted, the first step was 'to support the patient's strength,'[44] so that a way be prepared for the administration of medicine 'to remove the irritability of stomach and bowels,'[45] which was to be followed by the administration of evacuatives either as emetics or purgatives or both, in order 'to expel the morbid secretions'.[46] After this heroic regimen of stimulants and evacuatives, it was thought expedient to fall back upon conservative methods 'to restore the healthy action of the stomach before calling its digestive powers into action again'.[47] Basically, the mode of treatment entailed the use of stimulants and opiates—the former to restore confidence and the latter to prevent vomiting and purging. In between stimulants and opiates, evacuatives were to be used to get rid of the 'morbific matter'. Clearly, inconsistency and uncertainty were the chief features of the treatment plan, and this lent space for varied interpretations of the disease as per the after-effects of the confounding permutations and combinations of various drugs.

As the first step of the treatment plan, stimulants like spirituous liqours and, in urgent cases, spirits of hartshorn or ether were used. In common cases, a *Maderia*—glassful of brandy with an equal quantity of water—was used to revive the patient so as to halt the immediate danger of sinking.[48] Sometimes, undiluted brandy was also used or recourse was had to 'one drachm of aether or two of spirits of hartshorn in one ounce of water'.[49] These stimulants were to restore a degree of animation to the sinking patient. For respite from vomiting, stimulants were to be followed up by opiates. 'Fifteen drops of laudanum[50] in two teaspoonful of water'[51] was prescribed, and if vomiting did not subside, the dose was to be increased after every subsequent attack of vomiting. A 'second dose of 20 or 25 drops; third dose of 30 to 40 drops and so on after each attack of vomiting'[52] was to be administered. Opium moistened with water or spirit was applied externally to the stomach, especially the upper part of the belly, and was thought to help in stopping vomiting. Through the use of stimulants, the way was paved for purgative medicines that were administered 'with the view of expelling the morbid secretions of the intestines, calomel [the blue pill], readily suggested itself as an appropriate remedy'.[53]

As alluded to earlier, the risk of salivation did not deter the use of calomel in large doses. Sometimes, calomel was administered 'in smaller doses for its supposed chalogogue effects'.[54] In contrast, many advocated its full dose because, in their opinion, 'given in full dose [calomel] was often retained by the stomach and, though [it remained] inert during collapse,'[55] its latent therapeutic effects were to unfold during the time of reaction, and this was vital for the retrieval of the patient from the jaws of death.[56]

Further, in order to preserve the retentivity of calomel in the stomach, opium was combined with it since opium also acted as a binding agent.[57] So, a supposed purgative was cancelled by a binding agent for its supposed effects during the stage of reaction. Calomel and opium allowed the medical men to ride the tide of triumphalist medicine. A majority of them penned the efficacies of these sheet-anchor drugs with glee and gusto; only a few questioned their rationale. For most of them, it made the 'violent malady' admit to speedy remedy. A few cautious medical men expressed suspicion about the purgative effects of calomel but for the defenders of the drug, 'it was not used for its purgative effects'.[58]

In contrast, practitioners like Dr Craw were convinced that 'after bleeding and bath, a powerful purgative [and nothing more powerful than calomel existed] and a strong cathartic enema would have a much better effect than narcotics, the debility being imaginary'.[59] For some medical men, neither strong emetics nor purgatives were necessary to avert cholera, as their combination did not yield favourable results. Even doctors at the metropole sometimes expressed their suspicion. Dr Mackintosh of Drummond-Street Hospital was not clear about the use of purgatives, but refrained from stating 'the fact too strongly that purgatives [were] dangerous remedies'.[60] Other medical men, many a times, questioned the theoretical premise for the use of such remedies and, in their self-critical evaluation, admitted that the 'theory of disease which [had] chiefly led to its employment [was] not supported by anatomical facts, [and that] it was administered only on empirical grounds'.[61] In their evaluation, 'there appeared to be no argument in favour of its exhibition either from analogy or pathology'.[62] Such introspection, though valid, did not prove to be of much practical value because not many proven alternatives were available against this terrible fell disease. Even the free and frequent use of calomel was debated in the wake of the 1817 cholera eruptions. J. Annesley presented his observations regarding 'The Use and Abuse of Calomel' on 6 March 1824 before the Medical and Physical Society of Calcutta commenting on the divided opinion regarding calomel. He obliquely hinted at the limitations imposed by choleraic circumstance and the confusion fostered by and faced due to calomel among medical men—

> The most experienced are sometimes baffled, when they cannot satisfactorily account for its operation beyond what the eyes see:– the eye is generally a safe, but is not always a sufficient, guide, to those who are anxious to know the full and peculiar effects of whatever they use in medicine. *To this inconvenience we must submit*, till some fixed and established principle directs and governs our views of treating diseases, and of reasoning upon them.[63]

Annesley recommended the attainment of a sound and reasoned principle which was to 'be the object of every individual belonging to the medical profession, who sees the value of that profession to the community, and is resolved to give his unprejudiced aid towards its improvement'.[64] He cautiously and by convoluted logic of circumstantial utility and pragmatism, conceded and condemned his own 'partiality of judgment' and made a case in favour of administering large dose as against moderate use of calomel in cholera. Recounting in first person his advocacy of calomel, Annesley defended his 'propriety of administering it in doses more extensive than are commonly thought necessary, as the result of [his] own experience'[65] and delineated thus—

> I was in the habit of administering calomel only in moderate doses, till I perused the work of Dr Johnson, after which I began in my hospital in Trichinopoly to exhibit it in doses of one scruple each to a patient in the advanced stage of dysentery. Its action in this instance was so *strikingly manifest* in procuring ease and comfort to the unhappy sufferer, that, *although the case was not successful*, I determine to give it a trial at the commencement of those diseases which find most destructive and distressing in this country, dysentery, hepatitis, and fever; diseases which in general commence with great excitement and excessive irritability of stomach.[66]

It was in this manner that the ambit of the use of calomel was expanded. Having increased the use and scope of calomel in diseases like dysentery, hepatitis, and fever, 'which in general commence with great excitement and excessive irritability of stomach',[67] Annesley stated his general and blanket prescription based on calomel thus—

> in these cases,[68] the dose of calomel which I give is 20 grains, with one or two grains of opium: this, in seven or eight hours, is followed up with a smart purgative; and this system I continue daily till the secretions become healthy, when a tonic laxative is exhibited, and continued till the healthy functions of the bowels are restored.[69]

Basically, Annesley prescribed heavy doses of calomel for a shorter span of time with regular repetitions to produce miraculously curative and palliative 'salutary effects'. Salivation of the mouth as a symptom occasioned by the sustained use of calomel in small doses for a larger span of time was not considered by Annesley as a good line of treatment. Clearly, with heavy doses in a brief time span, the manifest salivation did not come to the fore and the blame of its abuse got masked.[70]

Nevertheless, the treatment of cholera by the heavy use of calomel, laudanum, and stimulants was termed as the 'rational method' of treatment. Many doctors in their heroic spirit to dominate and tame such a cadverizing and decimating disease, overemphasized the 'curative effects' of opium, and exhorted their professional brethren 'not [to] shrink from its use from the dread of its ulterior consequences'.[71] 'Ulterior consequences' in the form of secondary symptoms from all the above drugs were thought to be minor problems to be managed and targeted separately. These 'magic drugs' were often laced with many indigenous ones. *Cherayata*, rhubarb, and calombo root powder were simultaneously administered as part of 'rational medicine'.[72] Many more indigenous concoctions, expressed in native idioms, were added to instructions issued to native physicians who were to encounter the disease where European medicines and assistance were not procurable. The substitutes were 'watery decoctions of pepper, and such other warm aromatics and spices as could be procured, or any of such decoctions such as *punch-cole* and *dusmoolpaunchun*, or any of the stimulant medicines...such as *sawchagyo, chintamoney*, with *russasindoor* and juice of raw ginger'.[73] As purgatives, aloes, rhubarb mixed together as a pill from six rutties[74] of each, yielding up to five pills, could be administered at short intervals. *Senna* and *hureetoke* mixed and boiled with half a seer of water could also serve as purgatives.[75]

As it was difficult to account for the phases of cholera in every individual case during an epidemic, for quick results, doctors relied heavily on these blanket heroic doses based on hit and trial. 'Anything like **unmixed treatment** [was] never tried—**purgatives solely, narcotics solely, emetics solely**, [was never the case], [as] there was always a mixture of remedies'.[76] In their combative strategies, physicians, it was observed, 'should not rest content with the application of **any single remedy**; [results could be] accomplished most effectually and rapidly by a combination of measures. The warm-bath, blood-letting, and large doses of calomel and laudanum [were not only] to be immediately prescribed',[77] but if possible simultaneously prescribed. 'If bath be already prepared, the patient should be placed in it, and during immersion he may take the dose of medicine and have the blood-letting performed. One remedy, however, should not wait upon another; the first at hand should be administered first'.[78] No prioritization in the prescription was established. For bloodletting, a sufficiently large orifice was made in the vein; many a times it was advisable to open the vein in both arms and the patient was bled in the upright position.[79] Bleeding or venesection was not just a therapy, it was also a 'diagnostic tool', that is, from the amount and after-effects of bleeding, the stage of the disease and its prognosis was to be determined.

John Macpherson, the Deputy-Inspector General of Hospitals of the Bengal Army, on his arrival in India, found venesection as the common practice in Calcutta and, in an epidemic in 1842, he himself gave it a fair trial in a good number of cases.[80] Dr G. H. Bell did not give up the practice of repeated bleedings, until his death.[81] Some medical men were of the opinion that, for Europeans and robust natives, under the initial stage of attack, nothing helped like bleeding and that 'it was more successful than any other remedy, in cutting short the disease: usually resolving spasms; allaying the irritability of the stomach and bowels; and removing the universal depression under which the system laboured'.[82]

These gleanings from cholera treatises and reports convincingly prove that the remedial armament retained its arbitrary 'polypharmatic' flavour based on a few great 'sheet anchors' like calomel and laudanum laced with other purgatives and emetics for the larger part of the 19th century. If indigenous therapies and therapeutics were characterized by the sin of polypharmacy,[83] dominant Western or regular medicine's, or more particularly, allopathy's record was as sinful, if not more, where prodigious number of drugs, with sometimes opposing effects, were included in one prescription. Despite the triumphalist and combative stance of a majority of medical men, cholera epidemics acted as a leveller, in the sense that, both patients and doctors shared the same sense of anxiety—'In medicine we are like our patients, very apt to exaggerate the effects produced by our remedies'.[84] There was pessimism despite the rhetoric of heroic therapy. The triumphalist mode of articulation also acted as a defense mechanism to mask their anxieties. Limitations of heroic doses and anxieties due to moral and material unsettlement caused by cholera fed and accentuated each other. The cholera documents are, in fact, replete with anxieties of the 'embattled minority', but the anxieties of the vast majority plagued by this disease were underplayed by the cultural rhetoric invoked against them. The heroic history of cholera therapy and therapeutics allows us to understand the ways of 'colonizing the body'. Were the natives inherently slothful, fatalistic, and an enfeebled race, or did the 'absolute depots of pills'[85] found in their alimentary canals decimate them? Is there any assessment of the cases of debility accentuated and perpetuated by those opiates and stimulants? Do the crude census and culturally informed or misinformed cholera reports actually mirror the horrors of the mercurous compounds which dominant medicine poured down the throats of the vast native population? Do they provide any account of the extent to which native constitutions were ruined, or the number of the delicate and aged murdered by those 'efficacious drugs'?[86]

An attempt to seek answers to these questions explains the crudity of the process of 'colonizing the body'. Under the environmental paradigm in general, and the maismatic theory in particular, extensive statistical tabulation and analysis, with regard to cholera mortality and its relationship with seasonal and climatic parameters like humidity, temperature, and wind directions, were accounted for. Based on these, topographical maps were drawn for the selection of safe cantonment sites, but the 'rational' commitment of the dominant pathy did not engage itself with the statistical analysis of the effects of its treatment. 'Statistical results of treatment would have helped us,'[87] as some doctors realized and lamented. Nonetheless, the cholera archive does not provide us any proof that such hopes of some lamenting doctors were ever sought to be realized.

HAHNEMANNIAN REFORM AND LEGACY

At a theoretical level, it was understood and frankly admitted by regular practitioners of medicine that, in the case of cholera, as 'in many other diseases, the mode of practice has often originally been purely empirical and theory of its operation has afterwards been formed'.[88] Even then, medical men of the 'heroic age' dismissed the empiricist tradition present in their own medical thought and in the indigenous system of medicine with derision, as 'paraselcian adage'. Many a times, when allopathic practitioners could not explain the failure of a particular class of remedies employed, they attributed its unsuccessful use to the cardinal dogma of the empiricists, who were blamed with contaminating their medical thought and practice. Unable to explain their own reliance on the heavy use of the evacuative class of drugs in the cases of cholera, the rationalist strand shifted its blame to the empiricist strand. In the wake of unfavourable results of the evacuants in cholera, Macpherson pleaded for innocence on behalf of his professional colleagues, thus—'If, then, we adopt the evacuant treatment at all, it is not from our experience of its good effect in kindred diseases; it can only be on some ill defined notion of eliminating a poison, or by the practical application of dogma *"Similia Similibus curantur."*'[89]

This reveals how uncertain and inconsistent regular medicine was about its own therapeutic rationale and, to gauge how suspicious and vindictive the adherents of one strand of medical thought were about the other, let us briefly turn to Samuel Hahnemann's revolt[90] from the dominant and regular mode of pathy and his founding of a new pathy called 'homoeopathy', based on the maxim 'Similia Similibus curantur'—let likes be treated by likes. In contrast to this epithet, 'regular medicine generally prescribed *allopathically*, [where] treatment was based on principles *other* (from the Greek word 'allos') than symptom similarity. Typically allopathic medicine [tried] to remove or oppose disease causes, and to suppress or palliate symptoms'.[91]

For the entire 18th and a major part of the 19th centuries, most diseases were classified by the then prevailing regular medicine as inflammatory, and therefore, prescribed an anti-inflammatory regimen and treatment to counter them.[92] The heroic and repeated regimen of regular medicine, in a majority of cases, opposed inflammatory diseases systemically through the mechanistically, opposite, or anti-inflammatory effects of venesection, leeches, cupping, purges, emetics, mercury, opium, and blisters.[93] We have seen in our documentation of therapies for cholera, how allopathy prescribed powerful drugs in such potent doses to produce violent reactions in the patient, matching the power of disease with that of the remedy and the concomitant propensity of the body to manifest many secondary symptoms and iatrogenic complications.

In the context of prevailing heroic therapies with their indiscriminate purging, drugging, and bloodletting, Hahnemann had started to question his own convictions as an allopath, and about the crude ways in which medicine was being practiced. In his letter to a physician of high standing on the great necessity for a regeneration in medicine, Hahnemann poignantly revealed his feelings—

> It was agony for me to walk always in darkness ... and to prescribe ... substances which owed their place in the materia medica to an arbitrary decision. I could not conscientiously treat the morbid conditions of my suffering bretheren by these unknown medicines, which being *very active substances*, may so easily occasion death, or produce affections and chronic maladies, often more difficult to remove than the original disease. To become thus the murderer or the tormentor of my bretheren was to me an idea so frightful and overwhelming, that soon after my marriage, *I renounced the practice of medicine.*[94]

In an age when drug affliction had become a malady in itself, Hahnemann continued to articulate his feelings regarding the uncertainties of medical science and its practice, as 'in the practice of medicine a great deal that [was being administered to the patients] was not [yet] proved'[95] to be efficacious. 'Confusion in the laws of medicine [was] a continual source of annoyance'[96] to him. Moreover, it should be borne in mind that he was 'a thoroughly well-posted physician, skilled both in theory and practice, better read in various notions of the medical books of the time than most of his fellows'.[97] Besides being a physician, he also held the position of 'Stadtphysikus', that is, he had the power to supervise and control pharmaceutical chemists and their drug shops and stores under his jurisdiction.[98] 'He was also a surgeon; his treatment of necrosis by scraping the bone proves that',[99] yet, he was thoroughly disgusted with the mode of physik[100] of his age. 'How', lamented Hahnemann, 'can we complain of the obscurity of our art when we ourselves render it obscure and intricate?'[101]

Deeply concerned with the uncertainty, arbitrariness, and use of high doses of active agents as medicine, he began to raise fundamental questions regarding the philosophical underpinnings of dominant medicine. It should be remembered that Hahnemann's philological expertise[102] allowed him to become an exceptional scholar in the history of medicine, botany,[103] and chemistry,[104] and his larger intellectual commitment had a different pedigree and lineage. Instead of adhering to the rationalist Galenic tradition (which in his age was heavily influenced by the Mechanistic view of the human organism, leading to its mechanistic appreciation of pathology, and desiring powerful mechanical effects in remedies to oppose, dominate, and tame diseases), Hahnemann, in order to resolve his questions about heroic therapies and their murderous regimen, gravitated towards the faint and subdued empirical tradition of Greek medicine which based itself on the principle Similia Similibus curantur.[105] In the larger and dominant context of heroic therapy, and based on the retrieval and revival of the rational principle of Similia Similibus, Hahnemann sought to rationalize the practice of medicine which eventually culminated in his founding of a new school of medicine.

The Mechanistic and the Vitalistic

In order to appreciate Hahnemann's disgust with antagonistic therapies of the heroic age and his efforts to establish a higher and more sublime ideal of cure, in this section, we will briefly capture the philosophical underpinnings of the new therapeutic option which he promulgated.

The regular dominant medicine followed the Cartesian-mechanistic conception of the living organism which viewed the human body as a complex piece of machinery. The body was approached by what in today's parlance is called a systems approach. This mechanistic perspective also served as the basis of disease classificatory exercises, that is, nosology. As all 'human machines were essentially identical [and were] liable to common and recurring malfunctions of the constituent parts,'[106] the classification and elaboration of standardized categories of disease or class of diseases was made the basis of therapeutic endeavour and intervention. It is evident that in the mechanistic perspective, the body was not a whole and there could be no individuality accorded to sickness. This perspective, in a sense, refrained from according subjecthood to the body.

Conversely, Hahnemann rejected the mechanistic perspective and argued for a 'vitalistic' appreciation,[107] which emphasized on the wholeness of the human body.[108] Disease, as viewed by him, was a vitalistic problem affecting and implicating both physical and mental dispositions. Since the vital force is all-pervasive, both mental and physical symptoms as manifestations of the deranged vital force which primarily constitute the disease are important. Hahnemann elaborates that 'it is only the vital principle deranged to such an abnormal state, which can furnish the organism with its disagreeable sensations, and incline it to the irregular processes which we call disease'.[109] The physician's art constitutes the reading of these 'disagreeable sensations' which are manifest as morbid symptoms caused due to the derangement of the vital force. As this vital force in the deranged state is 'invisible in itself and [is] cognizable by its effects on the organism, its morbid derangement only makes itself known by the manifestation of disease in the sensations and functions of those parts of the organism exposed to the senses of the observer and physician, this is, by morbid symptoms'.[110] The empiricist strain in Hahnemann is more than evident[111] as, for him, through 'no other way can it make itself known',[112] and so the morbid signs and symptoms are to be collated with the sensations and sufferings articulated by the patient. These, in totality, constitute the disease. 'The affection of the diseased vital force and the disease symptoms thereby produced constitute an inseparable whole— they are one and the same,'[113] and the 'practitioners, therefore, only needs to take away the totality of the disease signs, and he has removed the entire disease'.[114] For Hahnemann, it was not conceivable, nor provable 'by any experience in the world, that, after the removal of *all the symptoms of the disease* and of the entire collection of the perceptible phenomena, there should or could remain anything else besides health, or that the morbid alteration in the interior could remain uneradicated'.[115]

Clearly, for Hahnemann, any disease was always the disease of the whole organism; it was individualistic. Treatment, therefore, needed to be focused on the whole person whose individualistic responses to the disease made allopathic 'nosology' redundant. Moreover, since the vital force was responsible for the harmony and equilibrium of the body, the morbid signs and symptoms of the body could be viewed as an expression of the body's attempt to restore normality. In his view, the task of the physician was to assist in the restorative process and not disturb the body violently by heroic intervention. As the body naturally reacted to morbidity, the aim of any therapy was to assist the body's own restorative and curative processes, and the treatment was to emerge from the observable phenomena of the 'signs and symptoms'. In Hahnemann's perception, therapy was actually subsumed within the diagnosis and, therefore, the morbid signs and symptoms were to be read positively. In contrast to the idea of conquering the disease by palliative and shortcut opposition, Hahnemann urged physicians to base their medication in such a way that it encourages the body's curative process, and to realize this goal, he argued, a similar remedy in small doses be administered in order to offer the vitalistic response a little extra aid to come to terms with the disease.

In the outlined vitalistic spirit with its empiricist philosophical underpinnings, Hahnemann started abhorring the suppressive, combative medical measures which entailed the administration of large doses and which fostered 'needless purgatorial suffering'. He was particularly critical of the employment of bloodletting[116] in cholera. Bloodletting was such an established practice that Hahnemann was 'denounced as murderer because he denied his patients the benefits of bleeding'.[117] For him, the bleeding mania of doctors was a disease in itself. He further disapproved of the general regimen of evacuant treatment for cholera (of which bloodletting was just a variety). Hahnemann was also against the use of calomel and other purgatives in such fatal doses. He had no direct encounter with cholera but, on the basis of the symptoms of the disease communicated by his followers, he advocated camphor, and was delighted by the fact that nature had provided this in abundance in the land from where cholera was supposed to have emanated.

In these initial years of his disenchantment with the allopathic use of heavy doses of medicine, Hahnemann started using only remedies called 'specifics', 'whose effects were in a measure known. [As] their physiological action was, however, but little understood,'[118] he indulged, in a big way, in what was called 'drug proving' on healthy human beings. Through this he wanted to ascertain the accurate account of the powers of medicine by assessing the physiological action they fostered and the consequent 'symptom picture' they generated. Hahnemann was always weary of and abhorred polypharmacy. He drew attention to the fact that it was unscientific for doctors to employ untried remedies on individuals who were diseased and to draw conclusions about the efficacy of the drug from the medley which results.[119] He exhorted to 'eliminate the cross-currents of disease' and then to note the pure and uncomplicated symptoms resulting from drug administration in a healthy human being.[120] On the basis of the maxim 'let likes be cured by likes', if a drug given to a healthy volunteer cause the presenting symptoms of the patient, that is, if the administered drug arouses the similar symptoms in health as is presented in a disease, that drug is administered in very low dilutions as a cure to the patient.[121] To revise and reform the prevailing practice of polypharmacy, Hahnemann proposed three cardinal principles—'(a) That the scientific mode of ascertaining drug action upon human being is by experimenting them upon a healthy individual, (b) That the healing properties of drug correspond to its disease-producing properties upon the healthy human organism, and (c) That as a necessary consequence of the above two propositions, the drug must be administered in such a dose that will not produce too great an aggravation of the exciting or natural disease'.[122]

So, for Hahnemann, 'Similia Similibus curantur' was the expression of the abovementioned therapeutic propositions. The 'drug picture' obtained, according to the above rules, was to be matched with the 'symptom picture' of the patient, for the selection of a true cure. The art of the healer was in his ability to match the 'drug picture' to the 'symptom picture' of the patient. In order to obtain 'drug pictures' of various medical substances, a reformed and revised materia medica was the need of the hour. With this in view, Hahnemann 'began the stupendous task of testing the materia medica of his day, the results are in the *Materia medica pura* in which are recorded the 'drug pictures' from the trials he made upon himself and his followers of the first 60 remedies'.[123] 'By the time Hahnemann died in 1843, he had supervised the proving of 99 medicines,'[124] and, as early as 1810–12, he had more or less laid down the cardinal principles of his 'radical' 'new' pathy—homoeopathy. They are—(a) Similia Similibus curantur (not *Sanantur*'), (b) the proving of medicine on healthy subjects, (c) the single remedy, and (d) the minimum dose. It is not incidental that all the cardinal principles of homoeopathy address one or the other vices of heroic and polypharmatic therapy.

CHOLERA, HOMOEOPATHY, AND SARKAR'S EXPOSITION OF HIS 'CREED'

The entry of cholera and homoeopathy in Britain was almost coeval. The terror of cholera and helplessness of regular medicine merged to instigate and accentuate cholera riots in some cities of Britain. The cadaverizing potential of cholera could not be curtailed by the 'scientific insanity' to 'bleach, leech and nauseam'. Doctors attending on cholera cases provided their patients with haphazard prescriptions heavily relying on calomel and particularly delighted if it bled the gums—for it was a proof that the medicine was working. They sometimes devised 'artful stratagems' to administer heavy doses,[125] though victims persisted in dying and doctors served as targets of contempt and sneer.

This was the opportune time for homoeopathy to make its mark felt, and by the early 1830s, homoeopathic physicians began to treat the terrible cholera with their mild specifics and according to the principles of their system.[126] As per the Hahnemannian dictum, 'the disease consist[ed] only of the totality of its symptoms'[127] and that there was no need to follow 'the old school's futile attempt to discover the essential nature of disease (prima causa)';[128] and so the physicians of the new creed did not embroil themselves with causation controversies beyond a point and remained aloof towards conflicting theories that were being propagated with regards to cholera. Instead, 'judging by the symptoms of disease and their knowledge of the action of medicines'[129] upon the healthy, they started using well proven drugs like arsenic, veratrum, ipecac, camphor, and cuprum, as prescribed by their therapeutic law. 'There was no propounding of ridiculous scientific pathology, no recommending of marvellous compounds on the part of homoeopaths'.[130]

Dr F. F. Quin,[131] a student of Hahnemann, found the opportunity to put his 'pathy into extensive action in 1831 against an epidemic of cholera in Moravia'.[132] Dr Quin along with Dr Gerstel and two other surgeons, Hanush and Linhart, had charge of all cholera cases in the town of Tischnowitz and its neighbouring villages. They treated the cases successfully with camphor. Dr Gerstel also found phosphorous useful in the stage of the collapse of cholera and its half-infected variety—cholerine.[133] So great was the success in Tischnowitz that its chief magistrate Ernst Dieble, on behalf of the authorities, sent a letter of thanks to Dr Quin stating eloquently their respectful acknowledgements.[134] Magistrate Dieble also sent his own statistics along with the letter of thanks which were in favour of the emerging pathy. According to him, out of 6,671 inhabitants, 680 had cholera, of which 331 had been under allopathic treatment and of whom 102 had died. In contrast, 278 were treated homoeopathically and only 27 died; of the 71 treated with camphor only 11 died.[135] At other places also homoeopaths were showing favourable results. 'Dr Peterson of Pensa treated 68 cases of cholera out of which 14 died. He used *Ipecac 20th*, *Chamomilla* and *Arsenicum 30th* dilutions. Dr Schubert of Leipsic, in 1830, recommended *Veratrum*, *Ipecac*, *Arsenic*, and *Chamomilla*'.[136] Doctors like Quin and Gerstel were in regular correspondence with Hahnemann. Though the latter himself had no opportunity of treating cholera, he took active part in advising his disciples through letters and pamphlets. In 1831, he wrote a pamphlet on the 'Cure and Prevention of the Asiatic Cholera'.[137] He distributed 30,000 copies of his 'Directions on Cure and Prevention' among inhabitants of Vienna, Hungary, Berlin, and Magdeburg. He recommended camphor as the principal remedy.[138] 'The patient must get [camphor] as often as possible (at least every 5 minutes), a drop of camphor (made with one ounce of camphor to 12 of alcohol) on a lump of sugar or in a spoonful of water'.[139]

Cholera was capable of producing contradictions in Hahnemann as well. As is clear, he gave camphor in quite large doses, though much less than the normal allopathic doses, but in contrast to his principle of minimum dosage. By Hahnemann's own admission, he gave large doses of camphor to produce an 'allopathic effect', or palliative action, so that the patient could be kept floating and the homoeopathic medicine may get time to act.[140] Camphor was recommended only for the first stage of cholera. After the first stage of the disease is passed, copper prepared from the pure metal, according to the methods and directions provided regarding the chronic diseases, and 'of which the patient is to get one or two globules every hour'[141] is to be given till he recovers. Hahnemann, however, advised against any other medicine to be administered simultaneously with copper. Camphor and cuprum were the new successful remedies that Hahnemann brought to light.[142]

The 'allopathic' contradiction in Hahnemann, with regards to the use of camphor, was also pointed out by Mahendra Lal Sarkar in his book *A Sketch of the Treatment of Cholera*,[143] first published in 1870. Clearly, by the 1860s, the Hahnemannian spirit had become well entrenched in choleraic Bengal[144] and doctors like Sarkar were creatively engaging with it. Sarkar, an accomplished allopath, who later changed his 'creed' to homoeopathy, was open-minded towards other therapeutic systems, laws, and remedies; for Sarkar, if judged on scientific basis, homoeopathy proved its worth to benefit humanity. Detailed drug provings, as practiced by Hahnemann, was one of the scientific basis of homoeopathy which attracted Sarkar towards this option. His conversion to homoeopathy was not a chance happening, nor was his engagement with it an amateur hobby that he developed. His 'change of creed' was very much a professional decision—a decision taken as a 'physician awakened to a sense of aweful responsibility of his calling'[145] and the 'physician's awakened sense' also demanded critical appreciation, not blind emulation. His veering towards homoeopathy was not without reservation. The context of cholera as a recurrent malady and its lack of treatment in allopathy, made Sarkar realize the lacunae in the then prevailing heroic therapies and also allowed him to appreciate homoeopathy in proper perspective.

Sarkar's mother 'who survived her husband for about four years, fell a victim of cholera'[146] when she was only 32 years and when Sarkar himself was barely four. Cholera epidemics rekindled the memory of his mother and challenged him as a doctor. By his own admission, allopathy was a '*signal failure in cholera*, scarcely less so in chronic diarrhea and dysentery, in fevers which were not amenable to quinine, and in vast majority of the diseases for which no specifics have been discovered'.[147]

As an allopathic practitioner, he gradually became alive to and concerned about the vices of drugging and rampant use of stimulants—the remnants of heroic therapy.[148] In this context, he regarded homoeopathy as a reform movement which tried to do away with the 'mischief of giving powerful drugs at random and in heroic doses and of the reckless use of such dangerous agents as the leech, the lancet, the cautery, etc'.[149] As a denouncer of homoeopathy in his initial days, he was challenged into witnessing and testing the efficacy of homoeopathic drugs by Rajendra Lal Dutt.[150] Further persuaded by Vidyasagar to comply with the request of Rajendra Dutt, Sarkar slowly came to terms with their challenge, request, and persuasion. Sarkar acknowledged the role of Rajendra Dutt and Vidyasagar in his veering towards homoeopathy—

> We ourselves, we must with gratitude acknowledge, owe our conversion to Baboo Rajendra Dutt, not exactly to his teaching, but to the pertinacity with which he used to urge us to look into the subject and give it a fair hearing and fair trial. The enthusiasm with which [he] laboured in the cause, the disinterestedness that he displayed throughout, the successes that he achieved, together with the conversion of such a man as Pandit Ishwar Chandra Vidyasagar who had derived personal benefit from homoeopathic treatment and whom no man could suppose capable of being duped;– all this induced us to lay aside our professional pride and professional obstinacy for a time.[151]

A few years before his conversion, Sarkar delved deeply into the available homoeopathic literature of his time.[152] As a volunteer-apprentice doctor, he not only witnessed the Hahnemannian principle of therapeutics at work at Rajen Babu's dispensary, but also compared his allopathic prescriptions with Rajen Babu's homoeopathic prescriptions and had the opportunity to assess the effects of those 'sweet globules' at the bedside of patients.[153] These were his years of 'trial'.

Convinced of the rationality of drug proving, and almost in the same spirit in which Hahnemann had written a letter to Hufeland[154] on the 'Great Necessity of a Regeneration in Medicine' where he gave vent to his anguish regarding the uncertainty of medical practice, Sarkar, too delivered a speech 'On the supposed uncertainty in medical science and on the relationship between disease and the Remedial Agents', before the Bengal branch of the British Medical Association on its fourth annual meeting in February 1867.[155] However, instead of any debate on his expressed views, 'hell broke loose' and, subsequently, he was expelled from the Association of which he was the founding Secretary. Overnight he became a quack. Rumours were widespread among the 'gossipy bhadralok' that Sarkar had 'lost reason and yielded to the seductions of Babu Rajendra Dutt'.[156] Orthodox medical journals like the *Indian Medical Gazette* printed slanderous accusations against him and this adversely impacted his medical practice. But despite being cornered, Sarkar decided to protest against the orthodoxy of the dominant medicine and started the *Calcutta Journal of Medicine* in 1868 on 'catholic principles' and without an 'exclusive' name.[157] In its very first editorial entitled 'Our Creed', Sarkar clarified that 'cures [were] affected in diverse ways,'[158] that is, there were diverse creeds of medical systems. 'If one system of medicine were successful in all cases, there would have been no emergence of any non-conventional or alternative system'.[159] The prejudices of dominant medicine were difficult to fight against. Sarkar not only stepped out of the pale of prejudice but invited and exhorted his professional peers to heed to the 'new creed' of professional conduct and higher ideals of cure—

> We have of course our own creed and our own opinions, but we shall not only tolerate but show due respect towards the creed and opinions of others, whenever sincere and temperately expressed. We do not pretend to have the monopoly of wisdom and truth. We shall not ignore facts which we cannot account for, or which clash against our pre-conceived ideas. Facts such as these will only serve to stimulate us to further and more careful inquiry, and we shall always allow them to exert upon us the wholesome influence of moderating our dogmatism….[i]n other words, *always to allow facts to modify opinions and not our opinions to distort facts*.[160]

The *Indian Medical Gazette* lampooned Sarkar's support for homoeopathy but the Catholic St Xavier's College mouthpiece, the *Indo-European Correspondence* or *Indo*, supported him. With humour, *Indo* alluded to Sarkar's erudition, but found the lengthy expatiation of his 'creed' a little 'unhomoeopathic'.[161] Re-emphasizing his stated creed of catholicity of being partial to none, Sarkar defended the journal's espousal of homoeopathy and the need to do so. Replying to the accusations, he made his position clear—

> The journal is looked upon as the accredited organ of homeopathic school. *We are not ashamed to own this*. On the contrary, we are proud of the honor. In advocating homoeopathy, we are not simply acting on behalf of an injured cause, but we sincerely believe that we have but ennobled ourselves by *being on the side of truth*, the greatest yet discovered by the intellect of man, and the most pregnant of the blessings of the whole human race. It is this conviction which has sustained us against the bad name we have acquired.[162]

Cholera always elicited Sarkar's attention. He indulgingly cited and expatiated on contemporary debates pertaining to the disease in his book on cholera which qualifies every yardstick of a classic textbook. As his book reveals, Sarkar was not a Hahnemannian in toto. In his probings on cholera, he was 'partial to none', neither to the 'old school' nor to the 'new school'. In choosing his therapeutic option, Sarkar reserved his right to be eclectic. This eclecticism was not to be a whimsical choosing but was to be based on the critical appreciation of lacuna of one system and the valid scientific and plausible options and explanations offered by other systems of cure. In the case of cholera, he based his etiological and epidemiological understanding as per the old school but drew his therapeutic resources from homoeopathy because here the 'proven drugs' offered a better possibility of constructing a pharmacopoeia for cholera. As regards cholera, 'the question for him was not *"system versus the life of our patient"*, but of *"cure versus disease"*'.[163]

Sarkar re-contextualized cholera in the light of the advancement made in medical science, but he did not prove to be a dogmatic blind follower of Hahnemann. Unlike Hahnemann, he underscored the importance of both pathology and the natural history of the disease. It was in this light that he wanted to see the physiological and pathogenic actions of the drug. As is apparent from the delineation in his book on cholera, Sarkar, while assessing the effects of the disease on the anatomy and physiology of the human body, adopted the Cartesian-mechanistic viewpoint. However, for the therapeutics of cholera, he explored the homoeopathic pharmacopoeia. In accordance to the mechanistic viewpoint, he dealt with the latest medical findings about the morbid anatomy in conjunction with the morbid physiology, which cholera occasioned. From the vast array of lesions and marks which cholera stamped on any organ or tissue, he tried to search for 'some link that will unite in a consistent whole the causes, symptoms and lesions of cholera'.[164] Sarkar was never dismissive of the pathology and nosology of the old school, but he understood the vices of polypharmacy and heroic doses and the havoc perpetrated by them, and in this context, he hailed Hahnemann's large-scale drug proving as a singular contribution. In his opinion, 'the great merit of homoeopathic system, it should be remembered, is that its foundation is laid upon a *materia medica* which consists of a detailed and systematic record of the pathogenic actions of whatever can disturb and disorganize healthy function and structure, which necessarily include poisons as well as less violent and milder substances'.[165]

The 'therapeutics' of cholera was Sarkar's prime concern and in the Hahnemannian spirit of drug proving, he endeavoured to compile all the drugs used in cholera to construct a ready materia medica for the disease.

This is clear from the last three pages of his book on cholera where he arranged 44 homoeopathic drugs and 12 allopathic drugs, according to their importance in the curative process.[166] While delineating on the different aspects of cholera causality and cure, Sarkar, unlike Hahnemann, was not unduly vitriolic towards allopathy, though he remained critical of it. Adhering to homoeopathic practice, he was aware of the shortcomings in both. His book on cholera reveals how he could bank on the strengths of both the schools against a humbling disease. Sarkar had the 'bilingual's confidence that a dialogue between different medical systems was possible'.[167] He stood for a more 'plural encounter' between the medical systems. Sarkar also read Ayurvedic texts and did not regard that system with contempt. We find him translating the Sanskrit medical text *Caraka Samhita* in 1879, from a handwritten copy presented to him earlier. Sarkar had great respect for his neighbour Ramanath Kaviraj and, mourning his death on 10 January 1879, he noted in his diary that 'we have lost a learned and a very popular Kaviraj'.[168]

Cholera even led him to develop an interest in a Tibetan text describing an ailment similar to cholera that prevailed in ancient India and China.[169] Sarkar, during a visit to Darjeeling met an old Lama, Sherab Gatscho, with whose aid, along with that of his (that is, Sarkar's) friend Sarat Chandra Das, he got 'translated some passages of a chapter in Tibetan medical work treating a disease prevalent in India and China.'[170] 'The description relat[ed] to disorder of the bowels with purging resembling cholera in some symptoms only'.[171] Sarkar also rode to Goom Pahar, on which was situated the 'Gomfa [monastery] of [the] old Lama, with the object of discussing with him the passages he said he had found relating to [the] disease characterized by vomiting and purging, and in which it has been prophesied [that this disease] will carry off 1/3rd of the population of the world'.[172] Sarkar was to return disappointed as that passage was not to be found.

We see in Sarkar a physician trying to make, as thorough as possible, an assessment of the prophylactic alternatives for cholera. Apart from his book on cholera, his diaries too are replete with references to the numerous cholera cases he attended. Astonishingly, his book does not find mention in any other contemporary work on cholera or fails to even figure in the footnotes of such works. Appreciative of the many virtues of dominant regular medicine in which he was trained, he explored the therapeutic alternatives offered by homoeopathy. He defended his position as a physician by asserting his right to choose the therapeutic principle on which he was to base his practice.

Sarkar, moreover, repudiated the exclusive and sectarian designation of a 'homoeopath' for himself, and claimed his place as a physician and his right to choose a therapy according to the ever soaring high ideals of therapeutics. Inherent in this exercise was the right to protest against the 'bigotry' of the old and new schools of therapeutics. Shunning sectarianism in medicine, Sarkar was of the view that in the domain of knowledge, professional trade unionism did not work, 'correct conclusions are easily reached by knowledge of all sides of a subject'.[173] Unlike Hahnemann, Sarkar neither professed nor preached homoeopathy as an absolute system of medicine. He did not subscribe to the Hahnemannian dictum that there was only one law of cure. He did not regard the vital laws of the organism as the be all and the end all. In his understanding—

> The human organism is governed by a variety of laws; its disorders therefore are manifold, proceeding from infringement of one or more or all of these laws; and consequently the therapeutics of these disorders must recognize the operation of all these laws. The great difference between the old and the new schools of medicine consists in the one generally ignoring the vital or dynamic laws and the other the mechanical and the chemical laws, which all combine in maintaining life.[174]

Against the exclusiveness of state patronage to allopathic or dominant medicine, Sarkar forged out his vision for a plural culture of medicine. According to him—

> In the present state of medicine, hospital ought neither to be exclusively allopathic nor homoeopathic. In an allopathic hospital every improvement in therapeutics would be admissible save one. In a homoeopathic hospital all improvement in therapeutics is shut save one. The medical officers of an allopathic hospital ought not [to] be tied down to a particular line of treatment, much less ought the medical officers of a homoeopathic one.[175]

In a self-critical assessment of his role as a physician, he saw himself as a sinner without being ashamed of being so, as far as the Hahnemannian dictums of high dilutions were concerned. In contrast to this dictum, Sarkar, in his own practice, used medicines in low dilutions and mother tincture forms. For him, the question of dosage was an open one. He did not accord canonical status to the maxim Similia Similibus because, in his opinion, according that status and interpretation was 'the most unphilosophical and painful straining of *Similia Similibus*'.[176] To proclaim it as the most superior law or that it should pervade all other laws of therapeutics was to preclude the possibilities of inquiry of science. But since it had refined and enriched the materia medica in many ways, and had many positive recommendations for the healthy existence of human beings, it was incumbent upon dominant medicine to recognize homoeopathy as one of the therapeutic systems.

In 1878, when the Faculty of Medicine protested against the nomination of Sarkar, objecting to their coming in contact with one who professed and practiced the absurd and obnoxious system of homoeopathy, he challenged the faculty to prove their objection to his practice of homoeopathy both qualitatively and quantitatively. Without ambiguity, he stated that the medical faculty was not qualified to do so. Exhibiting his masterly reading of history and the philosophy of medicine, he pointed out the persistent empiricist strain present in the medical thought from Hippocrates to Hahnemann. Sarkar cited many great names of dominant and regular medicine who were not only self-critical about their pathy, but were also alive to the claims of other pathies and their philosophical underpinnings in varying degrees. He quoted Hufeland who regarded homoeopathy as 'subsidiary to higher principles of rational medicine'.[177] Sarkar also alluded to Liston who, by his own admission, believed in homoeopathic doctrines to a certain extent.

As already indicated, in his appreciation of the plurality of therapeutic science, Sarkar did not give an exclusive name to his journal—it was merely called *The Calcutta Journal of Medicine*. Nor at a later stage did he venture to open a homoeopathic college, which he could have easily done like his peers, though he congratulated his physician brothers and philanthropists who contributed to the opening of homoeopathic hospitals at other places. He celebrated such instances as both service to society and service to science[178] and chided the wealthy of Calcutta to emulate similar examples. He greatly desired but could not open hospitals based on his vision of scientific and interactive plural medical systems and instead engaged himself with something loftier—the 'cultivation of science'—a general culture of science, where specialization would be a means and not an end.[179] In the exercise of an alternative therapeutic option and its practice in partial accordance with Hahnemannian principles, Sarkar had to face reprimand, 'ridicule and obloquy', but by the time of his death in 1904, homoeopathy had gained acceptance, respect, professional status, and avid practitioners who guarded and defended their role as physicians and ensured its further proliferation.

NOTES

1. Australia was perhaps the only exception which remained more or less immune to cholera. See, Briggs (1961:85).

2. Ibid., pp. 84–5.

3. Ibid., p. 77.

4. Interestingly, John Snow, whose contribution to the understanding of cholera causation and communicability remains a benchmark in the history of the disease, was also one of the founding fathers of anaesthesia. In 1853, he was the chosen doctor to administer chloroform to Queen Victoria during childbirth. See, Korner (1996:4).

5. Dr Mahendra Lal Sarkar was one of the earliest and famous converts to homoeopathy in 19th century India. Born on 22 September 1833, he graduated in medicine from Calcutta Medical College and obtained the degree of Doctor of Medicine (MD) in 1863, and declared his faith in homoeopathy in 1867. He lived as an accomplished and much sought after homoeopath all his life. He died on 23 February 1904. He founded an institution called Indian Association for the Cultivation of Science (IACS, 1876) for the promotion of scientific spirit and basic research in science among natives in India. Sarkar's journal *The Calcutta Journal of Medicine* which he single-handedly edited for more than 20 years played an instrumental role not only in the dissemination of homoeopathy but also in animating the medical debates of those times.

6. Sir Thomas Watson was a great commentator of the regular dominant practice of medicine—allopathy. His *Lectures on the Principles and Practice of Physic* published in two volumes in 1843 by John W. Parker, London, remained a widely circulated textbook in the 1850s and after, and acquired a high reputation. Watson was a fellow of St John's College, Cambridge, and of the Royal College. He was also the physician of the Middlesex Hospital. The lectures that comprise the book were first delivered at King's College, London in 1836–7. They were subsequently serialized in the *Medical Gazette*. It is interesting to note that Watson belonged to the generation just next to Hahnemann's.

7. Thomas Watson as quoted in Sarkar (1904:53–4). Emphasis added.

8. Lebert as quoted in Ibid., pp. 53–4.

9. Rogers (1928:8).

10. Arnold (1986:120).

11. Jameson (1820:27, 170–5).

12. Sarkar (1869:407).

13. Ibid., p. 407.

14. With the advent of annual sanitary reports for various presidencies in the post 1870 era, the mortality profile of cholera became more comprehensive, reliable, and based on firmer statistical grounds. In the last quarter of the 19th century, an average of 1.75 out of every 1000 population of British India died of cholera annually. Yearly regional variations with many high incidence years in several regions hinted at cholera's intimate links with the prevailing famine conditions in those years and regions. The high incidence in Bengal, its habitual domain, can be gauged from the fact that cholera death average among British soldiers in 1860–9 was 9.24 per 1000, though it dropped down to 2.49 in 1880–3. See, Cuningham (1884:33). The future of civil population definitely would have been worse. The diaries of Sarkar and his journal, *The Calcutta Journal of Medicine*, bear the stamp of choleraic times and the frustration fostered by the disease in the post 1870 era.

15. Scot (1824:iii).

16. Ibid., p. iii

17. Ibid., p. iii

18. Ibid., p. iii

19. Wise (1845:330).

20. A perceptive commentator on cholera and colonialism in India has succinctly suggested the growing incongruence and asymmetry in the dialogues between Western and indigenous systems of medicine—'They had little interest in entering into a dialogue with indigenous medicine, only in extracting from it what might be of use to their own practice. They saw all Indian medicine as innately inferior, confused Ayurveda and Unani with popular Hinduism and folk-medicine, and branded them all irrational and superstitious'. Arnold (1986:137).

21. Ibid., p. 137. Also, see, Gupta (1976:369–70).

22. Irvine (1848:2).

23. Ibid., p. 2

24. Another name for *Veshoo-u-geka* in Travancore was *Neer-comben*.

25. Scot (1824:xvi).

26. Ibid., pp. xvi and xvii. It is interesting to note that in another region of Kerela, after almost a century later, that is, in 1902, a vaidyan established his reputation and redeemed Ayurvedic tradition by facing the cholera calamity in and around Kotakkal. He roamed around the region ministering and consoling the sick and administering them a self-made tablet called '*Vishoochikari*'. For details, see, Krishnankutty (2001).

27. Letter from C. Chapman, Esq., Judge and Magistrate, Zillah Jessore, to W. B. Bayley, Esq., Secy. to the Govt. in the Judicial Department, Fort William, dated Zillah Jessore, 25 August 1817. Reprinted in Smith (1869:171).

28. Ibid., p. 171.

29. Ibid., p. 171.

30. Letter from C. Chapman, Esq., Judge and Magistrate, Zillah Jessore, to W. B. Bayley, Esq., Secy. to the Govt. in the Judicial Department, Fort William, dated Zillah Jessore, 28 August 1817. Reprinted in Smith (1869:172).

31. Calomel is nothing but mercury chlorides—1. Mercury (I) chloride, mercurous chloride, calomel $Hg_2 Cl_2$, a white insoluble powder, m. p. 3°C, used in medicine and as a fungicide. 2. Mercury (II) chloride, corrosive sublimate $Hg Cl_2$, a poisonous white soluble salt, m. p. 276°C, used as an antiseptic and to make other mercury compounds.

32. Opium was generally used as Laudanum which is nothing but an alcoholic tincture of opium.

33. Letter from R. Tytler, Esq., M. D., Asst. Surgeon, to C. Chapman, Esq., Judge and Magistrate, Zillah Jessore, dated Zillah Jessore, 23 August 1817. Reprinted in Smith (1869:172).

34. Letter from R. Tytler, Esq., M. D., Asst. Surgeon, to C. Chapman, Esq., Judge and Magistrate, Zillah Jessore, dated Zillah Jessore, 31 August 1817. Reprinted in Smith (1869:174).

35. Ibid., p. 174.

36. Letter from R. Tytler, Esq., M. D., Asst. Surgeon, to C. Chapman, Esq., Judge and Magistrate, Zillah Jessore, dated Zillah Jessore, 20 September 1817. Reprinted in Smith (1869:175-6). Emphasis added.

37. Extract of a letter from the Secretary to the Medical Board, dated 6 September 1817. Reprinted in Smith (1869:175-6).

38. Scot (1824:lvii).

39. Macpherson (1866:94).

40. Ibid., p. 94. Emphasis added.

41. Letter from R. Levy, Esq., Secy., Medical Board, to W. B. Bayley, Esq., Secy. to Govt., Judicial Dept. dated Medical Board Office, 23 September 1817. Reprinted in Smith (1869:188).

42. Letter from C. Chapman, Esq., Judge and Magistrate of Zillah Jessore, to W. B. Bayley, Esq., Secy. to the Govt. in the Judicial Department, Fort William, dated Zillah Jessore, 3 October 1817. Reprinted in Smith (1869:197).

43. Letter from R. Tytler, Esq., M. D., Asst. Surgeon, to C. Chapman, Esq., Judge and Magistrate, Zillah Jessore, dated Zillah Jessore, 1 October 1817. Reprinted in Smith (1869:196).

44. Memorandum from W. B. Bayley, Esq., Secy. to Govt., Judicial Dept. dated 23 September, 1817. Reprinted in Smith (1869:183).

45. Ibid., p. 183.

46. Ibid.

47. Ibid., p. 183.

48. Ibid., p. 183.

49. Ibid., p. 183.

50. Laudanum is an alcoholic tincture of opium.

51. Memorandum from W. B. Bayley, Esq., Secy. to Govt., Judicial Dept. dated 23 September 1817, p. 183.

52. Ibid., p. 183.

53. Ibid., p. 183.

54. Macpherson (1866:124).

55. Ibid., p. 124.

56. Ibid., p. 124.

57. Nicholls (1988:85).

58. Macpherson (1866:108).

59. Ibid., p. 108.

60. Ibid., p. 109.

61. Gull (1853:175).

62. Ibid., p. 175.

63. Annesley (1825:211). Presented on 6 March 1824. Emphasis added.

64. Ibid., pp. 211–12.

65. Ibid., pp. 211–12.

66. Ibid., p. 211. Emphasis added.

67. Ibid., p. 211.

68. That is, cases of diseases which in general commence with great excitement and excessive irritability of stomach.

69. Annesley (1825:212–13).

70. Ibid., pp. 211–17.

71. Macpherson (1866:114).

72. Memorandum from W. B. Bayley, Esq., Secy. to Govt., Judicial Dept. dated 23 September 1817. Reprinted in Smith (1869:184–5).

73. 'Instructions for Native Doctors in the Treatment of the Cholera Morbus, in the Mofussil, where European medicines and assistance are not procurable'. Reprinted in Smith (1869:192–3).

74. A contemporary unit of measurement and has been used intentionally

75. Ibid., pp. 192–3.

76. Macpherson (1866:105). Emphasis added.

77. Kennedy (1831:175). Emphasis added.

78. Ibid., p. 175.

79. Nicholls (1988:81).

80. Macpherson (1866:120).

81. Ibid., p. 119.

82. Johnson and Martin (1841:344).

83. It was generally alleged by European medical men that the indigenous system of medicine, especially Ayurveda, was 'chaotic' in its drug prescription owing to its adherence to polypharmacy.

84. Macpherson (1866:101–02).

85. Ibid., p. 95.

86. Ibid., p. 103.

87. Ibid., p. 103.

88. Ibid., p. 102.

89. Ibid., p. 107. Emphasis added.

90. The consideration of Hahnemann's revolt is important because the Hahnemannian questions will echo once again when we talk about M. L. Sarkar's conversion to homoeopathy. Both Hahnemann and Sarkar were trained doctors of the regular dominant medicine. Both had to grapple with cholera, the former in the first half of the 19th century had an indirect encounter with it; the latter in the second half of the same century had a direct encounter with the malady.

91. Nicholls (1988:3). Emphasis added.

92. Ibid., p. 87.

93. Ibid., p. 87.

94. Bradford (1970:33). This letter contains the seeds of Hahnemann's formulation of homoeopathy. Emphasis added.

95. Ibid., p. 33.

96. Ibid., p. 35.

97. Ibid., p. 35.

98. Ibid., p. 35.

99. Ibid., p. 35.

100. This term connotes the art of medical practice in 19th-century medical literature and is spelt as per its old usage. I have used the word intentionally to retain the flavour of 19th-century medical debates.

101. Woodbury, Jr. (1952:152).

102. At the age of 22, Hahnemann was a master of Greek, Latin, English, Hebrew, Syriac, Arabic, Spanish, German, and some smattering of Chaldaic.

103. Hahnemann always expressed gratitude to Schreber who taught him botany at the University of Erlangen.

104. None other than the great chemist Berzelius once said about Hahnemann—'That man would have made a great chemist, had he not turned out a great quack'. Quoted from Bradford (1970:29).

105. Both the empirical and rationalist perspectives were present in the eclectic Hippocratic corpus. At a practical level, it contained both the principles

of medicine, that is, the principles of 'Contraria Contraries curantur' and 'Similia similibus curantur'.

106. Nicholls (1988:58).

107. It is the vital force that animates the material organism in health and in disease and, for Hahnemann, 'the material organism, without the vital force is capable of no sensation, no function, no self-preservation; it derives all sensation and performs all the functions of life solely by means of the immaterial being (the vital principle) which animates the material organism in health and in disease'. Hahnemann (1979:98).

108. According to Hahnemann, '[I]n the healthy condition of man, the spiritual vital force (autocracy), the dynamics that animates the material body (organism), rules with unbounded sway, and retains all the parts of the organism in admirable, harmonious, vital operation, as regards both sensations and functions, so that in our dwelling, the reason-gifted mind can freely employ this living, healthy instrument for the higher purposes of our existence'. Hahnemann (1979:97–8).

109. Ibid., pp. 98–9.

110. Ibid., p. 99.

111. Hahnemann's rationalist urge to read the various symptoms in their connectedness to arrive at a diagnosis of the unique diseased state of the patient is also as much evident as his empiricist strain. In this regard, it is imperative not to talk in binary opposites of 'empiricists' vs. 'rationalists' in the context of Hahnemann in particular and homoeopathy in general.

112. Hahnemann (1979:99).

113. Ibid., p. 21.

114. Ibid., p. 21.

115. Ibid., p. 97. Emphasis added.

116. He drew the attention of his pupils towards the agonizing fact of how the regular allopaths were teaching 'to mistreat cholera and (to) make it fatal with blood letting to 30 ounces, quantities of leeches and calomel to the extent of three or four drachms, on a false theory and after the example… of *the best physicians in the world—the English*'. Bradford (1970:259). Emphasis added.

117. Ibid., p. 255.

118. Ibid., p. 35.

119. Ghose (1935:133).

120. Ibid., p. 133.

121. Vickers and Zollman (1999:1115–18).

122. Ghose (1935:136).

123. Woodbury, Jr. (1952:145–70).

124. Nicholls (1988:9).

125. Rosenberg (1962:157).

126. Bradford (1970:256).

127. Hahnemann (1979:20).

128. Ibid., p. 20.

129. Bradford (1970:257).

130. Ibid., p. 257.

131. Dr F. F. Quin was the greatest English disciples of Hahnemann with perhaps the most extensive experience of cholera. In his work *Traitment Homoeopathique du Cholera*, published in Paris in 1832, he recommended the alternate use of veratrum and cuprum from week to week as prophylactics against cholera and said 'that experience has shown that these substances have preserved numbers of persons exposed to cholera'. See, 'Prophylaxis of Cholera' (407).

132. Nicholls (1988:108).

133. Bradford (1970:266–7).

134. Ibid., p. 267.

135. Ibid., p. 267.

136. Ibid., p. 256.

137. Ibid., p. 261.

138. Ibid., pp. 262–3.

139. Ibid., p. 261.

140. Ibid., p. 262.

141. Sarkar (1904:67).

142. Ibid., pp. 67–8.

143. Ibid., pp. 67–9. Sarkar has shown similar other contradictions pertaining to other diseases as well.

144. In the 1830s, as Asiatic cholera took the metropole in its embrace, the 'new school' of medicine, that is, homoeopathy prevalent in other parts of Europe, found its way to the colony. Some military men practiced it as an amateur hobby from the 1840s. Some government medical officers stationed at Fort William were known to admire homoeopathy and practiced it. There are evidences that some missionaries also made this pathy a part of their 'do good ethic'. Dr Mullens of the London Missionary Society was known to distribute homoeopathic medicines to the people of Bhawanipore. Dr John Martin Honigberger, a German physician, who despite his use of homoeopathic medicines, did not consider himself a homoeopath.

As cholera was a recurrent phenomenon in India, many early homoeopaths encountered it. There are references that this mode of treatment was used by doctors in the General Military Hospital in Bombay, particularly in the treatment of cholera. One of the Judges of Sadr Dewani Adalat, Mr Ed D'Latour, sent homoeopathic medicines for free distributions to the inhabitants of diamond harbour where cholera was taking its toll. Dr J. Rutherford Russell, a medical officer at Fort William practiced homoeopathy. After his retirement, he returned to England to settle as a homoeopathic practitioner, and as a homoeopath he encountered the cholera epidemic of 1848–9, and even wrote a cholera treatise. Surgeon Samuel Brooking, a retired medical officer under the patronage of the Raja of Tanjore, established a homoeopathic hospital at Tanjore in 1847. In Bengal, in 1850–1, the Native Homoeopathic Hospital and Free Dispensary was established. Rajendra Lal Dutt and a French homoeopath Dr Tonnere were associated with this hospital, although the hospital did not last long.

For more examples and anecdotal accounts of this nature, see, Bhardwaj (1981:31–54). Also see the chapter 'Rise and Development of Homoeopathy in India's Past History' in Ghose (1935:27–83).

145. Sarkar (1904:iii–v).

146. Ghose (1935:2).

147. Ibid., p. 2. Emphasis added.

148. Biswas (2000:12, 15).

149. Ghose (1935:200).

150. Rajendra Dutt (1818–89): 'Born in Calcutta, 1818; educated at Drummond's school, and at the Hindu College; joined the Calcutta Medical College to be trained in Medical Science; after leaving the College, he opened a dispensary at his own house and commenced allopathic treatment, helped by Dr Durga Charan Banerji; In 1853, opened the Hindu Metropolitan as a protest against the laxity displayed in the Hindu college, and began to study homoeopathy; In 1857, started a business firm, Dutt, Linzu and Co., with Europeans as partners, which failed in 1861; there upon he established a homoeopathic dispensary; In 1864, Dr Berigny came to Calcutta, and with him began to spread homoeopathic treatment; In 1867, he converted Dr Mahendra lal Sarkar (q. v.) to homoeopathy; lost great wealth in business speculations; was very generous; died June 1889'. Taken from Buckland (1971:28).

151. Sarkar (1869:399).

152. Garnier's *Conferences upon Homoeopathy* and *Rights of Man in the Domain of Medicine* provided the initial influences upon Sarkar and many of his peers who were persuaded to take interest in homoeopathic literature. Morgan's *Philosophy of Homoeopathy* and Sharpe's *Investigation of Homoeopathy* aided in removing doubts and difficulties and placed homoeopathy in its scientific perspective before them. Hahnemann's *Organon* provided the grand intellectual ferment for the initial push which catapulted many, including Sarkar, towards a critical appreciation for the new radical view of medicine which had been proposed and prescribed by Hahnemann in his *Organon*. Sarkar recounts, vividly, in many instances in *The Calcutta Journal of Medicine* how these readings changed his opinion about homoeopathy.

153. Ghose (1935:50–70).

154. Bradford (1970:33).

155. Biswas (2001:46). Also, see, Ghose (1935:15). The speech titled 'Supposed Uncertainty in Medical Science and on the Relationship between Diseases and their Remedial Agents' was delivered by Sarkar at the 4th annual meeting of the Bengal branch of the British Medical Association at Calcutta on 16 February 1867. The full text of this speech is not available. It is not compiled even in Biswas (2003), which is otherwise an excellent and painstaking compilation. I have tried gleaning parts of it from the quotations of this very speech which Sarkar used in his other articles and numerous editorials in *The Calcutta Journal of Medicine*, which he started from January 1868. The authenticity that the quotations are certainly from the 'Uncertainty' speech comes from the fact that Sarkar has provided its reference in the footnotes of his numerous articles and editorials in his journal. The page numbers of the quoted 'Uncertainty' speech mentioned in the footnotes give us an idea that the speech was a rigorously written article of about 25 to 30 pages. The speech is very important because it was after this speech that Sarkar's life takes a turn.

156. Ghose (1935:18).

157. Ibid., p. 181.

158. Ibid., p. 180.

159. Biswas (2001:46).

160. Sarkar (1868:2,4). Emphasis added.

161. Biswas (2001:47).

162. Sarkar (1869:401). Emphasis added.

163. Sarkar (1904:iii–v). Emphasis added.

164. Ibid., p. 34.

165. Ibid., p. 42.

166. Ibid., pp. 143–6.

167. Visvanathan (1997:136).

168. Biswas (2000:56).

169. Ibid., p. 93.

170. Ibid., p. 93.

171. Ibid., p. 93.

172. Ibid., p. 94.

173. Ghose (1935:179).

174. Sarkar (1904:v).

175. Ghose (1935:182).

176. Ibid., p. 180.

177. Ibid., p. 177.

178. See Sarkar's reaction to the opening of Banaras Homoeopathic Hospital in *The Calcutta Journal of Medicine* (1868:467–70). Also, see, *The Calcutta Journal of Medicine* (1870:374–5).

179. Sarkar (1891:5).

7 Knowing Health and Medicine

A Case Study of Benares, c. 1900–1950

Madhuri Sharma

> *Bakula niyar inkar tang, khaini khale mang mang;*
> *sause pet, chot ba chati, ginli inkar bati bati;*
> *munh se biri chute na, kharchi kahiyo jute na;*
> *larika hole salo sal, nad niklal pichkal gal;*
> *T.B. ke hoiye sikar, aisan inkar karbar.*[1]

> Bony weak legs like a heron, always begging for tobacco,
> Bloated tummy, sunken chest, ribs one can count,
> Puffing incessantly, unable to make ends meet,
> Producing kids year by year, protruding belly, shrunken cheeks,
> Prey to T.B., this is how his life is.[2]

The above verse encapsulates the concerns of the 'educated section' about illness of peasant, poverty, and drug-addiction that affected the health of the rural population. It is one example of many interventions in newspapers, journals, and Hindi literature that concerned medicine and health care during 19th and 20th centuries.

There has been a substantial body of writings dealing with the 'maladies, preventives and curatives' of medicine, both in its 'western' and 'indigenous' forms.[3] Many of these studies tell us stories that are familiar to the scholars of History of Medicine, that is, of tensions between Western medicine and indigenous medicine, Western medical authority and expectations of health care. Though rich and insightful in their own approach, these authors have generally neglected the role and intervention of educated section in the sphere of health and medicine. This chapter seeks to explore the engagement of the 'educated section' of Benares at various social levels with Western medicine in the first half of the 20th century. This would also try to bring to light certain intricacies of the then existing health and healing practices.

Colonial sanitary and public health measures buttressed the authority commanded by Western medicine. At the cultural level, however, there was a complex dialogue between a variety of perceptions about disease and its cure. Along with engagement at various social levels with modern notions of diseases and their cure, this also involved encounters in many contexts with new medical sciences and medical technologies, such as the thermometer and stethoscope. How scientific knowledge about reproduction was invoked in public? What were the debates about norms of marriage, procreation, and pleasure? It argues that this intervention generated a rich corpus of medical tracts in Hindi which, in turn, popularized Western medicine among the masses. It further shows how educated people of the society were carving out a niche for themselves through these interventions at various levels. Last but not the least, the present study would elucidate the above arguments in the light of the experiences of Benares which has always been 'a major pilgrim centre for Hindus'.[4]

DAVA (MEDICINE), DUA (PRAYERS), AND DOCTOR

Premchand's *Godan* (Donation of a Cow) is an entry point to understand how the educated section in Benares perceived the possibilities of modern medicine. Munshi Premchand (1880–1936), a prolific writer, nationalist, and social reformer, tried to engage with this new realm of illness and medicine through the medium of the novel.[5] He was very receptive to modern medicine; what he tried to show in *Godan* was a situation in which those who needed the most were denied access due to poverty, and the rich could treat it like a luxury and a mark of social status. In *Godan*, we encounter a description of illness at three points, along the social spectrum. The first encounter is in a dialogue between a *zamindar* (landholder) and a peasant—

> Rai Saheb [landowner] says to Hori Ram [peasant]—'you know how it is, Hori! In a large family like mine some one or the other is always falling ill. But we are not expected to suffer from ordinary illness. If there is a slight temperature we are treated for pneumonia; a pimple is always a carbuncle. Frenzied telegrams are sent to the assistant surgeon, the surgeon and the chief surgeon. Messengers rush to Delhi and Calcutta to bring hakims and vaids. In the family shrine Durga is invoked. The astrologers get busy on

horoscopes. There is a tremendous to do to save the patient from the jaws
of death. On the slightest sign of indisposition the doctors get ready to
shake the pagoda tree…[6]

Here, getting treatment from renowned doctors and *vaidya*s for a simple
illness is a sort of status symbol for the landed gentry. The dialogue shows
the patient as willing to call upon both indigenous and Western medical
practitioners simultaneously, perhaps even to a ridiculous degree, and
also highlighted the variety of treatments, which the well-to-do could
draw upon, ranging from allopathic medicine to black magic and faith
healing. Illness, Premchand suggests, allowed the rich to demonstrate
that they could even call upon so important a figure as the civil surgeon.
Premchand also treats the medical professional with some irony as one
afflicted by greed rather than a concern for healing.[7]

In *Godan*, Premchand gives a narrative of illness at the other end of
the social spectrum, where medicine is longed for but is completely out
of reach because of the peasant's poverty. Hori Ram and Dhania, a poor
peasant couple, had six children born to them but three had died in infancy. Dhania [the wife] 'was convinced that with proper medical care
their lives could have been saved but she had not been able to buy even
an *anna* (1 anna equal to 6 paise) worth of medicine for them'.[8] Trapped
in debt to the zamindar and the village moneylender, they even did not
have enough food to survive.

The third scenario Premchand outlines is that of the rural migrant
to the city. Gobar and Jhunia had migrated to the city in search of job.
Jhunia had a two-year old son and she was pregnant again. Premchand
gives a heart-rending account of the situation she was reduced to by illness brought on by lack of food—

> Her [Jhunia] breasts were dry. Lallu [son] would howl to be fed and when
> no milk came he bit the nipples with his two-year old sharp teeth. She
> had not the strength even to push him from her…Lallu had diarrhea and
> stopped taking milk from her. She felt a great sense of relief. Within a week
> he was dead….[9]

Jhunia delivers her baby after a few months but again she has no milk
in her breast. A retired physician, after examining her exclaims, 'How
can she [Jhunia] expect milk when she is so anaemic? She would have to
take a long course of tonics before she hope to have milk in her breast.
How can this little bundle of flesh [new born baby] live without breast

feeding?'[10] There is a certain irony, perhaps, in this pronouncement about the need for a 'long course of tonics'.

Premchand's novel is one example of the variety of ways in which, through newspapers and journals, the educated section began to make themselves at home with knowledge about the body, and its well-being. They sought a new pedagogical role in public life by disseminating this knowledge in a paternalistic form to women, schoolboys, or the lower classes. Another aspect of this public engagement was the setting up of civic organizations to engage with sanitary issues and to mediate with government for 'improvements' in public health and sanitation.

Amongst the English-educated intelligentsia were the emerging 'professional classes' or doctors, lawyers, and teachers, seeking to carve out a niche for themselves in the society. They invoked their special qualifications to lend authority to the position they took in debates relating to eugenic health, medical practices, and sanitation. Sometimes this 'scientific' knowledge was proved in contrast to 'superstitious' beliefs. But sometimes, on a more persuasive note, an effort was made to represent it as an extension or a confirmation of traditional beliefs and practices relating to health.

One aspect of intervention was a quest to map new notions of sanitation onto the notions of ritual purity. Historians have shown how they sought to locate 'science' in the Vedic past, both to glorify the Vedic scripture and to suggest that modern science was not an alien or introduced form of knowledge.[11] Pointing to the crucial role which water played in the everyday life of Banarsis, they argued that concepts of cleanliness and sanitation were nothing new, but in fact, always integral to Banarsis life.[12] David Arnold has given one illustration of this endeavour in the formation of an organization called *Kashi Ganga Prasadhini Sabha*, in the last quarter of the 19th century, on the initiative of the Raja of Benares and his *diwan* (Chief Minister).[13] The main objective of this organization was to redirect the sewage of Benares, keeping the bathing ghats (bank of a river) free from 'pollution'. In his view, 'veneration for the Ganges, the traditional leadership of the Raja, and western (rather than Hindu) notions of cleanliness and pollution were in this conjoined'.[14] The word *'prasadhini'* means beautification. Their appeal to the public was '...Ganga is our mother and it is our prime duty to decorate her...'[15] The word 'prasadhini' was used to invest a sanitary project with a popular appeal, and to cast the endeavour as akin to an act of devotion. On the one hand, they sought to make people comfortable with terms like 'sanitation' and 'municipality' by framing them in well-known codes of religious practices. On the other hand, they also sought to refurbish notions of ritual purity by asserting that they were based on a sanitary rationale. Colonial officials looked upon such organization with approval as a sign of the awakening of a civic consciousness. Neville, in his 1909 District Gazetteer of Benares, sees the formation of a civic organization as 'Pollution-Prevention Society'—'...the pollution of river...so acute...in 1886 a **powerful** society was formed...*Kashi Ganga Prasadhini Sabha*... preventing pollution of the sacred stream...large sum of money was collected, and the assistance of government was invoked...the scheme... estimated expenditure of 24 lakhs was approved by municipal board in 1889...completed in 1892...'[16]

Along the same lines, the editor of *Nagari Pracharini Patrika* tried to correlate religious festivals and fairs with sanitation and municipal activities—

> ...*Gangaji nahane jate ho to pahele paani sir par chada kar tab pair dalne ka vidhan kyon hai? Jisse taluye se garmi sir par chad kar vicar na utpan kare. Diwali ise hetu hai kee saal bhar mein ek ber to safai ho jaye. Holi ise hetu ki basant kee bigadi hawa sthan- sthan par agni jalane se swach ho jaye. Yahi **tyohar** mano tumhari **municipality** hai...*[17]

> ...While going for a bath in the river Ganga why do we first put water on the head and then put our feet into the water? This is so that the heat from the feet does not rise to the head with harmful consequences to cause adverse effects. Diwali is celebrated so that at least once a year the surroundings get thoroughly cleaned. Similarly Holi is meant to clean the dangerous spring air by lighting up a bonfire at several places. Consider these festivals as your 'municipality'...

'PROFESSIONAL' AUTHORITIES IN THE PUBLIC SPHERE

Indian allopathic doctors employed by the sanitation and public health department as Health Officers played a vital role in transforming the people's perception about diseases and their cure. Through the medium of vernacular languages, such employees tried to disseminate 'scientific' ideas about the reasons for disease and their 'proper' treatment.[18] One such figure was Pandit Kali Charan Dubey, a Brahmin, employed as a Health Officer of Benares. He had a L.M.S degree and a Diploma in Public Health from London. Kali Charan Dubey sought to impart medical knowledge to the public via self-help manuals and primers. One of his medical tracts was titled 'Balako Ko Posharth Aavashyak Sikshayen—Essential knowledge about nutrition for young boys'.[19] Written in colloquial Hindi, it was meant to instruct school children. It drew attention to the fact that one-third of infants born in Benares died every year. The pamphlet blamed this on unsanitary conditions and on ignorant parents who did not take the right steps to protect their children against smallpox, cholera, and tetanus.[20] The solution was proper nutrition such as mother's milk, albumin, lime and barley water, and meat essence for the infants. The tract also explains to mothers the importance of clean and airy room for the delivery of the baby, and advises that if ever 'wet nurse' is required, she should be of clean habits and free from illness.[21] Here, we have an Indian doctor and a Brahman one setting out to dispense medical knowledge in a popular, non-specialist way in an orthodox religious milieu.

Dubey also published special tracts on smallpox, malaria, cholera, and plague, some of which were accepted for publication by the Public Health Department of the Municipal Board of Benares.[22] The tract on smallpox, a four-page booklet, stressed the importance of vaccination, in the form of a story. A son is born in two different families. While one family vaccinates their child the other does not. The unvaccinated child gets smallpox and loses his sight. The sufferer dies rebuking his parents' carelessness for not vaccinating him.[23] Concluding his story the author warns people that—

> ...yaad rakho ki chechak se bachne ke liye kewal teeka he eek upay hai... in panch baton ko yaad rakhna chahiye...1. teeka lo; 2. saat baras ke baad fir teeka lo; 3. teeka lagane walon kee baat maan lo; 4. jo teeka lagane se mana karte hon uski baat na suno; 5. teeka kee dava bachde se tayyar kee jati hai....[24]
>
> ...remember vaccination is the only cure for smallpox...keep in mind the following five points...1. Get vaccinated; 2. Get revaccinated after seven years; 3. Follow the vaccinator's advice; 4. Do not listen to those who advice against vaccination; 5. Vaccination is prepared from calf lymph.

In addition to the tracts published by the public health department, some medical practitioners got their tracts published at their own expense. The Nagari Pracharini Sabha of Benares and Munshi Newal Kishore Press at Lucknow were popular publishing centres.[25] The Saraswati journal launched by the Nagari Pracharini Sabha gave a lot of space to articles on health and disease, often worked by prominent medical practitioners of Benares, for instance, Dr Mahendulal Garg, Dr Murleedhar, Dr Pandit Ram Narayan Sharma, Dr Nand Kishore, and Dr Gadgil. These practitioners were trained in allopathic medicine; therefore the articles they wrote were based on the Western notion of medical science, that is, physiology of the body, for instance, blood circulation or the reproductive organs.

Disease, Causative Agents, and Cure

In *Plague-Tattva* (Element of Plague), Dr Mahendulal Garg explained the cause and spread of plague in the society.[26] He explained that the disease is caused by a special type of '*krimi*—microscopic organism', which enters into the body through wounds. The organism resides in the soil and is therefore called '*jamini bimari*—earthy disease'. The disease spreads through a dirty, unclean person, lying on earth, and also through rats, dogs, and flies. Citing various types of plague such as bubonic, pneumonic, and septicemia, the author suggests taking the patient immediately to the plague hospital and leaving the dwelling place.[27] Similarly, Dr Murleedhar explained about various 'microscopic pathogens' causing diseases in an article *Rogotpadak-Jantu Vijnan* (Science of Disease Causative Organism).[28] Lalli Prasad Pandey was one of the prolific writers on disease and human anatomy. In two different articles—'Malaria' and '*Malaria Ke Machhad* (Mosquitoes of Malaria)' the author, Lalli Prasad Pandey, showed the causes of malaria and its vector, and criticized various irrational views prevalent in society regarding malaria.[29]

Ayurvedic practitioners tried to persuade others within their group that the knowledge of science was necessary. So as to avoid humiliation from allopathic physicians, they should not lag behind in scientific knowledge and should learn some allopathic techniques. One of such Ayurvedic physician was Pandit Madhav Rai, who felt that vaidyas had to suffer humiliation many a time in front of allopathic physicians due to lack of understanding of what they said, so he persuaded the vaidyas to learn and practice some techniques of allopathic medicine—

> *Vaidya logon ko dacter kee baton ko bilkul na samajhne ke karan unka mukh dekhna parta hai…is vaste vaidyon ko bhi kuch toda bahut dactory vidya mein abhyas karma aavashya hee chahiye kyonki is vakt dactory vidya ka hee vishesh prachar ho raha hai aur dactory davayen sheegra fal bhi dikhane vaali hoti hain…*[30]

Vaidya being not able to understand the doctors' conversation had to face humiliation many a times...therefore vaidyas should also learn and do little bit practice of allopathic medicine because these days allopathy is specially promoted and these medicine also show quick results...

Pandit Madhav Rai had written a medical tract '*doctory chikitsa—* allopathic treatment' to give information about Western medicine to vaidyas. He had given detailed explanation of weights and measurements, how to check the pulse rate with a stethoscope, the analysis of urine, and the use of thermometer in checking the body temperature.

Ayurvedic physicians also sought to defend their special branch of medicine and its tenets of healing and to indicate that they were able to engage with issues of contemporary interest and concern. Shri Pandit Gurmukh Rai and Raisahab Vyas Tansukh were two renowned vaidyas (ayurvedic practitioners) of Benares. Shri Pandit Gurmukh Rai-*jee* based his description on the Western lines while explaining the concept of smallpox in his article '*Masurika*' (chechak).[31] Vaidya Raisahabvyas Tansukh, in one of his booklet '*Bachon kee bhishan mrityu sankya* (High Death Rate of Children)', explained the various causes for high infant mortality and also gave various remedies to reduce the same. The editor of *Saraswati* journal reviewing the booklet praised the author by describing him—'...*Raisahabjee Vaidya apne vishay ke purane lekhak hain. Aapne jo kuch likha hai usse sahitya ke sath lok kalyan bhi hua hai...*—is one of the old genre author on his subject. He along with benefiting Hindi literature has also benefited the society'.[32]

Physiology and Anatomy

Another line of engagement in the realm of medical science was the body and its parts. Colonial officials saw it as a triumph of Western medicine that high class Bengalis were able to touch dead bodies.[33] But it was Indian doctors who disseminated anatomical and physiological information about the body, seeking to displace what they now characterized as certain 'taboos' with a 'scientific' aptitude. Indian allopathic doctors disseminated this information by translating the English articles into Hindi. Dr Ram Narayan Sharma, a Licentiate Medical Surgeon, and Dr Gadgil, Doctor of Medicine, explained human physiology and anatomy in their articles.[34] Whereas in another article '*Manushya Ka Mastishka*' (Brain of a Human Being), Lochan Prasad

Pandey showed details of the physiology and anatomy of the brain.[35] In an article entitled 'Vivisection', Mahendulal Garg explained the importance and techniques of surgery, and in another article 'Rakt-Brahman', he explained the process of blood circulation in the human body.[36]

Attitudes to the Diseased

Some writers were also trying to change the attitude of people towards those suffering from contagious diseases such as plague. Dr Shri Bhagwan Das of Benares, an eminent academician, nationalist, and a very prominent figure in the social life, in his story 'Plague Ki Churail—witch of plague' wrote that plague was such a terrible disease that even close relatives of the sufferer abandoned him.[37] He advised them to be sympathetic to the sufferer.

INTERVENTION IN CIVIC AND MUNICIPAL LIFE

The educated people also felt they had to mediate with government authorities to demand improvements in sanitation and public health. To make their case, they invoked the authority of vital statistics. Munshi Ganga Prasad Verma, editor of the *Advocate* and the *Hindustani* (Lucknow), reviewed the sanitary condition of the United Provinces and showed the higher rate of mortality in the United Provinces as compared to other provinces. Giving fever as the main reason for higher mortality in an article 'Public health in the United Provinces', published in a local Hindi newspaper '*Zamana*', he declared that—'...Fever is mostly caused by the existence of mosquitoes near water pipes, so the drainage systems of large towns, such as Lucknow and Benares, should be improved... Narrow roads in congested areas should be widened and model houses for the poor should be constructed...'[38]

A correspondent of the Hindi newspaper *Bharat Jiwan* reported that the water was of deadly influence; the vapour from which filled the air with fever breeding miasma. He called for immediate steps to improve drainage in the vicinity of the ghats and also reported that the poor drainage allowed accumulation of stagnant water.[39] Complaints about the non-availability of pure drinking water and contamination of the sources of supply were frequently highlighted in the contemporary vernacular newspapers.[40] The editor of the *Hindi Hindustan* described steps being taken in Bengal to get the dirty water released by factories cleansed by 'Chlorinated lime' before it was allowed to run into rivers, canals, or from which people took water for drinking or other domestic purposes. He urged the necessity of similar steps in the United Provinces.[41] Colonial observers and British administrators perceived Hindu practices as unclean and blamed Hindu immigrants and their ritual acts as the main reasons for the propagation of disease and infection leading to high mortality.[42] But in contrast to colonial administrators, the educated class and employers, although imbibing the new terminology, protested that the condition in Benares was pathetic because the authorities were not taking enough measures to improve the sanitary condition and combat disease. A reporter of the Hindi journal *Saraswati*, by giving a translation of a report from *Sunday Despatch* and quoting that according to the British 'Hindus were the dirtiest people in the World', tried to represent himself as sanitary reformer and bearer of the new knowledge.[43]

NEW MEDICAL TECHNOLOGIES: FEAR AND ATTRACTION

New medical technologies were also a popular subject for public debate and discussion. Proponents of these new technologies like injection, thermometer, stethoscope, and x-rays, showed the advantage of accuracy in diagnosis and quick relief but they were also careful to point out their convenience in terms of maintaining certain norms and the social hierarchy. Dr Raghubir Sahaya Bhargav, writing on the benefits of the stethoscope, explained it as an instrument, which helps, in knowing the rhythm of heart and lungs.[44] He described the procedure for knowing the rhythm and commented that by analysis of the heartbeat and lung rhythm, a doctor could diagnose the symptom of various ailments.[45]

> *Stethoscope ke mukhya labh...jo streeyan seene ki paricha karana na chahti ho vah uska vah sira jo rogi ke sharir par lagaya jata hai swayam laga le aur doctor parde me se dono kano me lagane vale siron ko laga kar aawaj maloom Kare...maile-kuchale manushyon kee pariksha bhe kar lee jave aur kise prakar ka durgandh bhi na maloom ho. Rogi ke sameep kaan na lana pade...[46]*

Major benefit of stethoscope...those woman who wanted to get their chest examined hold the one end of the tool which should be kept on patient and **doctor behind the curtain** can put the both lead of the tool into their ear and can hear the rhythm...**person in rags can also be examined** and one can not feel bad body smell. No need to bring ear near to the patient...[47]

The stethoscope allowed medical access to women's bodies in a way, which showed an accurate diagnosis without any breach of purdah norm. Here, science is portrayed as advantageous because it allows the physician to distance himself from poor and dirty patients with accurate diagnosis without getting physicians in proximity to the patient. The thermometer used to measure the body temperature was also advocated with the same line of argument. Pandit Madhav Rai vaidya-*jee*, in his tract, had shown how to check the body temperature by using the thermometer and had also given names of various allopathic medicines, their uses, and prescriptions. He explained that just like the stethoscope, doctor did not need to touch the patient. The patient, according to his or her convenience, put the thermometer either in the mouth or under the armpit and after a minute could hand it over to the doctor. The doctor was able to view the body temperature on it.[48] Medical advancement, and especially the stethoscope and thermometer, gave access to bodies while maintaining the norms of purdah and of social hierarchy.

Ayurvedic physicians in defense of their special branch of medical knowledge argued that they these technologies were clearly described in the Vedas and other classical text but by the span of time these technologies had been lost for want of research. For example, one such vaidya Pandit Ramakant Tripathi alias Prakash, resident of Pratabgarh near Benares, outlined the reasons for the growth and popularity of injections in following lines—

Injection chikitsa pranali kee unnati ka vishesh karan uski upyogita aur sheegrah labhkari hona hee hai. Jo anya aushadhiyon se maheene me ache hote hain ve isse ek-adh saptah mein ache kiye ja sakte hain.[49]

Main reason for the growth of injection treatment is its importance and quick relief...other medicines which can treat in months can be treated within a week by injection...

Pandit Tripathi, justifying the importance of injections, also tried to authorize that this technology previously existed in Indian medical text but had been lost. No research in this field and a lack of efficient Indian medical practitioners was the main cause for the decline in this technology.

*...aajkal jo injection aur pichkari ka prayog kiya ja raha hai yeh hamare liye koi nayee baat nahi hai...**suchibhedan chikitsa** pranali vartman injection ka varnan bhi hamare ayurved mein bhalibhanti aaya hai...pracheen*

ayurvedyacharyon ne jo vidhiyan batayee hain un par na to koi anusand-
han ho raha hai aur na ham us par likhene ke shamta rakhte hain.[50]

Injections which are used now a days are not anything new to us...
skin piercing treatment called injection at present had been well described
in our ayurveda...there had been no research going on what ancient
ayurvedic expert had told to us nor we have capacity to write on it...

Coming back again to Premchand, we discover another facet of
representation and the way in which the new technologies enhanced the
'god-like' status of the doctor to give him an overwhelming degree of
authority over the patient. In his novel *Nirmala*, one patient in a situation
of severe illness accepted the frightening technology with utter docility—

Doctor ne sangidh swar se kaha...106 degree jwar hai...aakhir usne (doc-
tor) pichkari se koi dava bhaiya (patient) ke bajoo mein dal diya. Chaar
angul se kam kee sui nahi rahi hogi par bhaiya bhinke tak nahi...[51]

Doctor said seriously...patient has 106 degree temperature...doctor
inserted some medicine in the arm of patient via a syringe. Injection may
not be less than four inch but patient did not react...

There was other aspect as well about new medical technology where
one finds people yearning for new technologies. With the changing
time, people started giving due care to their hair, skin, and other things
related to their looks. In an article *'Chasma aur khubsoorti'* (Spectacles
and Beauty) in popular Hindi journal *Saraswati*, an unknown author
described the information about using spectacles.[52] He shows with the
help of various pictures of face the way spectacles increase the face
value and a person with weak eyesight could also easily read and write
by wearing a pair of glasses. Premchand has another depiction of a
light-hearted exchange of the way middle class was encountering with
technology. Premchand depicts the middle class yearning for certain
technology which was out of their reach.

Nayan:...jara apni surat banwa lo...yahan bijli ke dacter aaye hain jo bud-
hape ke sare nishan mita dete hain. Kya majal ki chare par ek jurri ya fir
siir ka koi bal paka rah jaye. Na jaane aisa kya jadu kar dete hain ki aadmi
ka chola hi badal jata hai...koi jadi-buti batao...bijli aur radium to bade
aadmiyon ke liye rahne do....[53]

Nayan, get your face overhauled...one electric doctor (x-ray or radium
or any current) had come here who removes all old age signs. There is
no possibility of remaining a single wrinkle on face or a white hair. Not

know what magic he does that whole make over (personality/appearance) changes…suggest me some herbal treatment…electric current and radium are meant for big people…

Above dialogues indicate that middle class were getting aware of new technologies and were very enthusiastic to experiment all things to remain young and beautiful. But the on-going dialogue also highlighted the ambiguous state of mind of the middle class. As technology was out of their reach due to high prices—'Totaram: how much fees he takes? Nayan:…500 rupees…' so they authorize that such expensive treatment was meant for high class people only—'if it's a matter of five or ten rupees then I can think…500 rupees is a big deal…suggest me some herbal treatment…electric current and radium are meant for big people…'[54] On the other side, their condition was like grapes out of reach from the fox. Due to incapable of availing the facility, they claimed the advertiser as a quack befooling people—'*Totaram: aaji koi pakhandi hoga, bevakoofon ko loot raha hoga. Koi rogan lagakar do-chaar din ke liye jara chera chikna kar deta hoga. Isthari dacter par apna vishvas hi nahi…*'[55] ('Totaram: he may be a quack, befooling peoples… smoothening faces by applying some colour or ointment for three-four days, and I have no trust on these advertising doctors'.) They wanted to have these facilities at minimal prices and at last they opt for cheap indigenous herbal products.

THE BODY AS A SITE OF PROCREATION

An important line of intrusion in the realm of medical science was the human body. This engagement was catering to a market which was not only eager to take knowledge of Western medicine but also knowledge of the body, not only as a site of disease but also as a site of procreation and pleasure. Here, the pedagogical role was sometimes very thin.

One section of the educated class was solely involved in imparting information based on modern scientific facts such as physiology and the anatomical description of sexual organs, the science of reproduction and child delivery, and the diseases related to sexual organs and their cure. They did not show the entire human body but only certain parts related to the medical sciences. For example, *Sachitra Guptarog Chikitsa* (Illustrated Treatise for the Treatment of Venereal Diseases) by Vaidy-abhushan Shaymlal was very popular. In its advertisement, Shyamlal claimed that the book was meant for curing *gupt rog*—venereal diseases.

He professed the use of Vedic and *Unani* methods for the treatment of venereal diseases. He had provided colour pictures of the sexual organs of women, the parts helpful in the formation of semen, loose breasts, healthy nipples, and so on.[56] Dr Baba C. C. Sarkar in his book *Stree Va Baal Rog Chikitsa* (Cure for Women and Child Disease) explained various kind of illness related to woman and child and gave instructions for their treatment.[57]

Women were advised on the care of the body, menstruation, neo-natal care, child birth, breast feeding, and child rearing. *Stri Subodhini* (Education for Women) published by Newal Kishore Press from Lucknow, contained topics like protection of the womb, women's health and diseases, the education of *dais*, medical care, and the treatment of illness of household members.[58] Women were constantly advised on how to take care of the child or child rearing. *Santan Shastra* (Scientific Treatise on Progeny), a book addressed to the mother, was on childcare, and dealt with birth, disease, food, and the health of the child.[59] Some literate women also played a pedagogical role. These women were drawing upon the pedagogical authorities of their degrees. One such figure was a postgraduate woman Nirmal Bala (M.A.). She wrote various articles about female body and women's curiosity about knowing their bodies and its activities.[60] It is not clear that in any way she was a medical practitioner or had any relation or interaction with medical practitioners. But the articles written by her in various issues of *Saraswati* were based on Western notion of medical science. In the article 'Kamini Kautuhul' (Curiosity of a Young Woman) she explained in parts, that is, the various stages of foetal development in the womb and the process of child delivery. Not only this but in another article she explained the concept of the menstrual cycle. Another writer, Hemant Kumari Devi, in one of her articles in the popular Hindi newspaper *Abhyudaya*, gave details of various exercises meant for women to maintain their body figure and health. *Abhyudaya* and *Saraswati* had a regular column in their issues related to women's health titled 'Matramandir—mothers temple' and 'Matramandal—mothers' association'. These articles in Hindi journals show that talking about the female body, the menstrual cycle, and delivery was no longer limited to women relatives only. Missionary women often talked with horror about the way the woman relatives discussed sex and sexuality among themselves, but here we find the intervention of a third person, an unknown woman in these matters. These issues gained importance and relevance as a part of an informative education. These women writers helped to bring these issues into the public domain.

BRAHMACHARYA (CELIBACY)—HEALTHY MIND AND HEALTHY BODY

Another section of the educated class, with their intrusion on the modern lifestyle, tried to give information for a healthy mind and a healthy body; such teaching based on the concept of *brahmacharya*, that is, abstinence from sex. Their modern discourse intertwined eugenics, childbirth, and a scientific 'rationality'. Healthy bodies ensured strong men who, in turn, were very important to a modern masculine nation. Brahmacharya became closely tied to the fears and hopes of modern times. The pervasive anxieties and tensions of the age of *kaliyug* were perceived as systematically undermining a healthy way of life—males were losing their physical and mental vigour. Many of these tracts used a highly sanskritized language and ran into pages. For example, Surya Bali Singh in his tract *Brahmacharya Kee Mahima* (Glory of Celibacy) claimed—

> *Virya anmol hai...mrityu, rog tatha burhape ka nash karne wala amrit roop bara upchar, brahmcharya.... Jo shanty, sundarta, smriti, jnan, arogya aur uttam santati chatahai, vah is sansar mein sarvottam dharm Brahmacharya ka palan kare....*[61]
>
> Semen is invaluable...nectar like big cure for death, disease and old age is (practicing) *brahmacharya* only...who yearns for peace, beauty, knowledge, good health and ablest progeny, should observe the of worlds supreme principle of *brahmacharya*...

Here we find him advocating brahmacharya to married men as well. There seemed to be a concern about eugenics as he suggested that men should release semen once a month for the ablest progeny. Justifying his statement according to classical texts, he wrote that the time period for the development of semen is one month; that is why *acharyas*—Indian preceptors—advocated sex once a month, because release of the semen before its full growth makes the body devoid of all elements which, in turn, makes the body weak leading to various diseases. The popularity of this tract can be judged on the basis of the number of copies it printed. Its second edition published 2,000 copies. Another tract on *Brahmacharya Vijnan* (the Science of Celibacy) was written by an advocate of the

Arya Samaj, Pandit Jaannarayandeva Sharma. He seems to be more concerned about the degrading condition of Hindus and tried to correlate brahmacharya as a tool for the cause of nationalism—'...*hindu jati ke samne jeevan-maran ka prashan upasthit hai. Par jeevan ya maran ka nirnayak Brahmacharya hai. Marnasan samaj ke liye brahmcharya hee sanjeevani vidya hai...*[62]

> (There is question of life and death in front of Hindu community. But Brahmacharya is the decisive factor for life or death. Brahmacharya is the life giver for dying society...)

Sharma, trying to motivate youths for the sake of nation, suggested that 'the more people understand the importance of *Brahmacharya* and as many as practice *Brahmacharya* in our society, the more the economic and intellectual level of our society will increase. The strength of *Brahmacharya* will only solve all our problems'.[63] Brahmacharya thus became a building block for claims to social and political power, cultural identity, and a 'scientific' way of life.[64] Other moral reformers and medical practitioners added to this discourse of celibacy. Print brought a flood of cheap self-help guides on brahmacharya; age-old instructions were repeatedly stressed and infused with modern definition. The male was inundated with treatises on brahmacharya,[65] against masturbation, and for the preservation of semen.[66] Instructions to the males were endless. He was to make all-out efforts to control his sexual urge from a very young age. *Hast maithun, svapn dosh, guda maithun*, homosexuality, and fornication were all encompassed as the major evils of male sexuality. Anything seen as involving orgasm and emissions was taboo and seen as leading to disease. Semen was the essence of life and its discharge was a loss of vital energy, regardless of how it happened. To ensure male purity, to see that not a drop of precious semen fell waste upon barren soil, the Hindu male was drilled into keeping rein over his fantasies, passions, and imagination. He was to desist from masturbation completely.

HEALTH, MARRIAGE ADVICE, AND SEXUAL PLEASURE

From another perspective, some of the reformers and established publishing houses felt that the intricacies of sex and conjugality life needed to be discussed explicitly because sexual pleasure was an important facet of modern married life. The discourse of eugenics was used but actually all sorts of titillating possibilities were explored, deriving a sexual intimacy from print. One theme was the way the sex life had to be organized for healthy procreation.[67] *Kamkala Rahasya* (Secrets of Sex) published by Hindi Sevasadan, Aligarh, in its advertisement, warned unmarried *brahmachari* boys to keep away but recommended itself to married women and men.[68] Such books claimed their legitimacy by highlighting the scientific 'facts' of sexual life. Many claimed to be prescriptive texts crucial for sexual compatibility and accomplishment. At the same time, to make their books attractive for their audience, they provided coloured pictures and carried out advertisements in prominent papers and magazines. The advertisement for *Kamkala Rahasya* claimed that it had attractive pictures which thrilled the heart, and that it was full of sexual desire. On the same line, the advertisement of *Kam Tatha Ratishastra Sachitra* (Illustrated Treatise on Sex and Sexuality), in the leading Hindi daily *Abhyudaya*, first established its 'scientific credential' and then said it had colourful and spicy photographs of women, not from India but also from Africa, Germany, France, Italy, and Australia.[69] Santram, an Arya Samajist and founder of the 'Jat Pat Torak Mandal', wrote an article in 1924 in *Madhuri*, in support of 'true' publications on sexual science, which was also publicity material for sex manuals.[70] He went on to write books like *Vivahit Prem* (Married Love) and *Rativilas* (Sexuality).[71] Abhyudaya Press published *Kashmir Kok Shastra* and Chand Press published *Dampataya Jivan* (Conjugal Life).[72] As these popular sexually explicit literatures were catering to the needs of an ascendant literate class, they were in turn attacked by Hindu publicist in order to sanitize them because they deemed these popular literatures as 'obscene' and 'degenerate'.[73] But the point of the controversy was how sexual pleasure played role in the technologies of birth control and how it could be used for sexual pleasure and yet maintains healthy procreation. During the mid-1930s, the popular press eagerly took up the issue of contraceptive practice terming it as 'marriage advice'. Marriage advice literature, which flourished during the 1920s, listed all the methods available to the 'modern couple'.

Pandit Krishan Kant Malaviya, nephew of prominent congressman Madan Mohan Malaviya, was one of the prolific writers on these issues. He wrote *Suhag Raat*, *Patiyon Ko Seekh*, and *Bahurani Ko Siksha* pamphlets advertised in *Abhyudaya*, a Hindi newspaper published from Allahabad.[74] Such articles and pamphlets listed the medical disadvantages of unrestricted procreation. Malaviya attacked the Puritanism of the

West pointing that it was not the part of Indian culture. The physical hardships of repeated pregnancies, the high maternal mortality rate, the lack of appropriate hygienic care during childbirth, and improperly performed abortions were denounced and blamed on 'popular ignorance'. So, on the one hand, some authors were supporting the use of contraceptive technology by modern couples to derive sexual pleasure and avoid unwanted pregnancy. Mechanical means of birth control were available in two forms—pills and '*rubber ke bane huye yantra*—instruments (condoms) made up of rubber'. Their main argument was that 'women become weak and lose their beauty and charm at a young age by delivering child year after year. A man loses his income and at last was not able to bear household expenses. To stop an increase in number of children, couples should use "condoms" and live a happy life'.[75]

On the other hand, some authors were, however, against 'mechanical' means of contraception, advocating abstinence as better for health and morality instead.[76] They argued that it would erode the characters of youths, and another reason put by them was that it would spill out of marriage. But in this too the authority of modern medical science could be invoked. Such discussions brought issues like sexual intercourse, sexual pleasure, and the means of birth control into the public domain. Indigenous medicine practitioners eagerly sought a place for themselves, their skills and their products on this new platform. They began to use the print media and advertising to sell their skill and products. The birth control debate had made a great impact on the society, which can be observed in the following Bhojpuri lore—'*Ka hoiyen lakh lai ke tarai taraiya,*

Ekthai thi bhaghirath lai ganga maiya.[77]
(What will one do with lakhs of sons?
Only one ablest Bhagirath was enough to bring Ganga on the earth.)'

Some reformers correlated the concept of health and used scientific explanations against the social evil of child marriage. With the changing time, people were against child marriage and were concerned about the health of the young. To promote these ideas, they had adopted the revivalist technique saying that certain practices were approved in religious texts and people should practice according to those texts.

...bahut si baaten jo samaj – virudh maani hain par dharmsaashtron mein unka vidhan hai unko chalayeia jaise...larkon ko chotepan hee mein shaadi karke unka bal, virya, aayushya sab mat ghatayia. Aap unke ma-baap hain

ya dushman. Virya unke sharir mein pusht hone deejeye, vidya kuch padh lene deejeeye...tab unka pair kaath mein daliye...[78]

Many things which are against social norms but are accepted in classical text...start practicing them, such as...do not degenerate the health, and semen of boys by marrying them at early stage...are you parents for them or their enemy...let semen develop in their bodies, let them have some education...then marry them...

Their modern discourse intertwined eugenics, childbirth, and a scientific 'rationality'. Healthy bodies ensured strong men who, in turn, were very important for a modern masculine nation.

MEDICINE AND SOCIAL WELFARE

Juvenile Health: Vice and Addiction

Juvenile health and the toxic effect of drugs were also some of the issues given importance by the educated section in the society. Here also we find them indulged clearly in the pedagogical role by disseminating the information regarding the effect of smoking ganja or chewing tobacco on one's health, and extended their role by mediating with government for the ban of toxic substances through columns in newspapers and articles in journals. *Bharat Jiwan* of 18 June 1906, through its column, argued for 'the prohibition of the sale of cigarettes and *biris* and liquor to persons below fourteen years in all provinces'. A correspondent of a vernacular newspaper *Arya Mitra*, referring to the sentence of transportation for life passed on a sadhu for willfully murdering a child at Allahabad at the Kumbh Mela, under the influence of some intoxicating drug, 'does not understand why government should not enact a law prohibiting the use of deleterious drugs which demoralize and ruined the health of those addicted to it'.[79]

The poetry cited in the opening paragraph of this chapter shows the eugenic concern of the educated class. Here, the poet emphasized the impact of smoking on the health of a migrant labourer or poor peasant, which results in weak generative power coupled with contagious disease such as Tuberculosis. Another bhojpuri poem warned the people against the use of drugs and tobacco. Poet addresses himself to the sadhus—

Please don't make [sadhus] your self-addicted, improve yourself. Tobacco from the dirt of cows ear and was mixed with animal excreta, it won't give you any pleasure. People will avoid you. You [sadhu] have nothing to eat even then smokes '*chilum*' along with young friends. You [sadhu] practice untouchablity but I think you as untouchable who smokes out the wealth of poor by which they are suffocated. [Sadhu] You are burden on this land and I [poet] pray that you go to hell.[80]

This kind of poetry depicts a transformation in society, that is, the sadhus who enjoyed social status were considered as burdens on the society. When a poet describes about poverty, family size, and diseases in his poetry, it seems that society was slowly imbibing the norms of de-addiction which was in totality a Western concept; whereas in India, addiction was not considered unethical or non-religious or blasphemous, as Shiva, who consumed all sorts of drugs, is worshipped by the Hindus. There was demand for de-addiction and poets were also promoting the utility and importance of small families. On the track of reforming the society, the poet shows the existing social hierarchy and practices of untouchability by the sadhus. He sarcastically remarked to the sadhu that they were untouchables rather than those they think, because they did nothing for the society and instead made youths addicted. This particular reference shows that the poet was very far-sighted. His view was that people were already suffering from poverty and famine and these sadhus, instead of doing some labour, went begging for alms, and if people were not able to provide anything to them they frightened them with harsh words. So the poet considered them as a burden on the earth.

MODERNITY AS MALAISE

On the one hand, modern medicine seemed to offer many possibilities for maintaining health whereas, on the other hand, many of the ills of the body were caused by a modern lifestyle for which modern medicine was not able to provide explanations. For example, a migrant labourer who lost his virility after leaving the village is described in the following Magahi folk song—

piya gailai Calcutta, lele ailai jatsaria,
seho jatwa garalkai rama sireestar,
jatwa na chalai rama, makario na dolai,
hathawa dhaile rama sunder nayanma dharai he lor,
ghrba charhal alai lachhman devera,
chhori dehu bhauji he jatsariya,

sasu je marai nanad gatiabai,
ohu parabhu bahar karai ekre balak binu.[81]

My husband has brought a grinding machine from Calcutta,
He has fixed up that machine under the sirish tree.
O, my god, neither the machine moves nor the handle moves,
The beautiful woman is holding the handle
And tears are oozing out of her eyes and says,
My younger brother-in-law comes on the back of horse
He asked me to give up the grinding,
Mother in law has beaten me, and sister-in-law rebuked me,
My husband has driven me out of house because I am barren.

In this folklore, the poet seems to be concerned about the women's situation in the family and tried to highlight the pains and sufferings of the barren women. The poet also seems to be well informed and knowledgeable about the impact of industrialization over a man's potency. Here, for the first time, it was shown that because of industrialization, the man had become weak and sterile. On the other hand, the poet eulogizes the purity of village air and lifestyle alluding to the vigour and vitality of the husband's younger brother residing in the village. In this folklore, the metaphor of grinding machine and its handle depict the husband's helplessness and impotency.

The authors of these contemporary popular writings had the advantage of mass print technology, photographic technology, and a commercial press. They could reproduce images, publish their books in substantially large numbers and ensure good sales; they were therefore bringing health-information to the masses and these had a higher visibility and reach. Their market was not limited to the literati—but extended to an increasing class of functionally literate people, including clerks, shopkeepers, traders, and students. This literature could now be found in the newly emerging book markets, local kiosks, and railway stations.

CONCLUDING REMARKS

The above analysis shows that the educated sections of the society were playing a vital role in dispensing new knowledge of diseases and their cure. In their engagement at various levels with the modern concepts of health, sanitation, and diseases, they invoked debates in the public sphere, sought a new pedagogical role in public life by disseminating this knowledge in paternalistic form to women, schoolboys, or the lower classes, and mediated with government for 'improvements in the public health and sanitary conditions'.

These educated sections of the society were using prescriptive texts while propagating new notions of health and medicine. For instance, they were supplying information in colloquial Hindi through newspapers, journals, medical tracts, or booklets. These people were drawing upon the pedagogical authorities, upon their educational qualifications, and official employment such as a health officer or sanitary inspector. Ayurvedic practitioners, in order to identify themselves in the new world of modern science and to avoid humiliation from allopathic physicians, also acquainted themselves with the new techniques of diagnosis. These technologies appealed both to patients and practitioners as it allowed near accurate diagnosis without any breach of the purdah norm. Hence, the physicians were able to distance themselves from the poor and dirty patients, and thus maintained their social hierarchy. But on the other hand, modern notions of sanitation and municipality were framed according to religious codes. They tried to locate 'science' in the Vedic past and in the veneration of Vedic scriptures. They emphasized that these techniques were not an alien form of knowledge, since these were explained and cited in the ancient Ayurvedic texts. In the course of time, these technologies were lost. Rather, they drew upon debates relating to eugenic health, medical and sanitation issues in order to carve out a niche for themselves. In doing so, 'science' and Western medicine were thus upheld by all practitioners of medicine. But this was not universally appreciated. Creative writers like Premchand and political crusaders like Madan Mohan Malaviya condemned them.

'Body as a site' was another important line of mediation in the realm of medical knowledge. One section was solely involved in imparting physiology and anatomical details of the body. However, another section intervened in the modern lifestyle by providing information for a healthy mind and healthy body. This multifaceted nature of medical discourse was based on modern discourse of eugenics, childbirth, and a scientific 'rationality'. Thereby, an attempt was made to correlate the discourses on nationalism with voices for male or masculine nation. Arya Samajist Surya Bali Singh and Pandit Jaannarayandeva Sharma advocated for brahmacharya. They used brahmacharya as a building block for claims to social and political power, cultural identity, and a 'scientific' way of life, and in order to motivate youths for the sake of building a strong 'masculine' nation. Whereas, Krishan Kant Malaviya, Santram, and Banarsi Lal Verma were in support of new technologies for sexual pleasure so to maintain healthy procreation. Some of them were also using mild pornography to meet the market demand. This rich corpus of Hindi tracts shows that there was concern only about men's health, thus marginalizing women. Repressive sexuality was widely preached against homosexuality even while accepting it as a part of male sexuality.

As healthy bodies ensured strong men who, in turn, were important to a modern masculine nation, issues related to juvenile health and toxic effect of drugs were also given due importance. Thus, medicine, on the one hand, seems to offer many possibilities for maintaining health, but this chapter also reflects upon a critique of colonial capitalism where industrialization, city, and machine had adverse effects. For example, it was thought that many of the ills of the body such as loss in virility, weakness were caused by modern lifestyle. While playing a pedagogical role, educated people were also trying to prove their authority over the masses. In addition, they were carving out a niche for themselves in the changing scenario by posing as their representative while mediating with the government. The above analysis shows that the educated sections were not passive recipients. They tried to internalize the modern notions, and thus securing their space in the newly-created professional structure along with social status.

NOTES

1. Poet Pandit Mahendra Shastri, '*visharad*', resident of Chhapara district of Bihar, was a nationalist and social reformer of the mid-20th century. The subjects of his poetries were poverty, peasant's condition, social reform, and nationalism. Sanskritayen and Upadhyaya (eds) (1961:167–8).

2. This is my translation of a folklore cited in Note 1. All translations from Hindi are mine, unless otherwise stated.

3. Arnold (ed.) (1989); 1991); Harrison (1994); Cunningham and Andrews (eds) (1997); Anil Kumar (1998); Kumar (ed.) (2001); Pati and Harrison (eds) (2001); Bagchi and Soman (eds) (2005).

4. There have been many studies about the religio-cultural aspects of Benares by Western and Indian writers. Although it was also a centre for Ayurvedic learning, the relation of medicine and imperialism is one of the yet unexplored themes. Lannoy (2002); Vidhyarthi (1979); Eck (1983); Sherring (2002).

5. Prem Chand was born at Lamahi village, about four miles away from Benares, on 31st July 1880. His original name was Dhanpat Rai. Some of his

novels were *Sevasadan* (1918), *Premashram* (1922), *Rang Bhumi* (1926), *Kayakalp* (1926), *Nirmala* (1928), *Pratigya* (1929), *Gaban* (1931), *Karmbhumi* (1932), and *Godan* (1936). Gupta (1968).

6. Premchand (1994:14).

7. Premchand in his short story, 'The road to salvation', described the doctor's pride in patients seated before him as equivalent to the pride the peasant takes in his flourishing field, the soldier in his red turban, or the coquette's in her jewels. (2001:19).

8. Premchand (1994:5).

9. Ibid., p. 224.

10. Ibid., p. 228.

11. Jones (1976).

12. *Nipatana-nahana* (latrine and bathing) go together. *Bhang chhanana* means both to grind and to strain the bhang very fine. *Safa lagana* is to wash clothes very vigorously, with a lot of soap, until very clean. These three sets of activities constitute the trip. *Bahri alang* is always described by a Banarasi as being the quintessential Banarasi activity. Nita Kumar (1988:83–9).

13. Arnold in Frietag (ed.) (1989:265); Neville reported that the project was completed in 1892. Neville (1909a:262–3); K. S. Muthaiah confirmed the failure of the scheme (1911:164).

14. Arnold, in Frietag (ed.) (1989:265).

15. *Bharat Jiwan*, 22 November 1886, in *Selections from the Vernacular Newspapers of the North Western Provinces*

16. Neville (1909a:262–3).

17. 'Bharat kee unnati kaise ho?' *Nagari Pracharini Patrika* (Reprinted article in *Bhartendu Ank*, Samvat 2007) (1952:127).

18. In the 20th century, Western medicine and medical system was well established and educated section of the society was internalized by Western notions. Here, the word 'scientific' is used as understood by the author described in the context during that period. The author viewed Western notion of health as 'scientific'.

19. Dubey (1913).

20. Ibid., p. 2.

21. Ibid., p. 4.

22. Pt. Kali Charan Dubey was a prolific writer of pamphlets for the Public Health Department of the Benares Municipal Board. In 1913, he published the following clutch of pamphlets—*Haiza Chinnh Nidan-Rokene Ke Upay* (Cholera, its symptoms and cure); *Malaria Ya Fasli Bookhar Ya Sheetjwar* (Malaria); *Taun* (Plague); *Chechak* (Smallpox).

23. Dubey (1913:1–4).

24. Ibid., p. 4.

25. Shri Gopal Prasad Khatri established *Nagari Pracharini Sabha* on 16 July 1893. Its main objective was the popularization of *Nagari* script and Hindi language. *Nagari Pracharini Sabha* published following health tracts—Jagrani Devi, *Chuut Wale Rog Aur Unse Bacchne Ke Upay* (Contagious Diseases and their Preventive Measures), 1909; Mahendulal Garg, *Paricharya Pranali* (Nursing), 1909; *Streeyon Ke Rog Aur Unki Chikitsa* (Women Diseases and their Treatments), n.d; Following two books published by Newal Kishore Press were very popular—Lala Baidyanath, *Plague Nivaran Upay* (Prevention and Treatment for Plague), 1909; Balak Ram Shukla, *Malaria Vijnan* (Malaria Science), 1939.

26. Garg (1908:208–10).

27. Ibid.

28. Dr.Murleedhar, 1908, 'Rogotpadak-Jantu Vijnant—Science of Disease, Causative Organism, *Saraswati*, Vol.9, No.9, 399–402.

29. Pandey (1908:492–4); (1911:68–72).

30. Madhav Rai (1947:preface).

31. Gurmukh Rai, 'Masurika', *Sudarshan Journal* (38–40).

32. Tansukh (1934:407–15).

33. In January 1836, at the newly established medical college in Calcutta, a Brahmin instructor, Pandit Madhusudan Gupta and four Indian students, performed a human dissection for the first time. Centenary of Medical College hailed it as the day when 'Indians rose superior to the prejudices of their earlier education and thus boldly flung open the gates of modern medical science to their country men'. The momentous day was duly celebrated in a militaristic fashion, by firing a 50-round salute from the guns of Calcutta's Fort William. *Centenary of Medical College*, Bengal (1935:13) cited in Arnold (1993:6).

34. Sharma (1912:301–4); Gadgil (1935:258–62).

35. Pandey (1909:221–3).

36. Garg (1908:430–2); "Vivisection", *saraswati*, no. 4, April 1906, pp. 201–2.

37. Bhagwandas, 1950, 'Plague hi Churail', *Saraswati*, 162–9.

38. Varma (1908:602).

39. *Bharat Jiwan* (1893:191).

40. *Hindi Hindustan* (1906:129); *Nasim-i-Agra* (1906:217); *Hindi Hindustan* (1906:129); *Almora Akhbar* (1906:217).

41. *Hindi Hindustan* (1906:129).

42. According to the Director of Public Health Department '...the immigrants act as a universal propagator of disease and infection. Aged and diseased persons wishing to die in the holy city Benares were the major immigrants. Due to overcrowding and unsanitary conditions, the Benares became the epidemic ground of cholera, typhus and plague and also suffered consecutively to chronic outbreaks of malaria and dysentery. Administration reports confirm the highest

mortality rate of the Benares through most of the 19th century...Benares was one of the most deadly cities in the northern India. With the onset of the monsoon, the mortality from fevers due to malaria, dysentery and cholera flourished. Small pox, "*Basant Rog*", reached its greatest intensity between March and June due to high temperature and low humidity. Benares suffered severe epidemics in 1878, 1884, 1889, 1897, 1926, 1930, 1934, 1942–5 and 1951–2'. *Annual Report of the Director of the Public Health of the UP*, Allahabad (1925).

43. *Saraswati* (1934:467–8).

44. Bhargav (1926:1).

45. Ibid.

46. Ibid., p. 2.

47. Ibid., Emphasis added.

48. Madhav Rai (1947).

49. Tripathi (1933:2–3).

50. Ibid.

51. Premchand (1923:116, 121).

52. "Chasma aur Khubsoorti -Spectacles and Beauty", *Saraswati*, part 23, no.1, 1922, pp.86–8

53. Premchand (1923:67–8).

54. Ibid.

55. Ibid.

56. Shyamlal,n.d, *Sachitra Guptrog Chikitsa*, Aligarh: Hindustani Book Depot.

57. Sarkar, 1937, *Stree va Baal Rog Chikitsa*.

58. Girdavar (1922).

59. G.S. Gaur, 1928, 'Indra', *Santan Shastra*, 2nd Edn.

60. Nirmal Bala, 1903, 'Kamini Kotuhal', *Saraswati*, Vol.4, No.8; 1903, 'Prasuti—Child Delivery', *Saraswati*, Vol. 4, No.11; 'Rajo Darshan', *Saraswati*, Vol.4, No.12.

61. Singh (1931:5).

62. Sharma (1927:1).

63. Ibid., p. 3.

64. Gupta (2001:69).

65. Suryabali Singh, (1928),*Brahmacharya Ki Mahima* – Glory of Celibacy, Benares; Gaurdas Maharaj, 1928, *Brahmachari Bano*, Agra; Pannalal Sharma, n.d., *Yuva Rakshak*, Agra; Lala Bhagwan Din, n.d., *Brahmacharya Ki Vaigyanik Vyakya*, Kashi Chimmanlala Vaishya, 1928, *Virya Raksha*, Meerut; Ganeshdutt Sharma Gaur, 1929, 'Indra' *Svapn Dosh Rakkshak*, Benares; Ramchandra Vaidya Shashtri, n.d., *Balopyogi Virya – Rahasya*, Kanpur, all cited in *Sexuality, Obscenity, Community*, pp. 69-70.

66. Ibid.,

67. I have drawn substantially in this section upon Charu Gupta's interesting Chapter 'Redefining Obscenity and aesthetics in print' (2001:39–65).

68. Advertisement of 'Kamkala Rahasya- secrets of sex', *Vartman* (18 March 1925:25) cited in Ibid., p. 53.

69. Advertisement of 'Kam Tatha Ratishastra Sachitra- illustrated treatise on sex and sexuality', *Abhyudaya* (26 April 1924:10) cited in Ibid., p. 54.

70. Santram 1924, 'Rati Rahasya', *Madhuri*, Vol. 3, No. 1, pp. 601–5, 5 December.

71. Ramnarayan Tendon (ed.) 1951, *Hindi Sevi Sansar*, Vol. 1, Lucknow, p. 307.

72. Banarsi LalVerma (1928), *Kashmiri Kokshastra*, Prayag.

73. Gupta (2001:39–65).

74. K. K. Malaviya, *Suhag Raat* Prayag (1930); *Manorama Ke Patra: Apne Patiyon Ke Naam* (1927). *His other works were Patiyon Ko Seekh* and *Bahurani Ko Siksha.*

75. Advertisement of Birth Control Techniques, *Abhyudaya* (8 January 1940:9).

76. Gandhiyan followers such as Santram, Banarsi lal Verma and Arya Samajist such as Pandit Jaannarayandeva Sharma and others advocated abstinence. For detail please see Gupta (2001: 69–70).

77. As told by an elderly woman of Benares, 22 December 2002.

78. 'Bharat Kee Unnati Kaise Ho Sakti Hai?' in *Nagari Pracharini Patrika* (reprinted article in *Bhartendu Ank*, 55 years, Samvat 2007) (1952:127).

79. The Arya Mitra, (24 May 1906:318).

80. NASHA NISHED
    Nasha na sadho sadhu sudhar karo,
    Jise jee se pasand na sang karo,
    Gai ke kano se jo paida hui khaini na kha,
    Janwar tak ke maladi mile na usse sukh sake,
    Thu thu karte karane na bhumi bharo,
    Chatne ko laar peete ho chillum chale liye,
    Kintu chua chut chaya tak chipi kyon puchiyae
    Koi nar na raha hai achhut naron!
    Funkte tu dhan garibon ka gala ghut gaya,
    Bharat bhar taruon , tum bhar paro
    (Pandit Mahendra Shastri Visharad, *Hillore*, Ramesh Printing Works, Patna, 1926:7–8). Sharma (1969:84).

81. Sharma (1969:84).

8 Healing the Sick and the Destitute

Protestant Missionaries and Medical Missions in 19th and 20th Century Travancore

RAJ SEKHAR BASU

On 4 September 1905, James Mcphail, while reading a paper at the Calcutta Missionary Conference observed, 'The medical missionary is one who seeks to serve His God and saviour as these men served their king and country. He uses the opportunities created by his professional skills not as they did to extend the bounds of the empire, but to advance the kingdom of God'.[1] As in many other respects related to missionary activities, South India led the way for medical missionary work. In the middle of the 19th century, Protestant denominations such as the London Missionary Society, the American Foreign Mission Board, and the Free Church of Scotland opened medical mission stations in different parts of this region.[2] The Protestant denominations fervently believed that medical mission was perhaps the most important agency to reach the minds of the rural poor. Such an enterprise was favoured, as all through the Church institutions had devoted their energies towards the conversion of the well educated and the 'high born'. There were strong assertions that a large section of the Indian population had remained outside the influence of the missionary schools. But, there had always been greater opportunities of interaction between a Christian missionary doctor and the native society. Indeed, some of the women missionaries involved with the zenana missions felt that medical missions could function like a kindergarten system for preaching the message of the Gospel. Thus, medical missions were believed to be institutions which would publicize the humanizing aspects of Christianity amongst a heathen population.[3]

Since the last decades of the 19th century, there had been a growing opinion that conversion had made the churches oblivious of the supreme Christian duty to heal the sick. It was also argued that medical relief work had been associated with the church from its ancient past. But, with the passage of time, the state had relieved the church from these set of responsibilities. Nonetheless, the church's role in arranging medical relief was sought to be revived. On several occasions, missionaries opined that the command of the Lord had always been to make arrangements for healing the sick and suffering population. In the words of a missionary, '......we are to preach by deed as well as by word and in the work of healing the sick that we are inspired not only by the example of Our Lord but also by His Express injunction to see in the sick and destitute, the impersonation of Himself'.[4]

Western medical missionaries also repeatedly expressed the opinion that prevalence of superstitions as well as unflinching faith in quack remedies had led to heavy loss of lives in different parts of India. The missionary characterization of the cultural terrain of the world had already come to be expressed in terms of two broad divisions—Christian and Heathen.[5] The heathen population was further subdivided into two distinct categories—'the cultured people and savages'. To most missionaries, India resembled Africa in terms of ignorance and backwardness. In their own analysis, overpopulation, lack of proper diet, and poor sanitation facilities had been responsible for the high incidence of mortality resulting from tuberculosis and smallpox.[6]

Such bizarre portrayals of India as a strange land reverberating with stories of mysteries and of deaths and horrors lent strength to ideas of Europe's civilizing mission. It buttressed the imperial claim that European colonial powers had brought Western medical science close to the doorsteps of the unfortunate nations. British official classes in India responded to such adulation by acknowledging the importance of medical work among the native populace.[7]

By the late 19th century, medical missions in India realized the potentials of their health and cure policy vis-à-vis the complex processes of Christianization. A European medical missionary, much later in the 1920s, interestingly observed—

for the continued preservation of Christianity to Hindus and Muslims, there is no more potent agency than the work of Medical Mission. The successful evangelization of a block of 320,000,000 may be regarded as the dream of an enthusiast. But the idea of let us say 320 medical missionaries, each ministering and witnessing to 1,000,000, no longer seems wildly impracticable.[8]

In other words, there was a belief that missionary medical enterprise which had essentially emerged from 'Christian humanism' could be utilized to promote Christianity in lands which had diverse faiths and cultural traditions.[9]

Nevertheless, throughout much of the 19th century, medical mission occupied a rather subdued position in the realm of missionary enterprise in India. The onset of famine and the heavy loss of human lives did bring about a change in the attitude of the missionary organizations. The large scale human despair and misery convinced them of the utility of medical missions. It came to be recognized that Christian medical institutions were powerful adjuncts to the missionary enterprise in India. Medical missionaries were seen as agents who would not only broaden contacts with non-Christian communities, but also provide a momentum to the preaching of the biblical teachings. The humanitarian opinion within the missions also stressed that the Christian premise to 'heal the sick', justified an important place for medical missions in every missionary programme. It thus became imperative on the part of the missionaries to develop medical work as an essential part of the Church ministry on the lines set forth by the founder Jesus Christ himself.[10]

In the present chapter, there would be an implicit attempt in unravelling the conditions under which medical missionaries, belonging to various Protestant denominations, sought to spread their message of Christian humanism through medical enterprise in late 19th and early 20th century Travancore. The establishment of Christian medical missions, barring some instances of local opposition, was made easy by the Maharaja's positive attitude vis-à-vis Western medicine. Unlike British India, where the primary object of the administration had been to ensure the health of the colonizers, the Maharaja's administration displayed an inclination to improve the health standards of the ordinary masses. This favourable attitude of the Maharaja towards Western medicine partly explicates the reasons behind the administration's decision to support Christian medical institutions. In course of time, these institutions were able to lessen the excessive burden that had been placed on the government run medical institutions in matters related to health, sanitation, and medical relief. However, the number of patients treated by the government run medical institutions far outstripped those who had undergone treatment in the Christian medical institutions. Despite these inadequacies, the Christian medical missions made significant interventions in the spheres involving medical relief to the lower castes.[11] The lower castes, such as the Pulayas, hardly had much access to government hospitals and their only option lay in seeking the help and support of the medical missionaries.

The narrative will essentially be based on the records and documents dealing with the medical mission work of the London Missionary Society (hereafter LMS), Salvation Army, and the Church Missionary Society (hereafter CMS) in Travancore. For all practical purposes, the chapter will broadly deal with the developments between 1870 and 1930. This sort of periodization is relevant especially since Christian involvement with medical enterprise assumed a great deal of significance in the years following the famine of 1875–6. By the opening years of the 20th century, the LMS and the Salvation Army not only competed with each other in terms of medical operations, but also in some cases proved to be rivals to the government run institutions. The LMS and the Salvation Army, despite being under staffed and poor in terms of finances, proved to be pioneers in the treatment of influenza, gastro-enteric diseases, and smallpox. The sincerity and devotion displayed by the missionary doctors in the dispensaries and hospitals made them particularly popular amongst the lower castes. This popularity of the missionary doctors accounted for the conversion of a large number of outcastes as well as loosening of the bonds of caste rigidities. Thus, by the early 1930s, the medical missionaries were able to reveal, beyond all doubt, the importance of medical mission work in the spread of the Gospel in a non-Christian land.

THE ENTRY OF WESTERN MEDICINE IN THE STATE OF TRAVANCORE

Western medicine did not find an easy entry into the princely state of Travancore. There was an initial resistance against the introduction of this new system of medical knowledge from the side of the local inhabitants. In order to thwart all prospects of this local resistance gaining ground, the state agencies initiated a series of actions. Sunitha B. Nair has argued that these initiatives on the part of the government run institutions were by no means solely responsible for the successful propagation of Western medicine. Missionary involvement has been singled out as an important factor behind the popularization of Western medical sciences. In fact, missionary activities instilled a new awareness about health and hygiene in Travancore.[12]

Missionary involvement with Western medicine in Travancore dates back to the early years of the 19th century. In 1811, the then ruler of Travancore, Rani Gauri Lakshmi Bai, had formerly permitted its introduction in the state. The introduction of Western medicine could be viewed more as an exercise in preventive health care against the growing incidence of smallpox epidemics. Colonel Munro, the Resident of Travancore, exerted a great deal of pressure on the Maharani to open a small vaccination unit under the supervision of a resident doctor. The Maharani finally yielded to Munro's insistence and this marked the formal acceptance of Western medicine within the territorial confines of her state. In the following decades, the sudden spurt in mortality figures resulting from smallpox epidemics, forced the state to enhance its patronage and support for Western medicine. Consequently, the vaccination rates underwent a steady increase. In the 1860s and 1870s, the vaccination figures registered for the lower castes were much higher in comparison to the figures available for the upper castes. All this undoubtedly proved that the state had succeeded in convincing the lower castes of the reliability of the new system of medicine.[13] It is in this context that the missionary involvement over issues related to health and hygiene should be analyzed in the case of Travancore.

The role of the medical missionaries as facilitators of a new system of medical sciences was solely premised on the logic of conversion. As has been argued, the members of the native population who got converted to Christianity in view of such missionary drives were expected 'to lead a totally different life armed with a new world view and different values'.[14] In the case of Travancore, medicine also played an important role in strengthening the bonds of informal collaboration that existed between the various missionary denominations and the government machinery. Both sides were believed to have been in agreement that dispensing medicine constituted acts of humanly altruism and philanthropy. Viewed from the Hindu Maharaja's zeal of a modernizing mission, missionary involvement with medicine held out possibilities for the growth as well as development of a charitable state. Thus, the missionaries were seen as worthy collaborators rather than potential rivals.[15]

THE LMS AND MEDICAL RELIEF IN TRAVANCORE

The first medical missionary, sent by the LMS to Travancore, was Archibald Ramsay. In 1838, realizing the demand for medical treatment on the part of the natives of Travancore, he started the South Travancore Medical Mission at Neyoor.[16]

But, he left the mission in 1842, to take up another job in India and the medical mission work was discontinued. Ten years later, the medical work was resumed in the Neyoor by Dr Charles Leitch, who built a good sized hospital.[17] The medical mission work was again discontinued after Dr Leitch was drowned while bathing in the sea near Neyoor. In 1861, Dr John Lowe, Surgeon and Padre, was sent to Travancore and from that time onwards there was substantial increase in medical work.[18] In the late 1860s, a medical school was started and six students were trained at Neyoor for the establishment of branch hospitals, within 16 miles its radius. In these years, more than 50,000 persons were treated by the LMS medical missionaries with the help of their native medical assistants.[19]

In the late 1860s, the 'untouchable' communities, comprising mostly of the Pulayas, were the major beneficiaries of the LMS medical mission work. The medical treatment provided to them in the branch dispensaries of Attur, Santhapuram, and Agastapuram, encouraged them to embrace Christianity. The medical missionaries realizing the potentials of medical work, particularly among the 'untouchable' communities, trained Indians in large numbers to serve as dressers. The Indian women converts were also provided training in midwifery. The medical facilities of the maternity hospital at Trivandrum were improved to meet the demands of the socially and economically deprived sections of the society.[20] The wealthy sections of the Hindu society as well as the ruling classes of Travancore supported the efforts of the medical missionaries to introduce medical training classes for the natives of Travancore.[21]

In the 1870s, the medical missionaries arranged door-to-door visitations. Such efforts led to their popularity among the lower castes. Subsequently, they accepted Christianity in large numbers and this gave rise to resentments among the upper caste landed groups. The South Travancore Mission Hospital and dispensaries provided treatment to lower caste patients. They were also requested to give up their religious superstitions and accept the teachings of the Gospel. The Bible women and the dressers preached the Christian ideals of love and humanity. They also provided famine relief in various parts of Travancore under the instructions of the missionaries.[22] The efforts of the medical missionaries to eradicate smallpox and cholera encouraged Christian mass movements among the Pulaya agricultural labourers in the following years.[23]

In the 1880s and the 1890s, the medical mission expanded. The LMS medical missionaries combined medical work with evangelicalism. They also requested the higher authorities of the mission to establish new dispensaries under the supervision of European missionaries. Dr Thomson's effort to provide medical aid to the indigent classes was appreciated by the Maharaja of Travancore. In 1884, the Thomson Memorial Fund was constituted with the Maharaja of Travancore as its patron. This fund proposed to collect Rs 20,000 for the medical mission in Travancore.[24] The medical missionaries also undertook a programme for the distribution of medicines manufactured in their dispensaries at a minimum cost price to the patients. In this case too, the medical missionaries received a great deal of support from the medical department of the Travancore government.[25]

In the 1890s, the missionaries received requests from the upper caste educated Hindus to expand their activities in new localities. Dr Fells, a LMS medical missionary, with the help of European nurses, made elaborate arrangements for the training of Indian nurses and midwives. The Martandapuram Hospital in Quilon also served as a training centre for the Indian dressers. Some of the wealthy Hindu landlords made monetary donations and also transferred revenue yielding rice tracts to the missionaries for meeting their expenses.[26] By the last years of the 19th century, there was considerable expansion of medical mission work in Travancore. The medical missionaries, encouraged by the lower caste interest in Christianity, established hospitals in Attingal, Trivandrum, and Vakkam.[27] In 1897, the Travancore authorities instituted a system of grants-in-aid for the medical institutions. The LMS hospitals made applications for such grants. The government only disbursed funds for the Neyoor hospital, since the other hospitals did not have men with the requisite qualifications. Nonetheless, the government provided financial support to the missionaries in eradicating cholera epidemics.[28]

In the early years of the 20th century, the medical missionaries devoted a greater deal of attention towards the treatment of leprosy. The Dewan of Travancore encouraged the missionaries to enhance the activities of the Leper Assylum at Neyoor.[29] In Attingal, Mrs Osborne, wife of a LMS missionary, looked after the children of the leper parents. These children were later sent to Quilon to acquire vocational training. The LMS missionaries with the help of the ruling groups in Travancore also built up a Leper Hospital in Trivandrum. This hospital was placed under the charge of a Darbar Physician.[30] The medical missionaries also opened Bible Classes for the Indian medical evangelists. A small group of six to eight young men were selected to undergo training for such purposes.[31]

In the years between 1900 and 1910, the medical mission expanded northwards and branches were established in Attingal, Kazhakootam, and Kundara. These three branches treated far greater number of patients every year than what was treated by the whole medical mission at the beginning of the century.[32] The mission hospital at Neyoor, which was one of the largest hospitals in Travancore, supervised 20 branches. At the same time, Indian medical assistants were trained in larger numbers to extend the benefits of Western medical science to a large humanity exposed to quackery.[33] By 1915, the medical mission opened 17 branch hospitals in Pareychaley, where the Pulayas and upper castes were involved in bitter struggles.[34]

In the late 1910s, the LMS appointed a larger number of medical evangelists to provide treatment to the Pulayas. The Pulayas showed a great deal of interest in the stories of the Gospel. Their interest in Christianity forced the LMS missionaries to utilize the services of Malayalam evangelists. The successful handling of leprosy patients also brought a large number of lower castes converts to the mission.[35] By 1917, the attendance in the hospital congregations conducted by the missionaries increased considerably.[36]

In the early 1920s, the LMS enhanced its budget on medical service. In 1921, the LMS hospitals and dispensaries treated 81,151 patients, of which 30,902 were surgical cases. There were about 2,738 gynecological cases. The number of leper patients in the Leper Asylum also increased. The LMS medical missionaries, in order to meet the demands of the patients, constructed new wards in the hospitals from the funds received from the native Christian and European owned industries.[37] The medical missionaries also maintained a European Nursing Home to attract funds from the European plantation industries.[38]

In the early 1920s, the Neyoor hospital remained the centre of LMS medical activities. Dr Pugh and Dr T. Somerville undertook plans and programmes to offer a high standard of treatment with modern equipments. Dr Pugh felt that since dyspepsia was common in South India and Ceylon, attention had to be devoted towards the treatment of gastric related diseases. The first X-ray machine was installed in 1923 and was the only one of its kind in South India, other than the one in Madras.[39] The doctors of St Thomas Hospital sometimes assisted the missionaries in performing critical surgical operations. Ian Orr, a medical missionary as well as a trained surgeon from Glasgow, was recruited by the medical mission to meet the increasing demands of patients for the treatment of stomach and other related diseases.[40] The LMS missionaries also introduced radium, diathermy, X-ray, and surgical implements for cancer treatment.[41] The LMS hospitals often treated cases for which the government hospitals had failed to provide treatment. E. A. Harlow, a medical missionary, observed in 1931 that 'the death rate in our surgical cases is substantially less than it is in the large hospitals in London and in the Presidency towns in India'.[42]

In the late 1920s, the LMS medical missionaries appealed to the European Companies of Travancore to provide them with funds for meeting their expenditure on medical services. The European Companies, such as Harrison and Crossfield and Malayalam Plantations Limited, agreed to pay the salary of an European nurse, who would look after the European patients at Neyoor. The medical evangelists also donated half the fees earned by them from their home visits.[43] The LMS medical missionaries also collected funds for the construction of hospitals in the northern and central parts of Travancore.[44] The extension of the LMS medical service in the northern parts of Travancore brought them into competition with the CMS.[45] The LMS branch hospitals in the Tamil-speaking areas also faced competition from the dispensaries and hospitals maintained by the Travancore Government and the Salvation Army.[46]

Nevertheless in the 1930s, the medical mission in Travancore was the largest of its kind set up by the LMS in India. In 1930, the LMS had 23 medical mission stations which treated 3,72,410 patients worldwide. The medical mission in Travancore alone provided treatment to 1,63,121 patients. In all, it treated 43.8 per cent of the total number of patients treated by all the medical missions established by the LMS.[47] The Directors of the LMS were determined to develop this work and qualified medical missionaries were constantly sent to Travancore.[48]

In the 1930s, the LMS medical missionaries utilized foreign funds to work among the depressed classes in India. European doctors were appointed in large numbers for the eradication of cholera, smallpox, and malaria, which were assuming endemic proportions among these communities.[49] Their efforts in this direction were strongly opposed by the Kerala Hindu Mission, which had been working with large funds for the uplift of the lower castes.[50] The Travancore Government, despite its support to the Kerala Hindu Mission, favoured the missionary programmes related to medical relief. The calamities caused by malaria epidemics in Travancore forced the ruling classes to grant additional funds to the missionaries.[51]

By then, the LMS missionaries had also planned to shift their centre of operations from Neyoor to some other place in central Travancore. They also planned to involve themselves in common programmes with CMS missionaries. There were several factors which were responsible for this change of attitude on the part of the LMS missionaries. Interestingly, their medical mission work in South Travancore, centred around Neyoor and Nagercoil, faced stiff opposition from the Salvation Army medical mission. Both the LMS and the Salvation Army entered into competition with one and another in matters relating to the establishment of branch hospitals and dispensaries in the rural localities. There was a growing apprehension in the missionary circles that overlapping of the two missions would lead to a lot of complications and rifts amongst Christian converts along denominational lines. The Neyoor hospital, apart from meeting the demands of the women patients, was also involved in dealing with patients of both the sexes of Travancore and from those of the adjoining princely state of Cochin. In fact, most of these areas had been previously under the jurisdiction of the CMS, which hardly ever had any programme of medical relief and rehabilitation. Incidentally, this informal understanding between the CMS and the LMS prevented an open confrontation with the Salvation Army. The confrontation could be avoided since the LMS utilized the tacit support of the CMS to enlarge its presence amongst the Malayalam-speaking population. This obviously left the Salvation Army to expand its influence amongst the Tamil speaking population of the region.[52]

THE SALVATION ARMY IN TRAVANCORE

The medical mission of the Salvation Army owed its inception to Harry Andrew, who was sent to Nagercoil in 1893 as a young boy of 17. Since his arrival, Andrew demonstrated his healing virtues, which soon gained popularity among the ordinary masses of the region. Emboldened by his success, he proposed the idea of a medical mission before the authorities of the Salvation Army in London. The authorities instructed him to return to London for taking up a dresser's course in a local hospital. After spending a year in London, Andrew returned to Nagercoil in 1895 and established the Catherine Booth dispensary.[53]

Subsequently, Commissioner Howard, the then Foreign Secretary of the Salvation Army, paid a visit to Nagercoil and supported Dr Percy Turner's plan to build a small hospital for the poorer sections of the society. Initially, this hospital comprised of an operation theatre, laboratory, and a small building which served as a ward for indoor patients.[54] However, the hospital faced financial difficulties from its very inception. The non-availability of funds posed problems for the supply of water, which was needed for meeting the demands of the hospital. After a considerable lapse of time, funds were available for sinking a tube well. Nonetheless, problems relating to water supply continued, because there was hardly much initiative to mobilize funds for the purchase of water pumps.[55]

Despite these deficiencies, the hospital which had been christened as the Catherine Booth Hospital was favoured by the royal household of Travancore. The Maharaja of Travancore on several occasions publicly appreciated the Salvation Army's medical work which intended to improve the health standards of his subject people. In 1901, he consented to be known as the Patron of the Catherine Booth Hospital and made a donation to the Salvation Army. This interest in the affairs of the Salvation Army on the part of the royal family of Travancore continued over the next three decades. In 1912, the Maharaja of Travancore, Rama Varma, personally paid a visit to the hospitals and expressed happiness that the activities of the medical missionaries of the Salvation Army had brought a great deal of relief to the suffering populace of his state. On this occasion, he made an observation, 'I am sure it must have been a heavy task for the Army and for its responsible officers to bring the institution to such perfection'.[56]

In course of the early years of the 20th century, the Salvation Army tried to enlarge the scope of its medical relief work by providing training to some of the Indian converts. These men and women were trained by young Indian Salvation Army officers so that they could meet the high professional and spiritual standards that had been set apart for Christian medical men. In most cases, the candidates chosen for such training found it too difficult to handle and this led to heavy dropouts. Finally, three men were able to qualify in the examinations held in 1907 and they were given charge of the new branch hospitals.

Nevertheless, it was fairly apparent that a larger number of paramedical staff was needed to carry on the ever increasing work of the hospital. In a short period of time, the Salvation Army decided to open a one year course for training young men as compounders and medical assistants. Men who successfully completed this course formed an invaluable support team to the European medical missionaries in running the various departments of the hospitals. Sometimes, private students were also invited to join such courses. The private students did avail such offers and paid tuition fees to receive instructions on medicine and first aid. The majority of these students came from Syrian Christian families. The wives of the students, on some occasions, also successfully qualified in the examinations.

The branch hospitals which had been established in the rural localities of Travancore tried to meet the needs of the poor and the socially despised sections of the society. These hospitals were built on a common plan comprising of a central block with provision for two wings. Their activities largely revolved around outpatient work and the cases related to chronic ailments. On the other hand, the indoor patients were ones who usually needed surgeries and had to spend a few days in the hospital for their recovery. In the case of the indoor patients, the Christianizing influence was more pronounced, since they were directly exposed to the evangelistic overtones of the medical missionaries in the hospital wards.[57]

By the year 1914, the Catherine Booth Hospital had came to gain wide popularity amongst lower caste groups as an institution which dealt patients with love and kindness. The rise in its popularity level influenced the Salvation Army to open up new surgical and maternity blocks. A new outpatient department was also constructed to deal with increasing groups of patients arriving from the northern parts of Travancore state. The medical missionaries also took steps to attract Brahmin and other higher caste patients. They issued instructions that a Brahmin indoor patient, who desired to maintain the dignity and purity of his twice born condition,[58] would receive every opportunity to reside in a private ward housing a separate kitchen. The relatives of the upper caste indoor patient were also requested to make their cooking arrangements in the kitchen that had been set apart for their use. This spirit of accommodation on the part of the Salvation Army medical missionaries attracted some of the upper caste patients and their attendants towards the message of the Gospel.[59]

The popularity of both the medical mission and the Gospel was related more to the concerted drives on the part of the missionaries to treat the women folk. The wives of the missionary doctors who served as nurses and were affectionately known as *ammals* carried out preliminary investigations about the causes of the illness afflicting the women patients. In course of time, sensing the possibility of a greater deal of conversion among the women patients, Indian nurses were employed to meet the growing demands of the women patients in the maternity wards.[60]

Subsequently, the activities of the medical missionaries shifted to other spheres of activities. Dr Percy Turner, who had been one of the founding members of the Catherine Booth Hospital, encouraged the medical missionaries to undertake the treatment of eye diseases. Dr Turner's training at the Central London Ophthalmic Hospital helped him to build up a team of trained ophthalmologists. At the same time, efforts were made to enhance the activities and programmes of the School of Medicine. This activity became a part and parcel of South Indian medical development. The graduates of the Nagercoil Medical School received recognition from the Travancore Government as qualified medical practitioners. They were authorized to take charge of grant-in-aid hospitals and to practice medicine, surgery, and midwifery as independent practitioners. Dr Turner also introduced training programmes for men who wished to serve as Hospital Assistant in the mission hospitals and dispensaries. The Travancore Government appreciated these efforts on the part of the Salvation Army to build a team of trained medical personnel who could offer their services in various parts of the princely state as well as in the adjoining parts of British India. The Dewan of Travancore sanctioned the appointment of a Senior Government Medical Officer who could assist the medical missionaries as a co-examiner in the final professional examination that was conducted for the medical students. The Dewan initiated this step in order to confer an official status to the medical graduates.[61]

The wide ranging activities on the part of the Salvation Army in Travancore had a whole range of implications. In the first place, the dedication and efforts on the part of the missionaries to introduce sophisticated medical treatment enabled them to establish the view that every individual was given a good treatment irrespective of his caste and class background. Second, the medical services offered by the Army convinced men and women of the efficacy of Western medical treatment, which the missionaries devised by combining allopathic practices with Christian practices of healing. In a sense, Western medicine, at the popular level, was seen as a system of knowledge which had its direct origins in Christian doctrines. The medical missionary was taken to be the representative of saviour Jesus Christ, enjoying the powers to treat people, both Christian and non-Christian. Thus, it was this humanitarian dimension of the Salvation Army's activities that led to growing interest in the healing powers of Lord Jesus Christ who was envisioned as a Greater Physician.[62]

By the mid-1910s, highly placed Salvation Army officials issued statements upholding the importance of medical missionary work in the overall programme of Christianization of the heathen population. Commissioner Booth Turner, in one of his addresses, made an observation—'It is in times of suffering and sickness that we appreciate as at no other moment, the kindly touch of sympathy and prayer. Then we realize that the most skillful ministrations are more successful when God's help has been invoked and His Name remembered and honoured'.[63] In this context, strong claims were also made that after the opening of the first Salvation Army hospital in South Travancore, the upper caste animosity towards the missionaries had considerably lessened. Medical work was believed to have generated public sympathy and interest for the missionary endeavours to improve the health standards of the ordinary people. The medical missionaries were also able to convince their authorities that the treatment offered to Hindu and Mohammedan patients had influenced a large number of them to read and study Bible for their own salvation.[64]

Such assertions were not wholly based on false premises. In South Travancore, medical mission work on the part of the Salvation Army led to sizeable conversions from the lower castes. In most cases, the villagers, influenced by the services provided by the mission hospitals, appealed to the Church authorities to depute an evangelist. The evangelists organized congregations comprising of people of several villages to spread the message of the Gospel. Sometimes, the inhabitants of the whole village decided on a mass conversion, while on other occasions, the huge enthusiasm for the Salvation Army left the missionaries bewildered. Nonetheless, the paucity of officers often stood in their way from gaining new adherents for the Church.[65]

In the early decades of the 20th century, the Maharaja's administration displayed a greater deal of interest in the medical work of the Salvation Army. The administration provided assistance in the form of grants to the hospital and its branches. The Maharaja also gave donations for the construction of new wards and other purposes.[66] In 1912, the Maharaja of Travancore donated a sum of Rs 3,350 for the erection of a new men's ward, which was to be dedicated in the name of the Maharani.[67] Almost a decade later, the thatched walls of the first ward were replaced by a solid masonry block for which half of the expenditure was borne by the Maharaja and the Maharani.[68] In the 1930s, the Salvation Army continued to receive donations from the Maharaja for its medical work. In 1934, C. P. Ramaswamy Aiyar, who was then the Legal and Constitutional Adviser to the Maharaja, inaugurated the new administrative and outpatients block, which had been built out of a donation of Rs 10,000 by the Maharaja.[69]

Undoubtedly, the state patronage encouraged the medical activities of both the Salvation Army and the LMS. Since the early years of the 20th century, the services provided by highly qualified doctors and other trained medical personnel had made the ruling classes aware of the relevance of medical missions. The state seems to have realized that the medical missionaries could perform a useful task by providing medical assistance to the poor, especially in places where government medical institutions had failed to establish themselves. At the same time, by patronizing the medical missions, the Maharaja could portray himself as a benevolent ruler, who discharged his duties in accordance to the norms of Hindu dharma.[70]

The medical work of the Salvation Army, in the course of the first three decades of the 20th century, also created conditions for mass conversions in the rural localities of Travancore. The successes of the mission doctors and their preaching of the Gospel led to regular village-level meetings, which mostly glorified the magical powers of Jesus as the saviour of mankind. On some occasions, the entire village converted to Christianity.[71]

THE CMS AND ITS DISPENSARIES IN TRAVANCORE

The CMS did not show much interest in establishing medical institutions in Travancore. Nonetheless, it did sometimes provide medical relief to the people, though admittedly on a much smaller scale. In the 1870s, the CMS missionaries established dispensaries in several parts of Travancore.[72] In the early 1870s, however, there was an opinion within the CMS that a medical agency could actually prove its importance, especially when headed by a European doctor.[73]

The CMS missionaries conducted medical activities mostly out of their individual interests. In 1884, Rev A. F. Painter distributed the medicines supplied by the Travancore Government and the Medical Missionary Association among the Arrians, a hill tribe settled in the highlands. He is said to have observed, 'the death rate among our people has been far below the average, due, under God, to my being thus able to doctor them'. Such instances of individual practices continued in the following decades. In the early 1930s, the Diocesan Council of the CMS lauded the efforts of the non-professional missionaries who out of their own individual concerns had tried to meet 'the simple needs of the sick around them'.[74] Subsequently, the CMS missionaries decided to build two floating dispensaries which could provide medical facilities to the people residing along the backwaters. A dispensary and maternity centre was also established by them to meet the demands of the common people.[75]

CONCLUSION

The narrative dealing with the activities of the medical missionaries belonging to the LMS, Salvation Army, and the CMS undoubtedly reveals the importance of the medical missions. These missions usually performed two major roles. First, they were organized with a zeal of proselytization and their obvious intention was to Christianize the lower caste Hindus. In the second place, the medical missionaries were also involved in stalling the reconversion of Christians to their original faiths—a process that was widespread during times of natural distress. As Koji Kawashima has pointed out that there were many instances when a number of Christians took recourse to heathen rituals and practices, especially when they were taken ill. In times of smallpox epidemics, Christian converts joined their heathen associates to propitiate the Goddess Mariamman, who was supposed to have brought about this havoc.[76] Thus, by combining the two rare elements of religion and medicine, the medical missionaries tried to be protectors of their faith as well as effective catalysts for mass conversion.

However, it is doubtful as to whether the medical missionaries endowed with such rare qualities could act as effective agents of mass conversion. Medical mission work hardly succeeded in creating situation for such conversion. Though the number of upper caste Hindus treated in the mission hospitals may have been large, this necessarily did not lead to their conversion to Christianity. The LMS medical missionaries were successful in converting a few lower caste individuals, but hardly met with success in converting the upper castes. The proximity of the LMS medical missionaries vis-à-vis the Pulayas brought them into confrontation with the upper caste Hindus.[77]

The opposition of the caste Hindus to medical mission work was much less when compared with their reactions towards the missionary educational institutions. Norman Goodhall, the compiler of the history of the LMS, candidly attested to the fact that medical missions probably provoked lesser controversies or raised fewer objections than the other activities of the missionaries. But, the medical missionaries had to toil hard to gain social recognition for their work. The strong anti-missionary campaigns launched by the Brahmin priests and the lower caste 'sorcerers' too, often impeded progress of the medical mission. Nonetheless, the successful treatment of infectious diseases on the part of the medical missionaries ebbed the popular aversion towards Western medical science. An increasing number of patients expressed their willingness to undergo treatment in the mission hospitals.[78] In Travancore, ruling groups as well as dominant caste groups appreciated the efforts of the medical missionaries and made substantial donations to the missionary run medical institutions.[79] Though the medical missionaries barely touched the peripheries of the local societies in South India, they were able to establish that they were only carrying forth the ideals of soul service and universal brotherhood of man.

NOTES

1. Mcphail (1906:1).
2. Ibid., p. 2.
3. Ibid., p. 9.
4. Ibid., p. 12.
5. Basu in Kumar, Deepak (ed.) (2001:180).
6. Mary Pauline Jeffrey, 1939, *Ida S. Scudder of Vellore: An Appreciation of Forty Years of Service in India*, Mysore, pp. 13-7.
7. R. Fletcher Moorshead, n.d., *The Way of the Doctor: A Study in Medical Missions*, London, p. VII.
8. Dr. Ernest F. Neve, 1928, *A Crusader in Kashmir: Being the Life of Dr. Arthur Neve, with an account of the Medical Missionary Work of Two Brothers and its later developments down to the present day*, London, p. 14.
9. Since the early decades of the 19th century, missionaries had emphasized the need to establish links between Christianization and civilization. Their ideas in this regard were guided on the lines of the biblical concept of sin. It was widely believed that the Gospel not only transformed individuals, but also enabled communities, societies, and states to live in peace and prosperity. Thus,

the hope of the backward non-European people lay in conversion to Christianity. For more details, see, Ibid., pp. 68–70. See, also, Simensen (1988:36–8).

10. Christian missionaries believed that since Jesus Christ had shown a great interest in relieving the sufferings of humanity, hospitals and refuges had to be built for the care of people infected with different diseases. They were greatly influenced by one of the sermons of Christ—'heal the sick and say unto them, The Kingdom of God is nigh to you'. See, Neve *op.cit.*, pp. 71–2, Manickam, Sundararaj (1977:169–70).

11. Kawashima (1998:120).

12. Nair in Kumar, Deepak (ed.) (2001:215).

13. Ibid., pp. 217–8.

14. Ibid., p. 218.

15. Ibid., p. 114.

16. Somervell (1940:11); Hacker (1887:54–8).

17. Ibid.

18. In the first Annual Report of the South Travancore Medical Mission, published in 1862, it was stated that 2,629 patients were treated during the year. In fact, 11 operations were arranged for the removal of tambours. There were 134 minor and 338 other related operations. The annual cost for running the mission was Rs 1100. See, Somervell, *op. cit.*, (1940:12).

19. Hacker, *op. cit.*, (1887:56–8).

20. For more details, see, LMS, Reports from Travancore, 1866, Box I, Medical Mission, Council for World Mission Archives, School of Oriental and African Studies (hereafter SOAS), London; See, also, LMS Incoming Correspondences, 1872–1878, Box No. 8, Folder No. 6, Council for World Mission Archives, SOAS, London.

21. LMS, Reports from Travancore, Box I, Council for World Mission Archives, SOAS, London, 1867, Medical Mission, Ibid.

22. In 1875, the South Travancore Mission Hospital and Dispensaries treated about 12,468 cases. In 1880, the number of patients was 23,936. In 1877, under the recommendations of the Committee and the Church Council of Travancore, a class was organized for catechists and Bible women. In these classes, they were given training in combating the common diseases as well as in midwifery. On an average, 15 men and 8 women attended these classes. See, LMS Reports from Travancore, Box 2, 1874–1882, Medical Mission, Council for World Mission Archives, SOAS, London.

23. Ibid., see, also, LMS Reports from Travancore Box 3, Medical Mission 1883–1887; LMS Incoming Correspondences, Mission, Box 9, 1878–1882, Folder 3 and Folder 4, Council of World Mission Archives, SOAS, London.

24. LMS Incoming Correspondences, Box 9, 1878–1882, Folder 2, Council for World Mission Archives, SOAS, London.

25. LMS Reports from Travancore, Box 4, 1888–1891, Medical Mission, Council of world Mission Archives, SOAS, London.

26. Dewan T. Rama Rao stated that the Puliars and Kuruvars suffered from want of medical treatment. He stated that for the treatment of fever and smallpox, they had to go to the hospital in Quilon, which was about 10 miles away. He donated Rs 100 for the construction of the building. He also expressed his desire to donate 220 *parahs* of arable land with an annual tax of Rs 200 to the missionaries. See, LMS Reports from Travancore, Box 15, 1893, Folder 1, Council for World Mission Archives, SOAS, London.

27. The missionaries took up projects to improve the conditions of the Pulayas in Pareychaley district. A European medical missionary was posted in Attingal. In Trivandrum, a hospital was opened at Nellikakuli with two wards. A medical missionary was also posted at Vakkam. See, LMS Reports from Travancore, Box 18, 1897–98, Folder 6, Council for World Mission Archives, SOAS, London; LMS Reports from Travancore, Box 19, 1899, Folder 2, Council for World Mission Archives, SOAS, London.

28. LMS Reports from Travancore, 1898–1901, Medical Mission, Council for World Mission Archives, SOAS, London.

29. The inmates of the Leper Asylum were baptized by Rev Hacker, a LMS missionary. See, LMS Reports from Travancore, Box 7, Medical Mission, 1898–1901, Ibid.,

30. LMS Incoming Correspondences, Box 19, 1899, Folder 4, Council for World Mission Archives, SOAS, London.

31. LMS Incoming Correspondences, Box 21, 1901–1904, Folder 3, Council for World Mission Archives, SOAS, London; LMS Reports from Travancore, Box 8, 1902–1907, Medical Mission, Ibid.

32. Somervell, *op. cit.*, (1940:14).

33. Ibid.

34. LMS Reports from Travancore, Box 9, 1908–1920, Medical Mission, Council for World Mission Archives, SOAS, London.

35. The missionaries treated the leper patients by using gynocardate sodium prepared from chaulmoogra oil by Sir Leonard Rogers. See, Ibid.

36. Ibid.

37. LMS Reports from Travancore, Box 10, 1921–1929, Medical Mission, Council for World Mission Archives, SOAS, London.

38. Ibid.

39. Kawashima, *op. cit.*, (1998:127–8); Somervell, *op. cit.*, (1940:16–7).

40. Ibid., p. 20.

41. Kawashima, *op. cit.*, (1998:128).

42. LMS Reports from Travancore, Box 11, 1931, Medical Mission, Council for World Mission Archives, SOAS, London.

43. LMS Incoming Correspondences, Box 28, Folder 3, 1926–27, Council for World Mission Archives, SOAS, London.

44. LMS Incoming Correspondences, Box 29, 1928–30, Council for World Mission Archives, SOAS, London.

45. LMS Incoming Correspondences, Box 30, 1928–30, Council for World Mission Archives, SOAS, London.

46. Ibid.

47. Kawashima, *op. cit.*, (1998:128).

48. Ibid., see also, LMS Incoming Correspondence, Box 30, 1928–30, Council for World Mission Archives, SOAS, London.

49. LMS Incoming Correspondences, Box 31, 1931–1933, Council for World Mission Archives, SOAS, London; LMS Incoming Correspondences, Box 34, 1934–36, Council for World Mission Archives, SOAS, London.

50. LMS Incoming Correspondence, Box 36, 1937–40 (ii), Council for World Mission Archives, SOAS, London.

51. LMS Reports from Travancore, Box 12, Medical Missions, 1935–40, Council for World Mission Archives, SOAS, London.

52. LMS Incoming Correspondences, In/2 1941–50, Council for World Mission Archives, SOAS, London; Church Mission Papers, G. 2 I.5/O, 1930–31, Church Missionary Society Original Papers, Church Mission Archives, Birmingham University.

53. Kawashima, *op. cit.*, (1998:133); For more details, see, Smith (1981:77–9); Jenkins (1995:52).

54. The Salvation Army medical work in Travancore was officially started in August 1896, following the disbursal of a grant from its headquarters in London for the purchase of some drugs and instruments. Initially, a room was set apart for medical relief operations in the divisional headquarters of the Army at Vadaseri. In January 1898, efforts were made to construct a special building which should serve as a hospital. For more details, see, *Light, Healing and Life : The Story of Catherine Booth Hospital*, Nagercoil (South Travancore), n.p., n.d., Catherine Booth Hospital, Nagercoil, India, File – I (preserved in the Salvation Army International Heritage Centre, London) pp. 3–7; Ratnam (1902:129–30).

55. Light, Healing and Life: The Story of Catherine Booth Hospital, *op.cit.*, pp. 3–6.

56. Ibid., p. 7.

57. Light, Healing and Life: The Story of Catherine Booth Hospital *op. cit.*, p. 12.

58. This is a reference to his upper class status.

59. W. Bramwell Booth, 1922, The Catherine Booth Hospital for One and Twenty Years : Being an Account of the Foundation and Development of the Catherine Booth Hospital, Nagercoil, Travancore India..

60. They were trained to serve as general hospital nurse under Mrs Turner and other European nurses. Prior to their postings, they had to qualify in the several tests and examinations conducted by the European doctors. For more details, see Light, Healing, Life, *op. cit.*, p. 16.

61. Booth, *op. cit.*, (1922:33).

62. Mrs Adjutant Turner, *In the Dark East Land, A Record of our Medical Missions*, AW February (preserved in the Salvation Army International Heritage Centre, London), File – I (1905:65); Brigadier Turner, *The Call of the East: Our Catherine Booth Hospital*, *op.cit.*, pp. 1–2.

63. Brigadier Sekunder and Devalee (Andrews), Salvation Army Medical Work in India (General) : Some Aspects of a Vast Opportunity (preserved in the Salvation Army International Heritage Centre, London), File – I, p. 14.

64. Ibid.

65. Travancore, Beginnings : *Memoirs of W. M. Stevens (Yesu Ratnam), India 1891–1913*, (preserved in the Salvation Army International Heritage Centre, London), n.p., n.d., p. 2.

66. Kawashima, *op.cit.*, (1998:135).

67. Ibid.

68. Ratnam (1922:24).

69. Ibid., Medical India A, Folder 2, International Heritage Centre; 'Light, Healing and Life', p. 8; 'Worthy Notes of Mention', p. 2, Turner 1, International Heritage Centre.

70. Kawashima, *op. cit.*, (1998:136).

71. Travancore, Memoirs of W. M. Stevens (Yesu Ratnam), 1933–34, (preserved in the International Heritage Centre of the Salvation Army, London), p. 2.

72. Koji Kawashima has pointed out that as early as 1870, the CMS missionaries had established dispensaries at Kannankulam, Mavelikara, and Tiruwalla. The dispensary in Mavelikara which was administered by G. J. Kuruwella, a medical evangelist, treated 1,134 patients in 1870. For more details, see, Kawashima, *op. cit.*, (1998:137).

73. Ibid., Minutes of Travancore Conference, 10 December 10 1873, Mission Book M-30, CMSA, University of Birmingham.

74. Travancore and Cochin Diocesan Magazine (November 1933:149).

75. Travancore and Cochin Diocesan Magazine (July 1935:90–1); Ibid., (March 1937:37–8).

76. Kawashima, *op. cit.*, (1998:138).

77. LMS Reports from Travancore, Box 9, 1908–1920, Medical Mission, Council for World Mission Archives, SOAS, London.

78. Kawashima, *op. cit.*, (1998:140).

79. Basu (2002).

9   A Mixed Record

Malaria Control in Bombay Presidency, 1900–1935

Mridula Ramanna

Indian responses to anti-malaria campaigns were not as vigorously oppositional, as to the interventionist measures during the plague epidemic of 1896–7. To the colonial authorities, in the words of Sir Leonard Rogers, it had 'this great difference that, with sufficient foresight and organisation, the greater part of the loss (from malaria) could have been prevented, because we have in quinine an invaluable prophylactic and curative drug whereas against plague we are almost powerless'.[1] In the background of encounters between epidemic control measures and Indian reactions was Indian medicine which the British medical establishment, with few exceptions, dismissed as unscientific. However, at the Imperial Malaria Conference, held in 1909, Sir Herbert Risley, referred to Ayurveda, which had designated malaria as the king of disease and had prescribed 'less primitive' remedies than charms and symbolic magic proposed by the *Atharva Veda*. Some recognition was due to this system, Risley urged, but it was hampered by erroneous theories and the lack of 'scientific techniques'.[2] In response to a resolution in the Imperial Legislative Council in 1916, the Bombay government gathered information, about the receptivity of Western and Indian medicine in the Bombay Presidency. By and large, it was found that Indians resorted to Western medicine for surgery and believed that it could act only for a short time, while Indian medicine, though slow to act, was considered effective, cheap, and locally available. It was preferred for the treatment of tropical diseases, for malaria, cholera, and for children's complaints. W. Dymock, in his *Materia Medica for Western India* observed that

English practitioners were impressed with the anti-periodic action in fevers of the tuber of *Aconitum Heterophyllum* (Atis), and stated that 100lbs were issued, annually, by the government store at Bombay.[3] Significantly, when quinine came to be recognized as the only effective method to combat malaria, only 17 lbs of this tuber was issued.

Discussions on malaria in Bombay figure in the writings of Charles Morehead, the first Principal of the Grant Medical College, which had been established in 1845. Morehead believed malaria to be the 'exciting cause' of remittent and intermittent fevers. Subscribing to the miasmic theory, Morehead held that 'it may be wafted by air from the spot where it had been produced and thus infected adjacent localities;' and observed that it was 'attracted by the foliage of trees', but lost its 'noxious properties', by passing over a surface of water and was 'lessened by cultivation'.[4] Henry Vandyke Carter, also Principal of Grant Medical College, endorsed the discovery of the parasite by Alphonse Laveran, which had been made in 1888 in Algeria. Then came the discovery of the vector, the female anopheles mosquito, first postulated by Patrick Manson and proved experimentally by Ronald Ross, who showed both the agent and the mode of transmission. The urge to define malaria in the third quarter of the 19th century, created a number of conflicting theories and understandings of the disease, as has been argued by Rohan Deb Roy.[5]

This chapter aims to evaluate the record of malaria control in Western India, in the first three decades of the 20th century. The analysis is based on the colonial records, contemporary newspapers, debates in the Bombay Legislative Council, and the detailed reports of the visiting officials of the Rockefeller Foundation.

In the 19th century, the distinction between malarial fevers and other fevers was not always clear to colonial health officials. Fevers figured, as the most frequent cause for deaths in the official statistics. By 1901, malaria was listed as being responsible for a large percentage of sickness, in Bombay city. Following detailed investigations by Charles Bentley, then Sanitary Commissioner of Bengal, preventive measures were recommended for Bombay. These included the covering of wells and introduction of fish to control mosquito larvae. However, resistance to these measures came from unexpected quarters. The Parsis, who had been in the forefront of the acceptance of Western medicine, had religious scruples about the covering of wells and Hindus and Jains had objections to using water which they regarded as being contaminated by the fish. These reservations were gradually overcome due to the efforts of activist health officials, Indian doctors, and civic leaders, as this review will show. The First World War and financial constraints put a brake on these efforts. Consequent to the commercial interests of the city making representations to the authorities to renew the campaign, it was resumed in the 1920s. By the 1930s, some measure of success in malaria control in Bombay was achieved. The anti-malaria campaign in the other cities of the Presidency was implemented through a scheme, passed by the Bombay Legislative Council, in 1924. Primary schoolmasters, called *upacharak*s were trained at civil hospitals, for two and half months, to provide elementary medical and surgical aid in villages and distribute quinine. They were taught to dress wounds, treat sore eyes, recognize and treat some diseases, and were provided instruction in elementary hygiene, in methods to protect the water supply, and in anti-malaria precautions. Thirty of these men worked in Poona, Bijapur, Sholapur, and Dharwar.

The picture was starkly different in the rural districts of the Presidency, where health care was negligible. Here, the difficulties of quinine propagation, according to Bentley, were the vendors, who campaigned against quinine and spread rumours that fever was liable to recur through its use, and practitioners who professed homeopathy and invariably decried the use of quinine. The Bombay government expected the municipalities to allot the resources, and while the latter funded curative medicine limitedly, they were reluctant to spend on preventive measures. The Sanitary Commissioner, T. E. Dyson, found that their implementation was both haphazard and half-hearted.[6] The conditions in the notoriously malarial North Kanara and Sind, and the poorly funded anti-malaria efforts, in these areas, would be the next theme of the chapter. It is significant that the contrast between the neglect of these regions and the better financed campaign in Bombay city were questioned by the Indian members in the Bombay Legislative Council. The last area of focus would be the princely state of Sawantwadi which sought and secured Rockefeller Foundation funding to combat malaria.

What emerges is a mixed record. The relative success in the city of Bombay could be ascribed to the proactive involvement of various agencies including the government. However, this was not the case in Sind and Kanara. The very candid observations of Paul Russell of the Rockefeller Foundation, who visited India in 1934–5, linked the severity of malaria in Sind to the defects in the Lloyd Barrage Scheme, while the representatives from Kanara attributed its persistence to the forest policy.

BOMBAY CITY

Police Surgeon S. A. Powell, in a paper read before the *Bombay Medical and Physical Society* in 1903, showed, on the basis of microscopic examination of blood in 3,413 cases of fever, that 2,542 cases had malarial parasites. The Bombay government appointed a committee, presided over by J. M. Cloghry, acting Surgeon General, and including H. C. Arnim, acting Sanitary Commissioner, Glen Liston, of the Bombay Bacteriological Laboratory, Pherozeshah Mehta, civic leader, and Dr Bhalachandra Bhatvadekar a prominent doctor, to investigate the cause of frequent occurrences of fevers in the city. But their enquiry of 1906–8 and the subsequent report laid greater stress on plague than on malaria.[7] Towards the end of 1907, there was an increase in malaria, which was attributed to the construction of the Alexandra Dock and Hughes Dry Dock. The victims included the governor's bodyguards, the crew of the Peninsular and Oriental Steam Navigation Company's vessels, which had docked in the Victoria docks, the nursing staff of St George's hospital, and guards and porters of the Great Indian Peninsula Railway. Both the hospital and the Victoria Terminus are located near the docks. The local press was unsparing in its criticism, alleging that there had been 'tall talk,' while malaria was 'deliberately' allowed to flourish'.[8]

In 1909, a committee of representatives of the Bombay Port Trust, City Improvement Trust, which had been set up in 1898 after the plague to clear slums, build sanitary *chawls* and broaden roads, the Railways, the Chamber of Commerce, and the Bombay Municipal Corporation, and A. G. Mc Kendrick, as expert malariologist, was appointed. House-to-house spleen census was carried out to map the severely affected areas. For the general improvement of the health of the city, the committee recommended the conversion of the intermittent water supply into a constant one, the abolition of the night soil system, the relocation of the sewage outfall, so that sewage could be treated before passing into the sea, and the opening out and development of areas like Tardeo, Mahalakshmi, and Worli.[9]

Mc Kendrick was soon replaced by Bentley, who carried out detailed investigations for three years, supported by John Andrew Turner, Bombay's energetic Health Officer, Liston, and W. B. Bannerman, Director of the

Bombay Bacteriological Laboratory. Writing in the *Journal of the Bombay Natural History*, about the results of his investigation of areas in the neighbourhood of the docks, Liston showed that 80 per cent of the children examined had enlarged spleens and 50 per cent of those had malarial parasites in their blood.[10] His study of the anopheles *stephensi* mosquitoes, breeding in pools and collections of water, which had not hitherto been recognized as malaria bearing, revealed that they were infected. Bentley confirmed Liston's discovery of the role of *a. stephensi*, while *n.rossi*, the commonest anopheles in the island, he held, had no part in the spread of malaria. Before Bentley's investigation, it was thought that drainage and flooding caused the disease, but he found that the years of excessive rainfall were not necessarily those of severe malaria and during long breaks in the rains, sporozoite carrying anopheles was found, while their proportion was reduced during continuous rain.[11] In his interim report on the southern portion of the island city, Bentley declared that the wells, the new dock yards, and railway yards were the breeding places. The Indian Sanitary Policy Resolution, 1914, found this conclusion, that the mosquitoes bred in wells, tanks, and cisterns attached to private houses and not in the swampy surroundings of the city, to be an 'unexpected fact' but conceded that conditions and causes varied from place to place.[12] Bentley averred that while the wealthier classes could protect themselves, the poor could not afford treatment and lost their wage-earning capacity when struck by malaria. He observed that while the centre of the island city, the 'best portion' of the city was affected, the outskirts escaped. By contrast, the centre of Calcutta was free from endemic malaria.[13] In his final report, Bentley, concluded that 60 to 75 per cent of all fever cases was due to malaria, and ascribed the intensifying of infections during the epidemic of 1908, which had affected all classes of the population, to the rise in prices in the previous six months. Contrary to widely held opinion, he pointed out that it was not the ignorant masses, which were an obstacle to malaria prevention, but the educated. Once the educated had decided that pure water supply, drainage schemes, and street lighting were necessary, they adopted these conveniences but were not so willing to accept anti-malaria precautions. A wealthy and influential house owner, who owned many houses in the 'best' parts of Bombay, threatened to take proceedings for trespass, in case any of his properties were inspected. On occasions when action was taken to cover wells, every conceivable excuse was put forth for non-compliance. It was well water and not piped water, that was regarded sacred enough to be used for religious ceremonies. Bentley regretted that many Indian doctors, practicing in Bombay, had little influence to persuade their wealthy clients to accept the measures.

As for preventive steps, Bentley conceded that education could be of great value but it was useless to talk of mosquito nets to the poor; instead they could be taught the value of quinine and trained to use it. Gratuitous distribution of quinine could be made by philanthropic agencies and the covering of unused wells promoted with inducements. For the implementation of these measures, he suggested that adequate funds should be voted in the Bombay Municipal Corporation, a special assistant to the health officer appointed, and legal powers given to carry out the necessary steps. He had confidence that Bombay, being the wealthiest and most advanced of cities, possessing a good administration and local self-government, with resources per head being larger than those of any other municipality in India, would achieve successful control over malaria.[14] The Bombay government sanctioned funding for the implementation of these measures and the Municipal Act was amended to give the Municipal Commissioner enhanced powers for dealing with mosquito breeding grounds. Research was carried out, by collecting statistics from areas in the vicinity of the city, both seriously and slightly affected by malaria. The results were summarized and the causal connection between accumulation of large quantities of water, arising from defective drainage, and the excessive mortality following the monsoon, established that malaria was the most important factor affecting mortality during this season.

PEOPLE'S RESPONSES

There was opposition to Bentley's suggestions, and 350 Parsi priests petitioned the Municipal Commissioner, in 1910, protesting the directive to close or cover wells. They contended that they could not use water, for religious purposes, if it was pumped from covered up wells, since it had to be exposed to the sun, to be regarded pure.[15] K. B. Shroff, Deputy Health Officer, who had qualified at the Liverpool School of Tropical Medicine, termed these as 'sentimental objections' including beliefs about the presence of 'saintly beings' in wells. Hindus and Jains also had objections, the latter being particularly opposed to the stocking of wells with fish.[16] The contemporary journal of cartoons, *Pickings from the Hindi Punch*, felt that women and priests were the main objectors and asked rhetorically, 'are religious prejudices and tears to be always respected at the sacrifice of the city's health?'[17] Turner's crusade against mosquitoes was caricatured by the *Pickings from the Hindi Punch*, depicting the Health Department as a woman in a sari, spraying disinfectant from a dish labelled sanitation.[18] Bentley's conclusions received endorsement from a committee of medical men, appointed by the Bombay Zoroastrian Association.[19] To bolster support for the campaign, public lectures were given at different venues by Shroff, and Doctors Constancio Coutinho and Hirji Gini. Sixty-five lantern slides, including those showing the discoveries of Manson and Ross, were prepared. Business magnate Jamsetjee Jejeebhoy exhorted his co-religionists to cooperate with the authorities. To oppose the closure of wells, he said, 'was as much against the spirit and teaching of religion as against the laws of health'.[20] The Anglo-Gujarati newspaper, *Rast Goftar*, recommended that municipal corporators should make house visits and counsel people to overcome prejudices rather than criticize Bentley.[21] Objections were ascribed to inordinate attachment to custom rather than to 'a proper appreciation of the spirit which runs through religion'.[22]

Other newspapers were not so supportive. 'Is the campaign to be of the same draconian and oppressive character which drove people mad exasperating them to a boiling point?'[23] Here, the reference was to the anti-plague measures enforced in 1896–7. An unnamed house owner wrote that Turner could require all owners to empty and clean wells, but to hermetically seal all wells was 'sheer *zulum*'.[24] One suggestion was the closing of wells with gauze as it would not offend religious scruples.[25] Most well owners seem to have ultimately borne the expense and trap doors were permitted in wells, in order 'not to wound religious susceptibilities'.[26] A weekly report of wells with larvae was even sent to local newspapers, *The Times* of India, *Jam-e-Jamshed*, *Bombay Gazette*, and *Bombay Samachar*, so that it would have a salutary effect in convincing the recalcitrant. While steps were taken to hermetically seal all cisterns in municipal buildings, it was observed that there was no supervision of docks, railway premises, military quarters, or the City Improvement Trust grounds.[28] It was also pointed out that dependence on well water was due to the inadequate water supply. There was public disappointment that the popular Liston had supported well closure, overlooking the fact that some areas had no water for days.[29] The rejection by the standing committee of the Bombay Municipal Corporation of the petition of

25,000 residents requesting a postponement of the proposed campaign was considered as having 'trampled' public opinion.[30] Described as a 'cold bloodedly colourless reply,' it was remarked, 'if the answer had come from the executive we could have understood it—but the answer comes from the corporation, in theory a body representing the public'.[31] The Bombay government's endorsement of the decision of the Bombay Municipal Corporation, came six months later.

ACHIEVEMENT OF CONTROL

Despite this resistance, the campaign worked. Turner and Liston described their efforts at the meeting of the General Malaria Committee, held at Madras in 1912. Turner averred that contrary to the general belief that malaria occurred only in rural areas, it had been found in densely populated regions, where *a. stephensi* bred in wells, cisterns, and tanks, some of them unused, and in docks and railway yards. The Health Department made diligent searches in their municipal wards, but had such pressure of work, that only a portion of their time could be devoted to anti-malarial measures, but private individuals could do their bit and see that there was no accumulation of water. Turner asserted that other causes of malaria were the climate, people's ignorance, illiteracy, religious susceptibilities among the educated and uneducated, both in the mainland and in the larger island of Salsette, adjacent to Bombay. Many owners of wells had given permission to treat the wells with pesterine, but the problems remained because of extensive building operations and unlicensed bullock stables.[32] Liston, in his speech, outlined the methods to ascertain the extent of malaria, through collection of statistics, examination of children for spleen enlargement, and the microscopic examination of blood sucking anopheles.[33] Liston and Sub-Assistant Surgeon, T. G. Akula, had found that *stegomyia fasciata* was widely distributed in Bombay, and bred in places closely associated with human habitation, where water had been collected for domestic purposes. This mosquito was the extra corporeal host of the virus of yellow fever. J. L. Marjoribanks, Deputy Sanitary Commissioner, conducted an investigation in 1912 of the malarial conditions in the island of Salsette, with the view of defining the direction and the limits within which residential development should proceed.[34]

A special malaria department was created under Turner's supervision, and Shroff was appointed Special Malaria Officer, with a staff of four inspectors, 38 sub-inspectors, and *begaries* (workers), and the establishment of a laboratory, equipped with two microscopes. 4,380 wells, 166 tanks, and 4,887 cisterns, were enumerated, with the sub-inspectors periodically visiting to check their conditions. The workers were taught to inspect larvae and distinguish between the culex and anopheles. Lectures were given at schools, with magic lantern slides, explaining the precautions to be adopted. The Bombay Sanitary Association propagated this information, through home visits, for which they were lauded. 'The city owes much to those who, under the auspices of sanitary associations, are quietly yet surely disseminating elementary hygiene principles among the poorer classes'.[35] The other measures adopted were listed. They were—(a) treatment of all pools and puddles with pesterine, (b) putting fish into tanks and wells, (c) filling of hollows and low grounds, (d) improvement of drains and gullies and of general conservancy, (e) taking action in cases where municipal action was defied, (f) collecting a weekly return of cases from all public and private dispensaries, conducting spleen census of children, and examination of the blood of patients attending dispensaries, and (g) the examination of all species of mosquitoes, found at different times of the year, and of samples of larvae, at the Bombay Bacteriological Laboratory.[36] Quinine tablets were purchased from Burroughs Wellcome, London, at a cost of Rs 1,200, for free distribution in the chawls.[37] Dr Adam's specific for malaria was advertised in contemporary newspapers as a vegetarian product.[38]

The Bombay government's initial sanction of Rs 30,000 per annum, to the Bombay Municipal Corporation, for this scheme, was raised to Rs 50,000, though this was still regarded inadequate to cover areas, located in the north of the city.[39] Liston delivered a course of eight lectures to prospective teachers at the Secondary Training College, Bombay, and the Poona Training College, on common diseases of India, which included malaria. Liaison was also established with sanitary associations in other cities. Leaflets printed in English and Kannada were distributed to members of the Dharwar District Sanitary Association and quinine tabloids sold through this organization. The Government of India conducted classes in 'practical' malaria work, twice a year, and 155 medical officers, of the civil and the military departments completed this course.[40]

There was such confidence in the success of this campaign that, in 1918, the special Malaria Department was abolished. This was soon found to be short-sighted 'false economy,' because malaria began to increase until it caused serious disorganization of business in the docks. Forty commercial houses in the Fort area subsequently sent a petition to the Bombay Municipal Corporation drawing attention to the serious situation. In 1923, the Malaria Department was reconstituted, with Shroff, again in charge. S. R. Christophers, of the Malaria Survey of India, who was asked to investigate, drew attention once more to the importance of dealing with cisterns and wells. The disease was severe till 1925, when it began to decline due to the reduction of the permanent breeding places by the vigorous action of the Health Department.[41] Nevertheless, the opposition to well closure continued, and the Hindustan Native Merchants' Association held a public meeting in 1929, to register their protest.[42]

A successful non-official initiative in anti-malaria work was the effort of Dr H. V. Tilak and reformer Gopal Krishna Devadhar, promoters of the National Baby Week. They purchased a three-reel film on malaria, for $100, made by the International Health Board of the Rockefeller Foundation. Distributed in 1925 by Educational Pictures Corporation, owned by Patel and Sons, Karachi, the film was designed for popular education on the nature, causes and the mode of transmission of the disease, the life cycle of the mosquito and the various methods of combating the mosquito, and controlling the disease. Advertised as indispensable for educational institutions, the film was a particularly successful combination of scientific facts and human interest material, with commendable photography, animation, and diagram work. The National Baby Week, which engaged in health propaganda, wanted to adapt the film, in the local languages, and use the drawings at lectures that they arranged in villages. The Rockefeller Foundation, on its part, seems to have been satisfied that the government was involved, bearing half the expenses and being represented on the committee of the National Baby Week.[43] David Arnold has referred to the anti-malarial self help movement, on the other side of the subcontinent. Launched in two villages in Bengal in 1917, it soon spread to 1,000 villages, by 1932.[44]

Bombay city was the focus of a survey made by Gordon Covell, Assistant Director, Malaria Survey of India, in 1928. He consulted Dr Sandilands, Turner's successor, J. S. Nerurkar, Assistant Health Officer, F. D. Mackie and S. S. Sokhey, of the Haffkine Institute, Challam Medical Officer, Development Department, P. A. Dalal, Health Officer, Sassoon Mills, and S. B. Mehta, officiating Police Surgeon. Like Liston and Bentley, Covell too concluded that *a. stephensi* was the carrier, found either in permanent breeding places, including wells, cisterns, fountains, water used in building construction, cellars with seepage water, and leakages from reservoirs or in temporary areas, like roof gutters, disused receptacles, unfinished buildings, and ill drained yards. Both Bentley and Covell noted that with the carrier, breeding inside houses, malaria in Bombay was unusually localized. Covell found that the tenements in the northern part of the island were unoccupied and the people, for whose benefit they were erected, did not favour them and preferred to live in their current crowded and unsanitary dwellings. He noted that there was lack of unity of control in the anti-malaria measures, insufficient staff to implement them, inadequate legislative powers to enforce preventive measures, and regretted that Bentley's recommendations had not been carried out in their entirety.[45] Covell recommended that textile mills, in the city, should also take anti-malaria precautions. These were the treating of ponds with Paris green, (first used against the Colorado beetle), roof gutters being swept out, larvicide being added to water in each dyeing vat, fire buckets being filled with sand, and scrap machinery stacked in such a way as not to prevent the accumulation of water.[46] Covell's recommendation that all breeding places be eliminated was pushed with vigour, and only 1,200 remained open out of 4,000 wells by 1933. *Gambusia*, fish to eat mosquito larvae, was used in wells with good effect and the incidence of malaria in that year was lower than it had ever been. From 403 deaths in 1923, the rate had declined to 71 in 1933.[47]

Paul Russell of the Rockefeller Foundation visited Bombay with his colleagues, W. P. Jacocks and W. C. Sweet. Dr R. K. Mhatre, Assistant Health Officer, who was in charge of anti-malarial work, showed them both the typical breeding places and the aquarium, where gambusia were bred. He related how he had experimented with indigenous fish, called 'khajuri,' *anabas scandens*, but he had found that they grew to such a size that they were unable to go into the crevices in wells, where larvae were embedded. A corps of sanitary inspectors had inspected the known breeding places; this programme costing Rs 1,70,000, in 1933. The Americans were impressed with these efforts. But Russell had a word of caution. He felt that the work was so effective that the danger was that with the comparative unimportance of malaria, the division might be closed down, though the threat from the disease remained, with the new constructions and the large influx of persons constantly coming into the city.[48]

QUININE DISTRIBUTION

The Indian Sanitary Policy Resolution had recognized quinine to be of great value, both as a prophylactic and as a preventive, and recommended that children should be given it during the season as a practical measure. Besides the remarks about Indian apathy and ignorance, there was noted the prejudice against taking the drug, when not actually suffering from the illness and for lengths of time. Though some enthusiastic civil surgeons would distribute handbills propagating quinine, on the whole, the population was left pretty much to its own resources. The provincial governments had from time to time ear marked resources to make quinine available at cost price meant to bring it within reach of the poorest people. But on inquiry, Bentley found that it was those who could afford to pay, including government officials, who availed of cheap government quinine. He contended that the existing quinine policy was a failure, since the class who could not afford it were not benefited in the least. He called for an increase of production to minimize risk of enhancement of price.[49] Bentley wanted all surplus profits of government to be devoted to making free grants to local bodies for the gratuitous distribution of quinine. He recommended suitable advertisements to be inserted in newspapers and placards to be displayed at railway stations.[50] Sanitary Commissioner F. H. G. Hutchinson endorsed Bentley's proposal and agreed with him that the sub-assistant surgeons had not been successful because their work involved touring in unpleasant weather and they were poorly paid. Hutchinson urged the need for free distribution of quinine, placing it within reach of every individual. Many patients received only palliative treatment. Therefore, instead of a mixture, disbursed through outpatients' dispensaries, he had recommended tablets. This would become practicable, when the Government of India, in addition to procuring it, would adopt a policy of state manufacture similar to that in force in Italy. Referring to the good voluntary work done by the Gujarat Sabha, in the Gujarat region during the influenza epidemic of 1918, Hutchinson suggested the use of itinerant lecturers, co-operative societies, charitable organizations, and missionary societies, to popularize quinine.[51]

What was the picture by the 1930s? Out of a total budget of Rs 187,372,000 for the Presidency, for the year 1933–4, Rs 7,358,000 was allotted for medical and public health purposes. Rs 70,000 was allotted for the purchase of quinine, of which Rs 30,000 was recovered from the

sale of the drug. In 1933, a new distribution policy was established, providing that the drug was to be supplied to those who were to supervise
their local use, that is, officers of the public health department, district
school boards, district local boards having a medical officer, and officers
of the revenue department.

SIND AND KANARA

Of all the regions in the Presidency, Sind and Kanara were repeatedly
recorded as notoriously malarial. Even though an experiment with a
mosquito brigade, which inspected wells, was started at Shikarpur in
1906, it seems to have been abandoned midway. At the Simla Conference,
Dyson explained that the overflow of the Indus river, at certain times
of the year, made Sind malarial, as were the forest tracts in Kanara.
Travelling dispensaries had been tried, but had to be closed because
the hospital assistants, in charge of the dispensaries, were found to be
incompetent, the cost of the experiment was excessive, and Western
medicine was unknown. Besides, there was no village site as such, the
village consisting of only isolated groups of huts, with no schools, post
offices, or shops.[52] High rates of stillbirths and infant mortality were
also linked to malaria. The *Sanitary Commissioner's Report* of 1913,
recorded the measures implemented in Sind. In Karachi, a mosquito
brigade, including an inspector, seven sub-inspectors, and 30 coolies,
inspected 400 wells and identified those with larvae. In Jacobabad,
water from canal beds was pumped out and disused wells treated with
kerosene, and in Thar and Parkar, the 'quininization' of school children
was adopted.[53] In 1913, Dr K. S. Mhaskar had conducted surveys in Sind
and Kanara. He had found the prevalence of *stegomyia* in Karachi and
suggested steps for its control. In Kanara, Mhaskar examined 70,000
children and found a general spleen rate of 20.6 per cent, and noted that
it was type *culcifacies* which was infected, breeding in river pools and
irrigation channels. But this comprehensive report only gathered dust,
as Paul Russell discovered 20 years later.[54]

As for curative measures in this region, the distribution of quinine was
in its infancy. It was sold in pice packets, till 1911, through small post offices, village headmen and school masters, and free distribution was also
attempted through zamindars, *mamlatdars*, *talatis*, members of district
local boards, and municipalities. Whereever quinine was given gratis,
people often stored it, or sold it in the bazaar for what it could fetch.

In the jungle tracts of Panch Mahals and Kanara, packets were found unopened and mouldy, and in such places, it was considered hopeless to overcome the apathy of the people. To overcome the difficulty of getting malaria sufferers to take enough doses to affect a thorough cure, a new system, which had been tried in East Bengal and Assam, was started. Small glass tubes, each comprising 20 tabloids of four grains, were distributed. Half a tonne of quinine, made up in this fashion, was issued to headmen, postmen, and school masters. The prices were fixed well below cost price and the retailers made a profit of seven *annas* on every parcel of 10 tubes.[55] The government deputed sub-assistant surgeons to tour, for five months, in selected areas, from 1910. In Hyderabad, Sukkur, and Larkana, they explained the use of quinine, the part played by mosquitoes in malaria, pointed out the defects in village houses and gave advice on general cleanliness and ventilation, visited schools, and examined children for spleen enlargement. In fact, it was found that the administration of quinine in Larkana had even increased the attendance of children at schools during the malarial season.[55]

In 1927, malaria was still responsible for 45,641 deaths in Bombay Presidency, the death rate being 2.38, with Sind having the highest rate. Paul Russell observing that the problem of malaria in Sind was of tremendous proportions, criticized the Lloyd barrage authorities for shelving the drainage scheme which should have been an integral part of the original barrage scheme, because of financial difficulties. In 1928, the Malaria Survey of India had warned the barrage authorities that the scheme, without proper drainage, would only increase malaria. 'It is not evident that any heed was paid to this hint'.[56] Covell's prediction of a rise in endemic malaria was confirmed. Besides the water-logging of hundreds of thousands of acres, was the very heavy rainfall in the two years after the scheme started. In 1935, 80–90 per cent spleen rates were recorded as against 15 per cent, in 1927–8.[57] Malaria was endemic throughout Sind but the incidence and severity varied; upper Sind facing more severe epidemics than lower Sind. There was found to be a direct relation between rice cultivation and the prevalence of malaria. It was not the fields, per se, but the badly kept irrigation channels and flooded areas formed by water escaping from the fields and channels that provided breeding places. Villages lying in a former bed of the Indus, and liable to flooding from the river, those situated on the banks of large irrigation tanks and in low lying tracts, where rice was grown, were the most malarial areas. The engineers had pointed out that Sind was always malarial, but the barrage scheme had definitely increased the incidence of malaria. In a scheme costing 45 million dollars, one might have expected budgeting for malaria control, especially if the scheme was planned to return 10 per cent profit. Russell maintained that it was doubtful, if there would be any profit at all, unless malaria was controlled, and urged the scheme authorities to undertake the responsibility of distributing quinine because neither the ruler of Khairpur nor the individual municipalities could be relied upon.

Questions about the prevalence of malaria were repeatedly raised in the Bombay Legislative Council by members from Sind and Kanara. Khan Bahadur Allah Baksh, from Sukkur, contended that though malaria came every year to Sind, the district local boards and government doctors did not have sufficient funds to distribute quinine. In fact, he felt that full advantage could not be taken of the perennial water supply as the cultivator, who was inevitably struck with malaria at the end of the agricultural operations season, did not have enough time for convalescence.[58] To his question whether malaria would increase with the Lloyd Barrage Canal scheme, the government answered in the negative, except on occasions, when water-logging took place.[59]

M. D. Kaiki, from Kanara, referred to the proposal of the forest committee (1925) which had recommended that the forests for two to four furlongs around villages be cleared to prevent mosquitoes breeding, but nothing was done.[60] G. S. Gangoli, also from Kanara, claiming that no other member of the legislative council came from as malarial a place as he did, pointed to the glaring contrast with Bombay city. With a population of 13 lakhs, the death rate from malaria in the city had fallen to 76 deaths, while Kanara, with a population of only one lakh, had 991 deaths. In Kanara there were no wells, only streams which had falling leaves from wild trees, and a forest policy, which prohibited the clearing of streams. Gangoli connected these factors to the high incidence of malaria. Teak cultivation had been increased by the forest department and Kanara had been de-populated. The officials of the forest department did not even stay in the region but claimed the allowance, for serving in a place with a bad climate, and resided in less malarial Dharwar or Belgaum. The government's response to this criticism was that they had spent Rs 1,625 in 1931–2 on anti-malaria steps in Kanara, the Governor's visit there had led to the despatch of two health officers to treat malaria and distribute quinine, and the Red Cross stationed at Belgaum had extended their activities to Kanara.[61] The decline of agricultural population in Kanara being caused by the increased pressure on forests had been noted in the forest report of 1917–18, as Subash Chandran has shown.[62] The member from Surat, Dr M. K. Dixit, complained that malaria was a constant companion in his district, reducing the resistance of villagers. The victims took two or three grains of quinine but their physical condition was so debilitating that they could not put in the hard work that was required for agriculture. He urged that government lend their helping hand, and attributed the improved conditions in Bombay city, to the municipality, which had spent more on public health than the Bombay government did on the whole Presidency.[63]

OTHER OBSERVATIONS OF PAUL RUSSELL

Paul Russell also filed a confidential report about the Andhra Valley Power Supply Company, at Bhivpuri Camp, 10 miles east of Karjat and 40 miles South-East of Bombay, in the western Ghats, where a power supply company of the Tatas was situated. The camp was part of a hydro-electric scheme, in which an artificial lake had been created. The construction was started in 1917–18 and the site chosen, without medical advice, was located under the hill near the clear waters of ravine streams and seepages. With rainfall of 125 inches a year, and high humidity, this place was malaria endemic, and saw an enormous amount of sickness and the company was put to enormous expense, but no real anti-malaria work was done till 1928. A half mile survey was conducted and all breeding places marked. The insecticide, Paris green oil, was used, and the programme was so effective that Covell reported in 1931, that the spleen rate had gone down to 30 per cent and cautioned that there should be no slackening of the campaign. The cost of the control measures had been relatively small. Russell had consulted the unpublished reports of both Covell and Dr Engineer, the Medical Officer.

Russell also visited Wadgaon Budruk, near Poona, a town practically abandoned by the population because of malaria. The inhabitants had moved to a site, a mile away on higher ground, where there were no streams. Wadgaon Khurd, near by, was similarly deserted. The cause of the malaria was *culicifacies*, breeding in the small stream running between the two towns. The inhabitants of both towns were relocated on the dry hill side with the assistance of the Rural Reconstruction Association of Poona.

The Director of Public Health of Bombay Presidency requested the Rockefeller Foundation for funding the building of a proposed malaria institute, promise of some funds from another unnamed private source having been secured. However, Russell was not supportive of this request as he felt that it could have no practical use.[64]

Making his comments on the all India malaria picture, Russell noted that malaria control was not like in Europe or in the southern United States. There were physical complexities, economic difficulties, the influence of religion, and indifference to disease and death in India. Rather than differentiating between urban and rural regions, Russell was of the opinion that it was simpler to divide into those areas, where it was economically feasible to control malaria, and areas where it was not. Controls would work in cities with population exceeding 15,000, in tea gardens, rubber plantations, railways, forests, cantonments, dams, hydro-electric plants, irrigation works, and pilgrimage centres. Russell lauded Bombay, Bangalore, certain tea gardens, and the Mettur dam in Madras for carrying out larval control. But in other regions official apathy was to blame, though funds were available. He particularly mentioned the forest reserve department of Bengal, which made a profit of $160,000, but did nothing to contribute to protect its personnel from malaria. He recommended Paris green and oil as the most potent weapons for larval control, but these could not be used in rural India, where it was not economically feasible. Instead, a wider and more intense distribution of quinine had to be pursued. As for the Government of India, he was unsparing in his criticism—'I can see no justification whatever for the Government of India to profit to the extent of several hundred thousand dollars annually from its production of quinine while a million of its citizens die of malaria each year'.[65] It was 'ridiculous' that Madras should spend only about $26,000 annually to control its chief cause of death and disability. He maintained that since all streams and irrigation channels belonged to the state, it must share the burden of malaria control. Russell held the irrigation engineers to be 'guilty' of increasing the malaria problem; not only had irrigated territory caused an increase in malaria but it had also put land out of cultivation by water-logging. 'Borrow pits' used to build roads and railway embankments were also a source of malaria in rural areas. Russell saw no hope of controlling malaria until farmer-made 'malariogenic' conditions were eliminated.[66] Russell lauded the Malaria Survey of India for its excellent work and regretted that it had no executive powers and its recommendations were frequently disregarded, as in the case of Delhi and Sind. He observed that labourers and even the higher personnel of the public works department, railways, or forest reserve had little protection.

In 1937, Rockefeller Foundation officials, M. A. Barber and J. B. Rice, made a study of malaria in the urban region of Poona and in certain adjacent rural areas. They found that localities in the irrigated region had far higher malaria indexes than those in the non-irrigated. The mosquito surveys showed a great variety of species of anopheles, *culcifacies* being the chief vector, plentiful in some localities even during the dry season. In other localities they found vivax or falciparum. But in the urban area, the malaria indexes were low except in the neighbourhood of one of the rivers which traversed the city. They concluded that similar blanket measures were hardly practical in urban and rural areas.[67]

ROCKEFELLER FOUNDATION'S ASSISTANCE TO THE STATE OF SAWANTWADI

A success story was Sawantwadi state, where malaria was the chief public health problem, particularly after the 1918 influenza epidemic. Hence, the government of Sawantwadi requested Dr C. Strickland, Professor, Calcutta School of Tropical Medicine, who had previous experience of malaria work in the Federated Malay States, to carry out a survey. He found *a. maculatus* and *a. culicafacies* to be the carriers, and recommended forestation along the hill stream for control of the former, and ditching, draining, and oiling for the latter. Anti-malaria work was carried on, from 1922. A qualified medical officer, R. M. Haldankar, was appointed and the campaign in the town resulted in the spleen rate coming down from 85 per cent to 12 per cent. But, the effort to control malaria in nine villages of the state was without definite result because of financial impediments and the extreme conservatism of the villagers. In 1928, Baburao, Sawantwadi's Minister of Revenue and Political Affairs, wrote to the Rockefeller Foundation requesting co-operation in malaria control. He pointed out that he had heard the latter was diffident to extend its activities to British India, since the Government of India expected subsidies, but he assured that Sawantwadi was independent and expected no such subsidy. The Governor of Bombay, Sir Leslie Wilson, who visited the state, recommended the request.[68]

The Rockefeller Foundation deputed Kendrick of the International Health Division to Sawantwadi, for two months, in 1929. His observations about the small state are interesting. The British had controlled the state from 1836 till 1925, through Sardesai Maharaj, who did not pay any tribute to the Government of India, but had his political dealings through the British political agent in Belgaum. As for public health, Kendrick found that with the exception of street sweeping, no sanitation work was done, and there was no facility for the training of sanitary inspectors or nurses. While piped water supply was available in the town, people in rural areas drew well water despite the proximity of perennial streams. The only educational health activity undertaken was the conduct of baby weeks. Smallpox had been controlled by the vaccination of all children before they reached the age of six months, and plague, by rat destruction and inoculation, but malaria remained the major public health problem. Five per cent of the revenue was spent on preventive medicine. Assistant Surgeon Barjorji Ardesir had noted that malaria was endemic in the state, even in the 19th century. Kendrick visited 15 villages and found the most malarial parts situated near the sources of the *nullah*s on the hillsides or at the foot of the hills. There was no control over the practice of medicine; many persons administered 'native drugs of various sorts, most of which neither do any good nor any harm'.[69] He felt the state had not kept pace with British India, yet he maintained that both Sardesai and his ministers were earnestly concerned with the people's welfare and the malaria officer worked despite handicaps.

Kendrick recommended to the Rockefeller Foundation that Rs 10,000 ($3750 at the time) should be granted, for malaria work, which was subsequently sanctioned. It was to defray the expenses of the salary of the medical officer, who was to be sent to the Ross field station at Karnal for two months study, to equip a laboratory, and provide a Ford motor car. The work commenced in July, 1930.[70] Attention was focussed on two particular villages, of Kolgaon and Akeri. Haldankar filed quarterly reports on the basis of his study of spleen examination, blood examination, larvae catches, adult mosquito catches, dissection of mosquitoes, birth and death figures, and meteorological data. Wells and nullahs were treated with Paris green, and locally available fish called *chand and fatki* were used to control larvae.

In the meanwhile, W. C. Sweet of the Rockefeller Foundation, who was based in Bangalore, made an inspection visit of Sawantwadi, in 1931. He found that Paris green control could not be 'economically practicable'.[71] Subsequently, experiments with small weekly doses of plasmoquine were started. Sweet's report confirmed the observation of Strickland that the greater part of the malaria was associated with villages situated at the foot of the hills. In villages to the north of Sawantwadi, where natural conditions were the same, government had given up its rights in similar reserve forests and the people had cleared the forests to grow crops, and subsequent to the clearing of the forests these villages reported to have 'lost' their malaria. From the studies and observations, Sweet concluded that it was not possible to recommend the use of oil, Paris green, ditching, or draining, due to the scattered nature of the villages in the state and the consequent high cost of these methods of control. Anti-larval measures were also not practical, hence, he suggested that the experiment of cutting the forest adjoining the highly malarial village would be the cheapest way of getting rid of the disease. An attempt to transport gambusia from Mysore to Sawantwadi had failed because it was done in the hot weather. Therefore, a more efficient gambusia hatchery was recommended. On the positive side, he noted that there was a laboratory building, the malaria department had been made a permanent part of the state administration, and the town now had a spleen rate of only 6 per cent.[72] One problem seems to have been the people's objection to have their blood tested, or to take plasmoquine. After much persuasion and explanation of its effects, most began to cooperate. However, when two or three chronic cases were given plasmoquine, as a curative, others too wanted it, but were refused, because it was experimented mainly as a prophylactic, and it was quinine which was promoted as a curative.[73] The Rockefeller Foundation's funding ended in December 1933. By this date, Haldankar had carried out the study for two and half years, and reported a decrease in malaria.

CONCLUSION

The review above has shown differing approaches and responses to disease control, in the urban and rural regions of western India. The success achieved in controlling malaria in Bombay city, before the First World War, was due to the collaborative efforts of malariologists, doctors, both Indian and British, community leaders, and the vigilant press. Significantly, the incidence of the disease increased, when controls were allowed to lapse, as a measure of economy. The vigorous implementation of anti-malarial measures was fortunately resumed, in the 1920s, and in the following decade, the *urbs prima in Indis* saw declining spleen rates. The reasons for this positive development was public involvement, adequate funds, and the fact that an important commercial centre like Bombay could not afford to have heavy mortality from a disease that could be checked and managed. Cities like Poona, Ahmedabad, and Karachi also made some efforts to promote drainage and propagate knowledge of preventive steps, but in small towns like Surat and Broach, where finance was the constraint, malaria raged. The case of the state of Sawantwadi, which showed enterprise in securing Rockefeller Foundation assistance to bring the disease under check, is an example of how effective could be local initiatives in health care.

The picture in the rural regions of the Presidency was markedly different. Rural sanitation had doubtless been handed over to local bodies, but they had limited funds at their disposal and had too many other heads of expenditure. Hence, Surendranath Banerjee had moved a resolution, in the Imperial Legislative Council, urging that government, which had both expertise and enormous resources, should put themselves at the head of the sanitary movement, and that malaria control should be above politics.[74] But little was done in the early years, beyond distributing quinine. Ira Klein has argued that though Sinton and others had maintained that it was not technically or economically feasible to control malaria among the rural population, the Indian Medical Service did regularly appeal for funds to reduce fatalities through reclamation and education, but these requests were denied by a government, which had other priorities.[75] The views of officials like Bentley, Christophers, Covell, and Hutchinson bear out the argument that the men on the spot and malariologists had better perspectives of the situation, but were invariably unheard or overruled by policy makers. Surveys were doubtless conducted, but were allowed to collect dust, as Russell observed about Mhaskar's report on Kanara. While commending the Malaria Survey of India for its recommendations, Russell regretted that it had no executive power, and that these were disregarded in Sind. His report on Sind confirmed what Covell had warned about, that malaria would increase after the Lloyd barrage scheme. Russell accepted that irrigation schemes were necessary, but contended that it should be possible, 'to educate or intimidate irrigation engineers and to guide farmers so that they would not create malaria'. In fact, he maintained that there was little interest aroused by malaria, though there was considerable incidence in the Presidency.[76] However, as shown in this chapter, the issue was indeed debated in the Bombay legislature, but with little follow-up action.

As for the overall picture, the observations of Russell about the complexities of the country are perceptive. He was unsparing in his criticism of the Government which profited enormously from quinine production but allowed its subjects to die of malaria. By the third decade of the 20th century, as Bill Bynum has argued, any comprehensive plan of malaria control still lay in the future.[77]

The author wishes to acknowledge the assistance of the Rockefeller Archive Centre, New York, which awarded her the Rockefeller residency grant, in 2003.

The names of Bombay and Poona have been changed to Mumbai and Pune, but have been used here as they were known in the early 20th century.

NOTES

1. Leonard, Rogers, 1930, 'Notes on a Proposal for Enabling Malaria Epidemics to be Foreseen and Mitigated', *Records of the Malaria Survey of India*, Calcutta: Thacker, Spink & Co., p.176.

2. *Proceedings of the Imperial Malaria Conference held at Simla in October 1909* (1910:95).

3. Dymock (1884:4–5).

4. Morehead (1860:6).

5. Deb Roy (2007:122–29).

6. *Report of the Sanitary Commissioner for the Government of Bombay* (1905:12); *Administrative Report of the Municipal Commissioner for the City of Bombay* (1906:12).

7. Covell (1928:7).

8. *Report on Native Papers, Bombay Presidency, Jam- e-Jamshed*, 24 August 1909.

9. Report of the Committee, Government Resolution, no. 1772, 23 March 1906, in General Department Volume, no. 46, 1909. Maharashtra State Archives, Mumbai.

10. Bentley (1911:24). Bentley's investigations were funded by the Government of Bombay, Bombay Municipal Corporation, Bombay Port Trust, and the Bombay Baroda Central Indian Railway Company.

11. Charles Bentley, 1918, 'Note on Sir Leonard Rogers Proposal for Enabling Malaria Epidemic to be Foreseen and Mitigated', RMS, 181. Sporozoite is usually a motile infective form of some sporozoans. Sporozoans are parasitic protozoans that have a complicated life cycle like malaria parasites.

12. *Indian Sanitary Policy, 1914: being a resolution issued by the Governor General in Council on the 23rd May, 1914*, p. 16. Calcutta: Superintendent, Government Printing.

13. Bentley (1910:28–9).

14. Ibid., pp. 153–6.

15. Ibid., pp. 138–9.

16. *Administrative Report of the Municipal Commissioner for the City of Bombay (ARMCB)* (1912–13:178).

17. *Pickings from the Hindi Punch*, (March 1910:401).

18. Ibid., (April 1910:443).

19. Report on Malaria Operations, April 1912–March 1913, in ARMCB (1912–13:171).

20. *ARMCB* (1912–13:180).

21. *Report on Native Papers, Bombay Presidency (RN), Rast Goftar* (20 August 1911).

22. RN, *Rast Goftar*, (7 July 1912).

23. RN, *Kaiser-I-Hind*, (8 August 1909).

24. RN, *Indu Prakash* (30 November 1909).

25. RN, *Indu Prakash* (15 July 1911).

26. *ARMCB* (1912–13:177).

27. RN, *Parsi* (20 August 1911).

28. RN, *Jam-e-Jamshed* (17 July 1914).

29. RN, *Kaiser-I-Hind* (6 September 1914).

30. RN, *Indu Prakash* (26 September 1914).

31. *Proceedings of the Third Meeting of the General Malaria Committee held at Madras, November, 18, 19 and 20, 1912* (1913:162).

32. Ibid., p. 163.

33. *Some Recent Sanitary Developments in the Bombay Presidency* (1914:2).

34. *Third Meeting, Madras* (1913:159).

35. Ibid., pp. 165–73.

36. *ARMCB* (1912–13:185).

37. *The Bombay Chronicle,*7 January 1919.

38. GD 476, 1916–18, GR NO 1474, 22 February 1913, 7 GR no. 1712, 26 February 1915; Municipal Commissioner's Letter No. 16834, 8 October 1917.

39. *Indian Sanitary Policy, 1914* (18).

40. Covell (1928:11).

41. *The Bombay Chronicle,*15 June 1929.

42. Rockefeller Archive Centre, New York, Rockefeller Foundation, Records Group 5, Sub Series1.2, Box 266, Folder 3362.

43. Arnold (1999:139).

44. Covell (1928:34).

45. Ibid., p. 63.

46. Rockefeller Archive Centre (RAC), Rockefeller Foundation (RF), Records Group (RG) 1.I projects, series, 464 India, Box 11, Folder 90.

47. RAC, RF, RG 5, Sub Series 1.2, Box 266, Folder 3362.

48. *Third Meeting, Madras* (1913:100).

49. Bentley in *Records of the Malaria Survey of India (RMS)*, p. 189.

50. Hutchinson (1919:190–2); (1920:193–5).

51. *Proceedings of the Imperial Malaria Conference* (1910:92–3).

52. *Report of Sanitary Commissioner, Bombay (RSC)* (1914:14).

53. RAC, RF, RG, 1.I projects, series, 464 India, Box 11, Folder 90.

54. *Some Recent Sanitary Developments* (1914:2).

55. Ibid., Patrick Hehir observed that Indian children had acquired some kind of immunity through frequent exposure to malaria. Hehir (1927:34–9).

56. RAC, RF, RG 1.1, Projects 464, Box 11, Folder 89.

57. Whitcombe (1995:257).

58. *Bombay Legislative Council Debates* (BLC), Volume 34 (1932:842–3).

59. Ibid., pp. 165–6.

60. *BLC*, Volume 19 (1927:1093).

61. *BLC*, Volume 37 (1933:950,1527–31).

62. Chandran (1998:698).

63. *BLC*, Volume 37 (1933:1540–2).

64. RAC, RF, RG 1.1, Projects Series 464, Box 11, Folder 90.

65. Ibid.

66. Ibid.

67. RAC, RF, RG 5, Series 3, Box 202, Folder 2472.

68. RAC, RF, RG 1.1, Series 464, Box 19, Folder 148.

69. RAC, RF, RG 2, 1929, 554, Folder 3723.

70. RAC, RF, RG 1.1, Series 464, Box 19, Folder 148.

71. RAC, RF, RG, 1.1, Series 464, Box 19, Folder 150.

72. Ibid.

73. RAC, RF, RG 5.3, Series 464, Box 208, Folder 2553.

74. Banerjee (1916:154–62).

75. Klein (2001:147–79).

76. RAC, RF, RG, 1.I Projects, Series 464, Box 11, Folder 90.

77. Bynum (2000:25–31).

10 Vulnerability of Women to Bacillus

Myths and Reality in India, 1890–1950

BIKRAMADITYA KUMAR CHOUDHARY

Increasing interaction amongst individuals and communities transforms economic, social, and cultural life of people at origin and destination both. Such transformation has positive as well as not so positive outcomes for different communities. The outcomes could vary based on the balance of power, willing and unwilling consent to the changes, and also the capabilities of individuals and communities to negotiate those changes. Owing to economic, social, and cultural changes, spread of different diseases, including tuberculosis, across the globe, has been one of many unintended consequences of exchanges across different parts of the world. India under the imperial rule did experience changes in the lifestyle of its masses along with enhanced movement through newly created network that consequently contributed to spread of the disease.[1] Changes in economy and lifestyle of population from 'open-field agrarian practice' to 'close-door crowded industrialization' did have an impact on spread of tuberculosis across country through regularly created disease networks. Tuberculosis, as a disease, has been as old as the human civilization in almost all parts of the globe, including India. There has been a plethora of literature on various diseases and their causes but for tuberculosis in early colonial period. It was only at the dawn of the 20th century, the real nature of tuberculosis could be identified, when it had already declined in the Western society.[2] The reasons for the decline of tuberculosis in the West are multifarious; ranging from nutritional improvement of people to improvement and implementation of public health.[3]

Contrasting theories are available about spread of tuberculosis throughout 19th and 20th century in India.[4] One reason behind such contradictory reality has been poor record keeping about deaths and causes of deaths in India. There were many reasons for reported inaccuracy ranging from cultural to economic and medical. On the cultural front, the fact remains that in dominant Indian tradition, human body was not considered of worth and there was no specific mechanism of keeping the death records. Apart from the cultural reason, during colonial period, the inaccurate account of diseases can be attributed to two main reasons—'purposeful negligence towards the population' and the 'inefficient' mechanism of maintaining the record'. For both of these, the government of the day, that is, the colonial British government was responsible. The prime motto of the imperial government had been the extraction of resources throughout the initial phase, and in an effort to justify its territorial expansion, later on they did manifest benevolence towards the population, especially through health-planning as evidenced by the Bhore committee report of 1946.[5] The report of a medical officer in 1899 quotes Dr Simpson, the late Health Officer of Calcutta, who recorded that at least 50 per cent of the mortality occurred without medical attendance of any kind.[6] This one statement in itself indicates towards a wilful negligence towards the health of humans in India, and also one reason for absence of record on morbidity. The second reason for non-reliable mortality and morbidity statistics remains as erroneous method of data collection. In 1947, the then Medical Advisor to the Secretary of State for India Lt General Sir Bennett Hance (1947) noted—the 'Indian statistics of morbidity and mortality are notoriously inaccurate, the method of their collection is archaic and the margin of error consequently very large'.[7] It is not that the British did not know the importance of maintaining the record of mortality and morbidity, as they were efficiently maintaining the same in Britain by 19th century. And there was no question of British being inefficient in administration either, as in India, they were able to maintain comparatively good governance in other fields that were crucial for running the empire, or say, for the existence of the empire. Nevertheless, British choose to be ignorant about this known crucial fact of maintaining the record for the population and Indian statistics of morbidity and mortality hardly considered adequate by professionals and policy-makers.

Still, the available statistics can be used for understanding the gravity of a particular disease or vulnerability of a particular section of population by a particular disease, as all of them are equally erroneous. The available statistics show that the nature and magnitude of death from tuberculosis and also from malaria was far in excess than even the most shocking outbreaks of cholera, plague, or smallpox. The deaths from tuberculosis were a reality and by 1916, it was widely accepted that tuberculosis in India was on the rise. One eighth of the population, that is, fifty million people of the sub-continent were reported suffering from malaria and the ratio between reported deaths and the reported cases was 1:50. While, for tuberculosis, the ratio between reported deaths and the reported cases was 1:5. It can be inferred that about two million five hundred thousand open cases of tuberculosis existed in India at any one time. And about 20 per cent of those suffering had the fate of meeting death due to the disease. Dr Hance compared the annual deaths from these two diseases with that of the deaths during the Bengal famine of 1943—

> when we consider that the Bengal famine of 1943, which shocked and hor-rified the world, and for the mitigation of which the charitable minded public all over the world subscribed vast sum of money, was responsible for an increase of the death rate of seven hundred and eighty thousand, that is only 78 percent of the annual death rate from malaria and *150 per-cent of the annual death rate from tuberculosis.*[8]

The higher deaths from these two diseases—malaria and tuberculosis, were attributed to several causes ranging from climatic to cultural, and later on to change in the lifestyle and economy.[9] The reasons that were advanced for this can be disputed but the fact was that the common men and women in the cities, towns, and villages were dying by tuberculosis, whether known as 'black magic of Bengal' or accepted as 'white plague'.[10]

VULNERABILITY TO THE BACILLUS

The vulnerability or susceptibility of a particular group, ethnicity, or gender, or a particular epidemiology has been an attractive and illuminating area of disease studies for two contrasting reasons—one, for 'putting the blame back on the sufferer', and other, for 'special care of the sufferer'. In the first case, a particular section of population, for example, here, women are painted as more vulnerable because of their own fault; while in the second case, efforts are made to understand the existing or past causes which have been responsible for higher morbidity and mortality in a particular section of society, and accordingly special care can be taken to eliminate the disease from the affected group. Whatever has been the outcome of such researches, the prerequisite, especially in historical context, is the availability of information. During pre-independence, the morbidity statistics for general population were hardly available. Definitely there was no question of having the epidemiological data or analysis of social epidemiology. In such a situation, one had to rely either on reports or the available statistics for different groups which can be taken as representative under defined conditions with known limitations.[11] Even without a reliable scientific analysis, various parts of the world and different sections of population invariably were dubbed as comparatively more vulnerable. Dominant streams of professionals suggested that Indians were more susceptible to the bacillus as compared to the British. For example, in 1938, Sprawson wrote in the *British Journal of Tuberculosis* that 'Indian population as a whole is more susceptible to tuberculosis than the population of England or Scotland and in India disease runs an acuter course…the immunity in India is low'.[12] The fact got established by the time that the virgin population and the virgin region, once exposed to the disease, becomes more vulnerable to the bacillus. This is not to suggest that there was no instance of tuberculosis in India before. As it has been noted several times that in India, from the earliest times, tuberculosis was known and a description of the same was found in the accounts of Hindu physicians.[13] The fact remains that the extent to which the disease was rampant was not known in India before the increased British encounter with the native population.[14]

The bacillus did not affect all with the same intensity. There was a marked difference in terms of susceptibility to the particular group and particular regions. Certain regions of India, like North-West Province and Punjab, were identified endemic regions for tuberculosis.[15] Certain population groups were considered more susceptible to the bacillus than others; important amongst them were interestingly the group of those who were preferred in armed forces. Lankaster in his report noted—'The most striking example of such people in India is the Gurkhas, who show in comparison with other soldiers of the Indian Army a greatly increased susceptibility to the mortality from tuberculosis. Similarly, it has been observed that the Pathans are also more susceptible than the ordinary Indian rural folk'.[16]

Moreover, he did not mention the reason for the reported higher toll from tuberculosis amongst Gurkhas or Pathans. The Gurkhas, who were the inhabitants of the virgin land, got exposed to the bacillus while working with the Europeans, and once they got affected the toll was larger amongst them. Similarly, it was highlighted that the prevalence of tuberculosis was higher among women. The death rate for the year 1896 among European soldiers serving in India has been reported as 86 per 10,000, while among European women the death rate was higher and noticed as 120 per 10,000.[17] Reports from the general population also suggest a similar situation prevailing with regards to the higher incidence among women. Lankaster in his report has stated that—'The fact that in India more than twice as many women as men suffer from consumption, and the still more serious fact that in Punjab there are only 17 adult women to every 1000 men (as contrasted with Madras where there are 1032 or the United Kingdom where the proportion is 1068 per 1000 men)'.[18]

It seems that in this part of his report, Lankaster was trying to establish a link between the differential sex-ratio and the prevalence of consumption while trying to compare that in United Kingdom, the sex-ratio was in favour of women, while in Punjab, it was disproportionately in favour of men. The reason of worry was that because consumption was a reason of death and was more among women, the already disproportionate sex-ratio would further pose a challenge to the government and society. In his report, he refers to the higher incidence among women in Calcutta, as female death rate from phthisis was 33 per 10,000, while the male rate was only 22. Further, the report noted that the phthisis death rate for Mohammedan women was 58 per 10,000 against 30 for Hindus.[19] A similar situation was reported from Lahore, where in each category, the female death rate from phthisis was higher. Table 10.1 shows that in each category of population, more deaths were reported amongst women than men.

Table 10.1   Deaths from Phthisis During Year 1913

Community	Mohammedans		Hindus		Others	
	Male	Females	Male	Females	Male	Females
Death from phthisis	150	299	59	86	15	21

Source: Lankaster (1916)

Nevertheless, another fact during the period was that women generally were dying without much of medical care and in most cases, cause of death remained uncertain and the deaths amongst women would be further high while taking into account this fact. The report that highlighted the differential death rate, however, did not probe in to the reasons of higher mortality amongst women or Mohammedans. Later on, committees were set up to investigate the reason for such a situation in India, who tried to compare India with that of West and also with other regions.

This statistics in the table is only a reflection of the reality that existed in different parts of the country during the pre-independence period. It was not only in India where susceptibility of women to bacillus was noticed, but also in the West. Greater susceptibility of women to tuberculosis in the West was also noticed more than once. In 1865, it was noticed that out of a hundred women, more than five would die by the age of 30 and more than eight would die by the age of 50. Multiple reasons were advanced for such a situation. The reasons for any kind of happening, especially for the occurrence of the disease, that too in 19th and early 20th century, are of two kinds—constructed and real. Even real cause are not true in all senses—how much convincing they may look, the fact remains that everything is subjective and subjectivity comes with power, and the balance always remains in favour of power. The reported higher incidence of tuberculosis in late 17th and early 18th century in the Western world was attributed to many causes. Two dominant but probably unfounded reasons can be highlighted here. First, women's greater susceptibility to tuberculosis was seen as proof of the inherent defectiveness of female physiology. Azell, in 1875, noted that, 'beyond doubt that consumption…is itself produced by the failure of the [menstrual] function in the forming girls…one has been the parent of the other with interchangeable priority'.[20]

Consumption might bring certain changes in the women's physiology but that is true for any individual irrespective of gender. However, at that point of time, women's specific physiological characteristic were blamed for the occurrence of consumption amongst women, and the negative effects on women's nature and on her reproductive system was given more importance than the other effect. In other words, the effect of consumption was considered as a reason for higher prevalence of consumption amongst women. The second unfounded logic for higher prevalence of tuberculosis amongst women was the feminine characteristics of the disease.[21] It was noted at several places that—'The association of tuberculosis with innate feminine weakness was strengthened by the fact that tuberculosis is accompanied by an erratic emotional pattern in which a person may behave sometimes frenetically, sometimes morbidly. The behaviour characteristics of the disease…not only were women seen as sickly—sickness was seen as feminine'.[22]

The rationale for propagating such a feminine characteristic of tuberculosis was based on subjective judgement of doctors. No 'objectivity', whatsoever, could be found for the proposed feminine characteristics of tuberculosis, except certain examples during the romantic age that had been categorized as feminine characteristics for being soft.

In India, during last 50 years of British rule, numerous reports on various aspects of tuberculosis became available. The similarities and differences in these reports with respect to the women's vulnerability could be of use as a window to see through the prevailing understanding about tuberculosis. Some reports suggested that women in India are comparatively safer than the European women; others argued that Indian women, due to several cultural and social practices, are more vulnerable to the bacillus. In 1899, Crombie in his report noted that in India, European women had higher prevalence of tuberculosis and also among the children of those affected women, since such children were not fed by the affected mothers. In case of the affected children of the European mothers, the doctors tried to establish a link between bovine to human tuberculosis through the practice of feeding cold milk (given that in the West, there was no concept of using warm milk) to children, as it was noted that, 'the European mother in India is very often unable to do so and her child suffers from improper artificial food and thus made more susceptible to infection and at the same time runs additional risk of being fed with probably tuberculous milk and butter not to speak of possibility of tuberculous meat'.[23]

Of late, it was established beyond doubt that cases of bovine tuberculosis and the consequent infection in India were rare. Sprawson noted in his report that—

> In one respect India can claim an advantage over the countries of Northern Europe in that it can apparently neglect the bovine bacillus as a source of infection. The Indian cow appears to possess a relative immunity to tuberculosis and though bovine tuberculosis is not so uncommon at any rate in Northern India as at one time it was thought, the bovine disease is believed to be so rare as to require no special public health measures so far protection of man is concerned.[24]

The higher prevalence of tuberculosis among Indian women got associated with several cultural practices like seclusion of women, child marriage, early pregnancy, unhygienic practices during delivery, and other related issues. The prevailing 'purdah system' (using a veil to cover the face) was understood as one major factor responsible for higher rate of consumption amongst women. Purdah system, in different reports, was understood in different senses. The most common ones are—one as the veil and other, as the place where women lived. Comparisons were made between men and women and it was noted that where purdah was not in use, men were more infected than women. Lankaster (1916) tried to explain it on the basis of cultural practice, and noted—

> There are some centers where there is more consumption amongst men than amongst women. These are invariably places where purdah system is not rigorously in force and where a large number of men whether as students or because of some special local occupation are living under conditions...such men are in fact living lives comparable in this respect to those of *purdah nashin* women and suffer accordingly.[25]

The Indian women were found living in separate portion of the house where guests and male members were generally not permitted. Such private enclosures were devoid of sufficient sunlight and open air by design. They were found living in one place known as *zenana*. H. M. Crake, Health Officer of Calcutta, noted his experiences in the annual report of 1913 that, 'in no fewer than six wards it was over 40 per thousand...*these figures constitute a terrible indictment of purdah system.* Surely the women of India have a claim to demand abolition of the custom which means premature death to so many of them'.[26] The purdah system remained prevalent in India, as noticed in the report of the then DG of Indian Medical Services, Sprawson, who in 1938, said that, '...oriental countries are those due to the Purdah system and the marriage of girls at too early an age. The evil effect...tuberculosis will attack successively the several members women and children who are living in one zenana'.[27]

The prevalent purdah system was also a condition that meant adopted leisure by women, as noted in one of the reports that, '...are living under the conditions which forbid exercise, and reduce to a minimum the opportunity of being in open air'.[28] These conditions were considered the reasons for higher prevalence of consumption. The purdah system for women, that meant that women would not work and stay back home to take care of family and child, was considered in most of the reports as an oriental practice as noted by Sprawson, in 1938. However, the tradition had its origin in the Western culture as noted by Ehrenreich and English that—

She was the social ornament that proved a man's success: her idleness, her delicacy, her childlike ignorance of reality gave a man the class that money alone could not provide. And it was the very harshness of the outside world that led men to see the house as a refuge – 'a sacred place, a vestal temple' a 'tent pitched in a world not right', presided over by a gentle ethereal wife.[29]

It was not that Western society has always been like that, rather, after certain stage of accumulation of wealth this practice came into existence.[30] There was certain acceptability of such tradition in the minds of the British, who were submitting the reports. The practice of such leisure is to be limited to a certain elite section of the society who can afford it. Lankaster in his report, noted that—

> The *victims of consumption belong for the most part to the lower strata of the purdah folk*, those whose husband keep them in seclusion because it is *a mark of respectability* so to do, without having either the will or the ability to provide the open air conditions under which alone such a manner of life might be compatible with a fair degree of health.[31]

The acceptance of purdah as a mark of respectability in Indian and many other oriental societies might be a cultural diffusion of such practice by the elite of the Western society. As these reports do accept that such practices (women observing leisure during day and staying back home) were not so prevalent in rural areas. Moreover, it can be read since early years itself in various reports that it was not the 'purdah system' *per se* that was responsible for higher prevalence of consumption but the unhygienic and unsanitary living condition of the population that was responsible for the higher prevalence. In his report, H. M. Crake, the then Health Officer of Calcutta noted that—

> The potent influence of this custom is directly responsible for a great deal of insanitary property in the native quarter of the city. To secure privacy efficient lighting and ventilation are absolutely disregarded, the zenana or women's apartment is being usually the most insanitary part of the house. No wonder that tuberculosis, which thrives in damp, dark airless corners, plays havoc in the zenanas.[32]

The study of the etiology and epidemiology of the disease has highlighted that bacillus survives longer in the dark and humid corners of the house than in the open. The ideal condition for the cultivation of the bacillus was ready in each of the households and the most affected ones were the women as they stayed longer in the house. In 1913, the health officer of Calcutta noted that—'Intolerably bad as the housing conditions are in many of the slums of Calcutta, it is only when the inmates are constantly exposed to these insanitary surroundings days and nights that they suffer so severely. Amongst males who can escape during the day the rate of mortality is little more than half than amongst females'.[33]

Child marriage was another factor that was considered a reason for higher vulnerability of women to bacillus. Lankaster, in his report has noted that, 'a social custom which is only second to…in prejudicial effects upon the health of Indian women is that of child-marriage'.[34] Indian reformers did launch a campaign against the early and child marriage at different levels. However, it was widely prevalent in different parts of the country as even now rampant incidents of child marriages can well be noticed in spite of legal restrictions. Sprawson, in 1938, in his report highlighted that, 'the evils of too early marriage are seen in the undue prevalence of acute tuberculosis following childbirth or lactation. These are evils of the middle and upper classes'.[35] The reports of the doctors from different parts of the country did suggest a direct relationship between child marriage and the incidence of tuberculosis. Lankaster, during preparation of his report on tuberculosis, contacted several doctors from different parts of the country at various centres and noted in his report that—'At some of these there were upwards of 50 medical men present and at all the question of child-marriage as a contributory factor in the spread of tuberculosis came up for discussion. With only one single exception it was regarded as being a most important cause of the prevalence of the disease amongst young girls'.[36]

Child marriage is not a direct reason for the occurrence of tuberculosis but the consequences that follow used to make women more vulnerable. The consequences were noted more obviously in two ways—one, that after marriage women had to observe strict purdah, and other was that after marriage there were frequent cases of successful and unsuccessful pregnancies amongst newly wed women. The understating about the reproductivity of women and relating reproductive health with that of tuberculosis was based on the fallacious principles. Fallacy behind this was that, it was the availability of the nutrition during pregnancy that make women more vulnerable to disease than the mere use of reproductive capability.

One doctor raised another aspect—the issue of the level of exposure as the reason for higher prevalence of tuberculosis amongst women. He compared rural and urban population of the same age group and of same cultural background. Observation of the doctor, in 1916, regarding the difference in the prevalence rate of tuberculosis between rural and urban population was noted—'at the one meeting where a contrary view was expressed the one argument that was pressed was that early marriage is as frequent in villages as in towns, and yet consumption is far less common in the former'.[37] The difference between villages and towns in early 20th century can be understood in terms of lower level of exposure to the bacillus. Girls before marriage were not directed to observe purdah but immediately after marriage the seclusion was to be imposed on the women, especially the newly-wed ones. This was practiced at both the places, in towns and villages, probably more severe in villages, as villagers were more traditional. However, comparatively higher levels of exposure to the insanitary conditions in the towns were the one reason that was recognized later in various reports for women being more vulnerable in towns. Apart from this, professionals continued to accept repeated childbirth as a dominant reason for higher prevalence of the disease amongst women.

Women, who generally used to live in the back portion of the house, where there was hardly any sunlight, were found doing so religiously, especially during the period of childbirth. It was a known practice in India that during the period of childbirth and immediately after that, women are impure, and during this period of impurity they should not be seen in the open. Higher incidence of fever amongst newborn children was attributed to exposure of the children to the open air. The child and mother, therefore, needed to be protected from the exposure of the *sheetal vayu*, that is, cold wind. During the period, when mothers were weak and needed extra protection, they got an environment that was favourable to the growth of the tubercle bacillus.

The reasons, which were advanced as real for Indian situation, need further scrutiny. As discussed above, certain cultural practices were seen as a cause of higher prevalence of tuberculosis. However, it was not taken into consideration that such cultural practices might have protected the population from other diseases from time immemorial. There also is a probability that when these cultural practices were adopted, deaths and morbidity from tuberculosis was not alarming. Rather than going into the intricacies of cultural practices, it was conveniently used for 'victim blaming'. While looking at it in retrospect, one feels the need to go for critical analysis. The pertinent question in this regard would be in whose interest such 'victim blaming' was done. The other associated reason for an increase in the number of the patients can be attributed to the opening up of sanatoria in virgin locations and the introduced changes in the lifestyle of the urban and rural population due to the change in the economic structure of the country during colonial period. These factors like industrialization and sanatorium, in combination and in isolation, affected women's health in a negative manner. Cummins highlighted the effect of these aspects beautifully—'...the effects of contact with a new industry on traditional life of an agricultural or pastoral community tend to be such as to emphasize the harmful aspect of poverty, to impose new standards and desire, to diminish simplicity and content and to produce the type of psychological background which favours misery and aggravates infective processes'.[38]

The change in the lifestyle and the change in the working conditions in the urban area affected the men folk initially, and consequently the women back in the rural areas. Rural folk went to work in the industries, and returned to their village, once they were declared not fit to work. The movement of people did result in spread of diseases, like tuberculosis, as Jeffery pointed out that people travelled by railway to fairs and religious festivals were also transported some distance to work and often back again. Short-term movements probably increased the problems of controlling a number of communicable diseases.[39] Though Jeffery chose not to mention tuberculosis in these lines, nevertheless, the spread of tuberculosis in the rural areas and amongst the women of the household had been established by others.[40] These return migrants infected with the bacillus came to villages and infected the wives and mothers unintentionally. The opening up of sanatoria at virgin locations also contributed to this as the local population, especially women, came in contact with the infected person in course of the supply of the essential commodity for daily use. Women, once infected, remained confined to the household. With lower nutrition and less exposure to the open air and sunlight they became the worst sufferers. Another damning reality during colonial India was that the doctors were not permitted to examine the women patients physically. The infection seems to be transmitted to them from outside, something like STDs (Sexually Transmitted Diseases) in recent times, and the reasons often given were unhygienic conditions and unawareness. Women, otherwise, were considered as the gatekeepers of health as they were responsible for keeping the home clean and bacillus-free. They played a key role in the prevention process inside and outside the household through their function as wives and mothers inside the home, and as nurses and midwives in hospitals and sanatoriums.

The customs that were associated with women in India were found to be better explanations, even by British medical experts, who were giving different explanations in Britain. The reason may be that in India—a colony—the cultural practices needed to be corrected according to the British way; thus, the prevalent practices can be found in the books and reports of the doctors and other professionals as the reason for higher prevalence of the disease. The justification for such logic can be found in the diffusionist approach to development. Petras, using diffusionist approach, highlighted—'the diffusion theory represents a much more sophisticated rationalization for imperialist activities that the old doctrines of "manifest destiny" and "white man's burden". Yet in its final analysis, the theory underlines a form of cultural imperialism that accompanies economic imperialism'.[41]

The diffusionist approach believes that development is largely the result of the spread of certain cultural patterns and material benefits from the developed to the underdeveloped nations, and within each underdeveloped nation, a similar process of diffusion takes place from the modern to the traditional sector. In a similar way, Lankaster noted that 'the only hope of bringing a real change in the conditions obtaining amongst very poor is by first making them popular amongst those of a higher social level'.[42] Nevertheless, the accounts that were found discussed mainly about the upper and upper middle-class women.

SANATORIA FOR WOMEN

The available treatment does motivate the patient to report the symptoms. The different etiological factors called forth divergent ways of treatment. The initial treatment efforts remained limited to opening up of sanatorium and other preventive measures, as there was hardly any reliable medicine available for the treatment of the disease. Identification of the bacillus and recognition that it is an infectious disease by Koch in 1882 remained a landmark in the combat of the tuberculous disease in a scientific way. It was in 1840 that sanatorium treatment was initiated, but actual operationalization of this therapeutic means started in 1890, when confinement of the patients was thought necessary and the recuperation process required a 'change in weather'. Sanatorium treatment remained a key to tuberculosis control programmes throughout the world.

In India, too, the initial governmental and charitable efforts remained concentrated on the opening of good sanatoria in different parts of the country and their management in good hands. One such effort that shows the attitude of the then colonial government can be seen from the following address to the Madras government—

> The government of India are advised that the treatment of phthisis in the early stage of the disease in sanatoria, in which patients can receive the most minute daily attention of specially experienced physicians, affords the only hope of cure, and they believe that many *valuable lives* will be saved if suitable institutions for the treatment of tuberculous patients are established in this country.[43]

This kind of initiation was noticed often in the official correspondence of the British empire throughout the last 50 years of its operation in India. After the submission of the report by Crombie in 1899, the fact that tuberculosis in India had become widespread was almost an established fact and professionals started discussing the possible and probable combative measures. Back in Britain, the fight against tuberculosis was at its best after achieving the expected lowering in its incidence, and now the empire had to protect the life of British nationals in the colonies, outside the motherland, from tuberculosis. The concerns in various papers and reports did not get translated into action until repeated reports and resolutions from the British Congress in London exerted adequate pressure on the imperial government to take action against the menace. Once the argument was accepted that the valuable lives were to be protected, the sites for sanatoria were identified. These sites were generally located in the regions which otherwise were having low prevalence of the disease. Interestingly, some of the regions where prevalence was low were identified as most favourable for treatment of the disease due to their location.[44]

The first government sanatorium was opened only in the year 1917. Private and missionary efforts prevented the situation from getting completely out of hand. With permission from the government but without any support from it, the first sanatorium in the country was opened at Dharampore near Shimla in 1909, thanks to the keen interest of Mr Malabari of Patiala. But, after his death, the institution suffered a financial setback and by the year 1916, its future seemed bleak without more generous support.

The first important sanatorium for women was established at Tilonia, near Ajmer, under the auspices of the American Methodist Episcopal Mission, but this was limited to girls of the school and orphanage run by the mission in North India. The second important institution for women patients was initiated during the same time. This missionary-run sanatorium was established at Almora under the auspices of the London Missionary Society, but the access was again limited to Christian women only. These were two important sanatoria exclusively for women but they remained limited to a particular group of women excluding most native Indian women. Bhowali was probably the first institution set up under the provincial government's auspices, but built and financed mainly by private endowments to treat tuberculosis patients. Lankaster compared it with the best of sanatoria in the West. Apart from these, there was one sanatorium at Madanapalle in South India run by various missionary societies working in Madras and another at Lonavla near Pune. Various other institutions were in operation and were run either on a complete philanthropic basis or some, with an aim that combined profit with philanthropy. A majority of the beds were available on payment basis only, and there was no facility available in the form of open-air treatment for those people who were unable to pay the charges. There were a few seats available free of cost in Bhowali sanatorium, but the charges incurred for food and accessories, while staying in the sanatorium, were too costly and unaffordable for the common man. The argument explaining the limited number of beds for the common people was that the beds remain vacant, as the common people did not come for the treatment, because either they were ignorant about the treatment or simply were unable to pay the charges of the sanatorium. Whether beds were available or not for the common people, sanatorium came to those regions, which were suited for the treatment of the tuberculosis patients.

In India, there was no sanatorium exclusively for women where Indian women could be admitted. One was opened for European women but Indians were not permitted there. Further, Indians were against the idea of their women being admitted among the men of different origin. The upper and middle class resisted it more strongly as they would have to stay with the army personals of a different caste. The lower caste might not have such strong resistance against going to the sanatorium, but affordability was a big question. Though most of these sanatoria were philanthropic efforts, staying there meant a high cost and very few in the country could afford at that point of time.

CONCEPTION OF TUBERCULOSIS

The variation in the prevalence and the perceived reasons for higher prevalence amongst women was also an outcome of the way tuberculosis was conceptualized in India as well as elsewhere, especially in Britain. The conception of the disease in India, or for that matter anywhere in the world, varied along some of the key variables. Important among these were the causation and association factors like climate, heredity, nature of disease (that is, contagious or non-contagious), and so on., Heredity and weak immunity of individuals often becomes the prime explanation for diseases like tuberculosis. Questions of individual behaviour and social structure remained embedded in the epidemiological responses to tuberculosis before and after the discovery of tubercle bacillus. Even the test of rationality or the explanation of the cause-effect relationship also remained centred around the culpability of urban life, moral lassitude, individual action, and other individual behaviour.[45] Most important among the other explanations was the contagious character of the disease. It was this nature of the bacillus on which the everyday movement of people in the household and outside the household was dependent. Indian understanding of tuberculosis in the 19th and early 20th century was not dissimilar from that of the British understanding, as policies in India, whether economic, public, or health, were directly guided from England.

The contagious character of phthisis was known since the 16th century, but this view, and the extreme measures against the disease, died by the late 19th century, due to the unsupportive character of British physicians.[46] This affected the British attitude towards the disease and the measures that were taken to control it in the United Kingdom as well as in the colonies. They did take punitive action against the spread of other infectious and contagious diseases like syphilis. India also got affected with this situation at large, as reflected in Crombie's report of 1899, which put on record that—'Tuberculosis is a communicable disease, but it is not infectious in the popular sense of the word, in the sense in which scarlatina, mumps, and typhus fevers are infectious although the only *scientific distinction* is that the infectious material of tuberculosis is not so easily diffused, as is that of the disease named'.[47]

During the next decade or so, this view regarding the contagious nature of tuberculosis prevailed in India, as is obvious from various archival records, despite British physicians accepting the infectious nature of the disease as evident from one of the resolutions of British Congress on Tuberculosis for the Prevention of Consumptive. The resolution, passed at the general meeting on 27 July 1901, recorded 'that tuberculous sputum is the main agent for the conveyance of the virus of tuberculosis from man to man, and that indiscriminate spitting should therefore be suppressed'.[48] There were repeated requests from annual meetings of the British Congress on Tuberculosis in this regard, yet the government did not make an active effort in combating the disease or making it compulsory to notify the incidence of tuberculosis as was done in case of other diseases like cholera or plague or syphilis. Despite higher incidence amongst Europeans, the Government of India did not do much because of its conception of the disease, as even in Britain, it was only in 1913, when notification of all cases of phthisis was made mandatory. They remained skeptical about taking such measures against tuberculosis, even after the establishment of the infectious nature of the disease. Dubos attributed this inaction to different factors and put on record that this inaction was '...in part because certain physicians were not entirely convinced of the contagiousness of phthisis, in part because the strict application of the edicts was too costly, also because so many personal interests were involved'.[49]

The knowledge about tuberculosis in colonial India can not be questioned. The prime problem areas were the intervention by the state and the limitation of the colonial government in taking the appropriate measures to contain the spread of the disease and provide the therapeutic measures to the affected population.

The two dominant views regarding prevalence and spread of tuberculosis was widely debated in India as well.[50] Other factors, including habitual and customary ones, were often referred to as the causes for the infection and its spread. The various conceptions of the disease made different sections of population vulnerable in different ways. In the entire situation, women became more vulnerable. The contagious character of the disease was not considered worst, so when the male member of the family returned from the town and city, the responsibility of taking care of their ill health was on the women. Most wives and mothers unwittingly did not take appropriate precaution to prevent infection. Where the contagious character of the disease was known, the cost of meeting the preventive expenses proved deterrent. The women in Indian set-up, culturally, have been the last consumer of most of the commodities, right from food to the most needed health care facility. They remained the last to go to the doctor, and late detection does not have any treatment. Mortality amongst women remained higher.

CONCLUSIONS

The unavailability of data for the mortality and morbidity of the common population does show a kind of insensitivity. The majority of the surveys were done in the urban areas, and only a few were done in rural areas. The problem was that in rural area, the surveyors were never allowed to interact with Indian women and the male members generally reported. There was hardly any account about the situation that was prevalent amongst the lower strata of the society in India. Efforts of the British rulers towards combating tuberculosis remained confined to European men and women. Native Indians were left on charity; that too was hardly available for common rural women. Still, the key question here remains that why women remained or became more vulnerable to the bacillus, or it was the circumstances in which women's body became more susceptible to the bacillus. Accounts from different parts of the world suggests that there is no logical ground to conclude that women were more susceptible to the tubercle bacillus, though number of writings including the reports on tuberculosis during the colonial period in India argues the same. General interpretations of the Indian family system suggest that the Indian women used to be the last to eat, girls were never preferred over boys, and wives and mothers kept working even when they were unwell. These situations, in combination, meant lesser nutritional intake and higher strain for ladies of the household, even when they were generally not working outside the household, especially in the industrial sector. In India, industrialization has been identified as the major reason for the spread of the disease in the rural hinterland owing to the newly created disease network with main actors as invalidated industrial workers returning to their native land.[51] Along with industrialization, the increased movement of the patients due to improvement in transportation remained the key reason.[52] This was the condition in British India under colonial rule. The major concern of the academicians and social scientists have been that whether the situation for women in independent India improved in conception of their susceptibility of a particular disease or still they fall pray to the culture of 'victim blaming'.

NOTES

1. Imperialism—a complex ideology that had widespread intellectual, cultural, and technical expression in the era of European world supremacy, rather than a mere set of economic, political, and military phenomena. The intention of this expansion was nothing but the accumulation of wealth and the occupation, or rather exploitation of the so-called 'unclaimed' land full of mineral and other resources. There were unintended consequences also ranging from cultural amalgamation and the 'creation of disease network', which spanned the world. For details on expansion of disease and imperialism see, Watts (1999).

2. Scientific nature of the bacillus that confirmed the real cause of tuberculosis was determined only in 1890 by Robert Koch, however, the prevalence of tuberculosis in Europe by then had already declined. For details on the prevalence and the decline of it during 1854 to 1901, and the comparison of decline of the same in next 70 years, see, McKeown (1976:50–6).

3. Fairchild and Oppenheimer (1998:1105–17).

4. Medical professionals from different parts of the country during early half of the 20th century argued about the faster growth of disease in their areas; however, Director General Medical Services, as well as different reports submitted to the then Government, like Lankaster (1916), reported that disease was already rampant, only increase was in reporting such cases from different regions. For details, see, Choudhary (2008:1–4).

5. Similar arguments had been noted from different parts of the world about the way colonizers dealt with the native. '…western medical science, being part of the oppressive system, has always provoked in the native an ambivalent attitude. This ambivalence is in fact to be found in connection with the occupier's entire mode of presence. With medicine we come to one of the most tragic features of the colonial situation'. For the details of the argument, see, Fanon (1978:229–51).

6. Simpson (1897), quoted in Home/ Medical- A / No. 95 / October 1899. New Delhi: National Archive of India (NAI).

7. Hance (1947) in an address to the *Common Wealth and Empire: Health and Tuberculosis Conference*, London: National Association of Prevention of Tuberculosis (NAPT).

8. Ibid. Emphasis added.

9. The higher incidence of malaria in the filthy cities, in the wetlands, change in the working hours of population in different regions, in the regions where irrigation projects were taken up, were reported. Similarly, association

of tuberculosis was shown with that of climate, crowding, various cultural practices, and so on. For details on these aspects, see, Akhter, Dutt, and Wadhwa in Noble, A. G., Costa, F. J., Dutt, A. K., and Kent, R. B. (eds) (1998:151–68); Arnold in Scott, J. C. and Bhatt, N. (eds) (2001:186–205); Turshen (1977:55–60).

10. In common vernacular language, tuberculosis was known as 'Bengal ka Kala Jadu' meaning 'black magic of Bengal'. In Bengal, tantrik practices were popularly known as 'kala jadu'. Later on, when at an advanced stage of tuberculosis, workers who used to return from Calcutta used to look pale and sometimes vomit blood, and initially it was thought to be the outcome of black magic as the nature and cause of the disease was not known. Dubos and Dubos (1952) have referred to tuberculosis as 'white plague'.

11. The statistics were available for army, for jail, and sometimes for the population, on the basis of a survey like of Lankaster's Report of 1916. These statistics revealed that in jail, the persons who remained for longer time had higher prevalence. The limitations are like one has to think that population who are going to jails are offenders. When we look at the records of crime, what is noticed is that more of the confinement in jails was for the reported robbery of food grain. However, when at same point of time, different level of morbidity was reported from different groups, one can analyse the situation and can ascertain if they were more vulnerable or the social and political conditions were against them that made them more susceptible to the disease.

12. C.A. Sprawson, 1938, 'Peculiarities of the Tuberculosis Problem in India', The British Journal of Tuberculosis.

13. Walker (1955).

14. For details on this interaction and spread of disease, refer to Choudhary (2008 a).

15. For details, see, Lankaster (1916); Sprawson (1938).

16. Lankaster (1916).

17. Crombie (1899).

18. Lankaster (1916).

19. Ibid.,

20. Azell Ames (1875) quoted in Ehrenreich and English in J. Ehrenreich (ed.) (1978).

21. The higher rate of infection amongst the poets, novelists, and so on, has been seen as the disease goes to those who are emotional, and women were considered more of an emotional being than a rational being. It is another fact that the so-called emotional identity of the women was also created by the then male dominant society, especially the middle class that could afford a non-working wife who was only supposed to protect her beauty and fertility. For more details on this refer, Ehrenreich (ed.) (1978) and Dubos and Dubos (1952).

22. Ehrenreich (1978:127).

23. Home/ Medical- A / No. 95 (October 1899)

24. Sprawson (1938).

25. Lankaster (1916).

26. Ibid., (emphasis added).

27. Sprawson (1938).

28. Lankaster (1916).

29. Ehrenreich and English (1978:122–4).

30. The withdrawal of elderly and children from the labour force is considered a characteristic of economic advancement; the same was true for women in the 19th century when their leisure was considered as status. Otherwise, there were phases when women worked in factories and fields in Western society as well—'This was a period of America's industrial revolution, a revolution base on the ruthless exploitation of working people. Women and children as young as six worked fourteen-hour days in factories and sweatshops for subsistence wages', Ibid., p. 123.

31. Lankaster (1916). Emphasis added.

32. Health officer quoted in Ibid.

33. Quoted in Ibid.

34. Ibid.

35. Sprawson (1938).

36. Lankaster (1916:70).

37. The doctor quoted in Ibid.

38. Cummins (1932) Health, No. 79/32 – H, 1932.

39. Jeffery (1988).

40. For the details of the spread of disease in India, see, Choudhary (2008 a).

41. J. Petras, quoted in Berberoglu (1992:13).

42. Lankaster (1916:74).

43. Home / Medical –A/ May 1912 / No. 40-64. Emphasis added.

44. Lankaster op. cit. (1916).

45. Armstrong (1983).

46. Muthu (1922:4).

47. Home / Medical-A / No. 95 (October 1899). Emphasis added.

48. Home / Medical-A / No. 96-103 / October 1901, New Delhi: NAI.

49. Dubos and Dubos (1952:30).

50. According to the first, 'the seed make soil—the constitutional diathesis is the result of bacterial infection' that is dependent on the constitutional character of the human body, while according to the latter, 'the strumous or scrofulous diathesis was a primary condition which instead of being caused by the toxin of tuberculin bacillus was the result of bad living and poor nutrition'. For details on this, see, Muthu (1922).

51. Author has dealt with in detail the newly created disease network and the outcome of it. See, Choudhary (2008).

52. Haggett (1990:95); Jeffery (1988).

11 Negotiating Subalternity in Everyday Life

Social Construction of Tuberculosis in Colonial and Post-colonial India

ARABINDA SAMANTA[†]

In this chapter, the term 'subaltern' is employed to convey a limited meaning. It essentially relates to a social category, which is primarily informed by classes other than the more entrenched and dominant ones. This may amount to a position of de-elitization of history, but more appropriately, it negotiates a story of the 'other'. Moreover, the idiom of 'rebellion' or 'defiance', which is celebrated in the subaltern perception with much fanfare, is not conceived in this construction of subalternity.[1] In fact, the study seeks to situate tuberculosis, 'the disease of civilization', in an appropriate Indian societal situation, and view the ailment from multiple sites, keeping in mind the process of 'othering'.

The study will indeed approach the history of tuberculosis on four levels. In the first section, it will seek to present an epidemiological biography of the disease, followed by an analysis of the reasons behind its emergence as a 'modern epidemic' in the late 19th and early 20th century. It will also examine the ways contemporary medical practitioners perceived the causes of the malady. Globally speaking, four etiological models appeared to have dominated the medical thinking in this context—(a) theories that emphasized contagion; (b) those which attributed the cause

[†] The author wishes to express his gratitude to the Wellcome Trust Centre for the History of Medicine at UCL, for giving him adequate financial support to work on this chapter at British Library, London.

to physiological disorders; (c) those which found the origin in hereditary predispositions; and (d) those theories, which observed a link with
behaviour and lifestyles.[2] The study will show how one of these theories—the hereditary theory—eventually triumphed over the others and
became the dominant for the better part of the 19th century. It would
also argue that while the disease was endemic to the country from earliest
times, it became epidemic only after the country began to industrialize in
the early 20th century. Mortality from tuberculosis began to rise in about
1880, but the disease really took off between 1900 and 1919, when India's
textile, jute, mining, and other industries began to show off. And finally,
the moot question is how did the people, as also the patient, perceive this
disease? What was the response of the society at large? Larger than this is
the crucial question—how did the sick tend to evaluate a doctor?

The study would also consider the community, sex, and age incidence
of the disease. Taking the community incidence, the disease is found to
have been rather more frequent among the Muslims than in Hindus in
proportion to their relative numbers in the total post-mortem records.
On examining the frequency in the two sexes of either community, it
appears that the greater incidence of tuberculosis was among the females than in males, and that this feature was especially marked among
Muslims. The question is why was it so? Was it because of the well known
less open-air, out-of-doors life of females than males in India, which was
more particularly the case among Muslim women, shut up in the too
frequently ill-ventilated zenanas? There had been an impression at the
beginning of the 20th century that pulmonary phthisis was a disease
from which old people were practically exempt. But one is surprised to
see in India the large number of cases admitted amongst people above
the age of 50. Was it symptomatic of a process of long-term malnutrition
perpetrated by an exacting colonial power?

Contrary to what Dr A Crombie, Indian Medical Service (IMS), argued in 1899 at the International Congress on Tuberculosis in Berlin,
that tuberculosis was rarely found in India, we have evidences to believe
that the killer disease was not only present in the country during the first
50 years under the Raj, but in fact, increased its intensity by the opening
decades of the 20th century. But the moot question is what exactly was
the rate of mortality? Contemporary statistical evidences vary so much
so that it is extremely difficult to arrive at a reasonable estimate. The
study would therefore seek to compute the proportion of active and

latent tuberculosis disease in Bengal from the Calcutta Medical College Hospital's earliest post-mortem records, as is left to us by Dr Leonard Rogers, comprising 2,783 medical and 558 surgical autopsies.[3]

Again, of the miscellaneous classes, the highest incidence appears to be amongst the sweeper class. The other classes among whom the disease is most prevalent are the goldsmiths, tailors, carpenters, tea sorters, and the Gurkhas. Does it have anything to do with the nature of their job? Or does it indicate an approximation of the two proximate categories of disease and subalternity? As regards age incidence, the largest number of patients was between the ages of 26 and 30, and children between the ages of 1 and 5 furnish the fewest admission.

At a different level, the focus will also be shifted to other regions of Asia, Europe, sub-Saharan Africa, and the US, and a comparison would be instituted to comprehend the differential perceptions of the disease at different cultural zones. Experiences from other parts of the globe indicate that the disease appeared with vengeance in the wake of industrialization, or closely associated with an accelerated process of urbanization. For the last 400 years, the disease was arguably spread by European empire building, colonization, and crowding in the European cities. India in the 19th century had hardly experienced any industrialization, nor did she embark on a course of colonization. But the disease assumed an alarming proportion in India during the colonial period. How would we explain this phenomenon?

Finally, tuberculosis has, roughly speaking, three stages, namely, phthisis, consumption, and tuberculosis. Admittedly, each stage has its own meanings and characteristics. In the second stage consumption, tuberculosis was thought to be responsible for the patient's beauty and creativity.[4] This kind of romanticization can be seen both in the West and East, not only in literature but also in paintings. The question is what about the Indian experiences? The present chapter would therefore arguably seek to explore how the proliferation of tuberculosis and the consequent medical intervention had been interrogated, interpreted, understood, and constructed in the context of people's collective imagination and cultural tradition.

Diseases have indeed had a salubrious effect on contemporary Western historiography. In the past 20 years, a 'germ school' of public health history has followed Charles E. Rosenberg's *The Cholera Years* (1987). Books like Allan Brandt's (1987) study of syphilis[5] and Sheila M. Rothman's (1994) account of tuberculosis[6] have brought to bear the notion of 'social construction' of disease to perceive how the people of the West understood, coped with, and even tried to prevent various infectious diseases.[7] The emergence of such a school of public health historians in the past 15 years has, of course, legitimized the recognition that infectious disease still poses a major threat to public health, which needs to be informed by our historical experiences.

In contrast to the abundant crop of scholarship now available on the social history of disease in Africa, Europe, and North America, disease in South Asian history remains a relatively less addressed agenda. Again, despite widespread prevalence of epidemic diseases in India during the entire colonial period, we still lack a comprehensive biography of any epidemic disease and its social consequences.[8] Though we have a few monographs on some of the epidemics—malaria, cholera, plague, smallpox,[9] and so on, tuberculosis, the country's national peril and a veritable 'scourge of Bengal', is yet to find a social historian to tell its tale in a proper historical perspective. Mark Harrison and Michael Worboys' study, though otherwise extremely useful, concentrates by and large on a comparative analysis of the British, African, and Indian situations, and that too, for a relatively shorter temporal space of three decades.[10] And as such, a social history of tuberculosis in colonial and post-colonial India still remains an important desideratum.

BIOGRAPHY OF THE DISEASE

Mortality

Before streptomycin was discovered in 1945, outbreaks of tuberculosis (TB) were responsible for the destruction of the greatest number of people in history. TB has existed from the very dawn of civilization. Records of TB in mummies were found in Egypt as far back as 5,000 years ago.[11] Although considered by many to be less aggressive than smallpox, bubonic plague, and leprosy, TB is responsible for the largest number of deaths in history. It is estimated that one billion people were destroyed by TB in the last two centuries.[12] Known as 'consumption', an appropriate name for this destructive process in the lungs, TB was observed to have passed on from one member of the family to another and from one worker to another in crowded European plants. Before discovery of the cause of TB, it was suspected that particles of sputum ejected into the atmosphere by 'open' cases of TB were likely to be aspirated by healthy individuals. Many conditions were thought to be responsible for TB—one was a familial 'weakness'; another was the mythical explanation of 'predisposition'—these were accepted as reality.[13] The tragedy of TB, apart from the fact that it destroyed large numbers of people, was that the disease frequently affected young adults in the prime of their lives. Greek historian, Herodotus, expressed the situation very poignantly when he said—'In the time of plague it is the parents who bury their children'.[14] The young would depart long before they were able to make a contribution to the society.

Koch's discovery, in 1882, that the cause of TB was a bacterial infection, and the subsequent findings that tiny globules of secretion expelled from lung cavities contained live bacteria, solved the mystery of the 'epidemic spread of consumption' among crowded sections of the European population. Obligatory isolation of patients with TB was instituted only in the last century. Notwithstanding numerous remedies proffered by physicians over the millennia, there was no definite treatment for TB. Fortunately, natural resistance to TB contamination prevented development of clinical disease in the majority of individuals in the Western population. About 20 per cent of patients who contracted active TB would recover spontaneously from the illness with the help of natural resistance. The majority of patients with TB, before antibiotics, would be at the mercy of the advancing disease. Before the discovery of artificial pneumotherapy and thoracoplasty, the patients with advancing disease merely languished, awaiting death.

In India, TB appears to have been prevalent from the Vedic civilization. Indian medical records, as old as the second millennium B.C., contain directions for diagnosis of the disease based on symptoms; we have also evidences of therapies based on herbs, metals, minerals, and the general managements of daily life.[15] Nevertheless, the ailment in all probability had never assumed an alarming proportion. Prior to the year 1840, we do not find much mention made regarding the existence of TB and phthisis pulmonalis among the indigenous population of India. In 1844 and 1845, Dr W. A. Green proved the existence of phthisis among the indigenous inhabitants of Howrah and Midnapore.[16] In 1845, Dr Edward Goodeve made similar observations among the people frequenting the civil hospital and dispensary at Cawnpore.[17] Dr Allan Webb recorded in 1848 that he had diagnosed phthisis among the Hindu *paharrees* (hill men), and at Burdwan in Lower Bengal.[18]

But during the second half of the 19th century, the picture drastically changed. TB appeared with vengeance, and it took an alarming proportion. In 1856, Dr Morehead related his experiences of phthisis at the European General Hospital, Bombay, from 1838 to 1853, and among the 'natives' admitted into the Jamsetjee Jejeebhoy Hospital, Bombay, from 1848 to 1853.[19] In the former, the admissions amounted to 184, with 79 deaths, while in the latter, to 445 with 268 deaths.[20] From 1857 to 1867, 454 cases occurred among the indigenous people treated in the Calcutta Medical College Hospital, of whom 285 died. In many of these cases, the history has pointed to repeated recurrences of malarial fever, with enlargement of the spleen, resulting in confirmed anaemia.

Some of the doctors with Indian Medical Service in the colonial government, however, tried to shout down the best arguments in some of the findings of their own officials. Dr A. Crombie is a case in point. At the International Congress on Tuberculosis in Berlin in 1899, Dr A. Crombie submitted a report on the prevalence of the disease in India in which he asserted that it was quite rarely met in 'natives' of this country as compared with temperate climate. Only three per cent of the deaths, he argued, which had been inquired into in the province of Bengal, had been returned as due to phthisis.

During the 1920s, there had been a widespread impression among the medical men that TB was rapidly spreading in the country. By 1920, Lankester had adduced numerous evidences from the statements of medical men in various parts of India about the increased incidence of the disease during his laborious enquiry undertaken several years ago.[21] It became evident that the disease was chiefly urban in its distribution, for the frequency of the infection or spread of this disease depended on whether the people lived huddled together under bad hygienic condition in towns or were well separated to avoid repeated or massive inoculations from source of infection.[22] This was the reason, argued A. C. Ukil in 1826, why nomadic people rarely and the inhabitants of thinly populated rural areas less frequently got it. A few decades ago, it was argued, the disease was practically unknown in the rural areas and was much less prevalent than now even in urban areas in this country, as had been shown by Lankaster from evidences of medical men all over India.[23] It was popularly believed that the vitality of the race was at a much lower level then than it was 50 years ago, and that TB, like many other diseases, was increasing by leaps and bounds.

Statistical Evidence

The death rate from TB, chiefly of the lungs, was 2–3 per cent in the cities of Calcutta, Madras, and Bombay. The following comparison (Table 11.1) of deaths from TB speaks for itself—

Table 11.1   Comparison of Deaths from Tuberculosis

	Year			
Towns	1904	1919	1921	1924
Calcutta	1608	1889	NA	2232
Madras	348	1309	NA	NA
Bombay	3548	2780	NA	NA
Karachi	NA	210	223	447
Bengal	NA	NA	4055	5577

Notes: NA = not available

Source: Ukil, A. C. (1926) 'The Problem of contacting Tuberculosis in India', The Calcutta Medical Journal, Vol. XXI, No. 5, p.216.

However, one can hardly judge the exact situation from the statistical returns for the simple reason that the methods of registration of diseases were more often than not faulty. For instance, a large number of cases returned as 'fever' had been found to be really due to TB. Dr Rogers once found 9 per cent of such deaths to be really due to TB.[24] Dr U. N. Brahmachari found 10.8 per cent of cases returned as 'fever' to be due to TB. Bentley thought that in rural districts of Bengal, as many as 5–35 per cent of deaths registered as 'fever' was really due to phthisis.[25] If we take over 10 per cent from the number of annual deaths from 'fever' in Bengal (a little over 900,000), the figure for deaths from TB in Bengal comes to 90,000, whereas the Sanitary Commissioner's Reports register the figure somewhere between 5,000 and 6,000. The health officer to the city of Calcutta estimated the total number of men suffering at any given time to be five times the number of deaths.[26] This is perhaps arguably too low an estimate and the number would probably be more than double. From information elicited from the District Health Officers in various places, it seems that in the 1920s there were over 200,000 open cases, that is, discharging tubercle bacilli, of lungs tuberculosis in Bengal alone.[27]

From an analysis of 3,300 post-mortem reports of cases that died in one of the biggest hospitals in India, Calcutta Medical College Hospital, Sir Leonard Rogers, Professor of Pathology, Medical College, Calcutta, had shown the disease was more prevalent among the Muslims, goldsmiths, tailors, carpenters, tea sorters, and the Gurkhas.[28] The disease was spreading rapidly among the lower middle class in towns. It was also increasing among mill hands but seemed to be rare in boatmen in rivers. In 1904, Dr Rogers had enquired into the causes of deaths attributed to 'fevers' in Dinajpur, which constituted 90 per cent of the total deaths.[29] He obtained clear histories of phthisis in 9 per cent, which he believed must have been an underestimate of the total mortality of this disease.

The great mortality produced by TB was also well brought out by the post-mortem records of the Calcutta Medical College, in spite of accommodation being available for only a very limited number of suitable cases applying for admission. In the earliest Medical College Hospital records, even before the epoch-making discovery of tubercle bacillus by Koch, cases of phthisis were returned in two classes, namely, tubercular, and non-tubercular. Perusing through the records of Medical Series from September 1886 to September 1906, comprising 2,783 cases, it appears that *active* tubercle during the period amounted to 18.3 per cent and *latent* old tubercle 7.2 per cent, the total of all forms being 25.5 per cent. The Surgical Series comprising 558 autopsies indicate that *active* tubercle, including phthisis, was present in 10.2 per cent cases. In the Combined Series *all* forms of active tubercle amounted to 17 per cent.[30]

The striking figures reveal the terrible prevalence of tubercular disease among the indigenous people of Bengal who formed about 95 per cent of the post-mortem subjects. Thus, no less than 17 per cent of the total deaths were from tubercular diseases, or if only the medical series are taken, which more truly represent Calcutta deaths, the figure rises to 18.3 per cent. Further, 7.2 per cent more shows old latent tubercle in the lungs, making a total of 25 per cent of the whole being found to be tubercular. The frequency of latent or healed tubercle in the lungs is of great interest, if only as showing that the early stages of the disease may commonly be recovered from even in Bengal.

The subjects of old tubercle included a considerably larger proportion of persons over 40 years of age than either the total number of cases or the active tubercular series. They were also considerably less frequent in females than in males, in proportion to the relative numbers of each, namely, 17.7 per cent of old tubercle against 28.5 per cent of recent Ptubercle among females. This might well be connected with Indian females being more shut up in their houses than males, with consequently less of open air, which was so essential to the recovery from this disease. The extreme rarity of recovered tubercle in Muslim women bears out this view, only two such instances being met with out of 92 recoveries in Dr Rogers' observation.

Race and Sex Incidence

The prevalence of TB among the Hindus and the Muslims has been worked out for each sex, and the results are compared with those of 1,040 post-mortem subjects in three volumes, selected as illustrative of different decades.

Taking the community incidence, the disease is found to have been rather more frequent in Muslims than in Hindus, in proportion to their relative numbers in the total post-mortem. On examining the frequency in the two sexes of either community, it appears that the slightly greater prevalence in Muslims is entirely due to the exceptionally high incidence of tubercle among Muslim females; 25.0 per cent of the disease in this community having been in females, although only 15 per cent of the total Muslim subjects belonged to that sex. Among the Hindus, there was a similar, although less marked, excess among the females, namely, 29.8 per cent against 26.0 per cent of total subjects. On combining the two communities it appears that tubercle was found in 28.5 per cent among females, against 23.5 per cent of subject of that community.[31] The striking feature of Table 11.2, then, is the greater incidence of tubercle among females than in males of the Indians; this feature being specially marked among Muslims. These facts are in accordance with the well known less open-air, out-of-doors life of females than males in India, which was more particularly the case among Muslim women, shut up in the too frequently ill-ventilated zenanas.

Dr G. A. Harris, Professor of Materia Medica, Medical College, Calcutta, argued that of 666 cases of TB admitted to his wards since 1900, the males largely outnumbered the females (469 to 197).[32] Europeans and Anglo-Indians taken together, numbered 235, and Hindus 281, Muslims 105, and Indian-Christians 45. Of the total, 539 had been discharged as relieved, and 135 had died.[33] If it be permissible to draw any conclusion from these figures, it would appear that the conditions

Table 11.2   Race and Sex Incidence

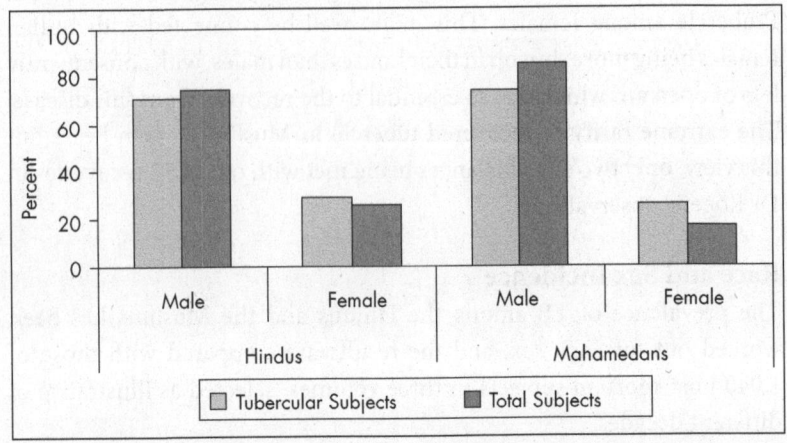

Source: 'Gleanings from the Calcutta Post-Mortem Records: II. The Incidence of Tuberculosis Disease in Bengal'. Rogers, Leonard in *Indian Medical Gazette*, February 1909.

favourable to the development of phthisis among Hindus on the one hand, and Europeans-Indians, Anglo-Indians taken together on the other hand, were about identical, while the disproportionately large incidence among the Muslims was noticeable.

Occupation of Patients

Dr Harris observed that 34.5 people followed no occupation at all, 19.2 were of the coolie class, and 19.2 were of the clerical class.[34] Of the miscellaneous classes, the highest incidence appears to be among the sweeper class, and when considered their careless and filthy habits, one is only surprised that they do not show a higher percentage of incidence. However, contemporary vernacular literary tracts indicate that office-bearers, peons, *chaprasis*, *durwans*, hotel-boys, *bawarchis*, motorcar drivers, rickshaw or cart-pullers, sepoys in the police force, food-venders, *goalas*, dhobis, factory-workers, prostitutes, and slum-dwellers were the most frequent victims.[35]

Age Incidence

The distribution of tubercle among the Indians in each decade is shown in Table 11.3, together with those 1,040 cases of all kinds, for comparison. Further, the ages of those dying of other diseases, in which old latent tubercle of the lungs was found, have also been given, as they differed considerably from those of active tubercle.

On comparing lines 2 and 3 of the above table, it will be seen that tubercular diseases were met with at all periods of life, but 61.5 per cent of the deaths took place between the ages of 20 and 40 years, being in much the same proportion as the deaths from all causes in those two decades. On the other hand, fatal tubercle was relatively more frequent up to 20, and less so after 40 years. The later partial immunity might possibly be due to earlier weeding out of the most susceptible subjects, and to some

Table 11.3   Age Incidence of Active and Latent Tubercle

	Age					
	0–20	21–30	31–40	41–50	51–60	Over 60
Old Latent tubercle	28.6	23.9	22.9	25.9	15.3	3.3
Active Tubercle	20	36.7	28.3	9.5	3.6	1.8
Total Subjects	15.8	36	25.5	15.3	6	1.4

Source: 'Gleanings from the Calcutta Post-Mortem Records: II. The Incidence of Tuberculosis Disease in Bengal'. Rogers, Leonard in *Indian Medical Gazette*, February 1909.

degree of acquired immunity in those who had recovered from attacks of the disease.[36]

Dr Harris's observations also corroborate the above statements. As regards age incidence, Dr Harris argues, the largest numbers of patients were between the ages of 26 and 30, and children between the ages of 1 and 5 furnished the fewest admissions, as one would expect with a chronic disease like pulmonary phthisis.

The most outstanding feature of the table is that it demonstrates that the largest number of cases admitted amongst people are above the age of 50, as there was a prevalent impression that pulmonary phthisis is a disease from which old people were practically exempt.

NEGOTIATING THE DISEASE OF CIVILIZATION
Between 1882, the year of the discovery of the tubercle bacillus by Robert Koch, and 1900, Indian medical fraternity had been very occasionally publishing papers on the subject. But the problem of prevention of TB in Bengal does not seem to have informed them adequately until the

early years of the 20th century. It was thought that TB was essentially an urban ailment, rampant among all classes of people in Calcutta, that

Table 11.4   Age Incidence of Tuberculosis Spread over Years

Age Group	1900	1901	1902	1903	1904	1905	1906	1907	1900–1907
1–5	0	0	1	0	0	0	1	1	3
6–10	1	1	1	0	3	1	1	1	9
11–15	3	5	4	4	5	5	3	4	33
16–20	12	11	10	10	11	10	12	7	83
21–25	13	23	11	14	14	12	15	15	117
26–30	16	22	22	13	25	25	10	14	146
31–35	9	18	8	6	11	9	2	16	79
36–40	8	6	6	8	10	7	6	6	57
41–45	2	13	4	6	4	5	11	6	51
46–50	2	6	6	1	3	6	2	5	31
51 and above	9	12	5	3	8	6	6	8	57
Total	75	117	78	65	94	85	69	83	666

Source: Harris, G. A. 1908, 'Tuberculosis Disease in India', *Indian Medical Gazette*, Vol. XLIV, p. 41.

approximately 10 per cent of the total deaths were due to TB, and that the prevalence of this disease was far more than that of any of the purely tropical diseases.[37]

From the post-mortem records of the latent and healed TB, as provided by Rogers and Pilgrim in 1909, it was considered that 'under proper conditions of treatment in the sanatorium in the early stages, the prevailing rate of mortality could be largely prevented'.[38] Towards the early part of 1909, the Medical Section of the Asiatic Society of Bengal took a prominent part in addressing the TB problem from various viewpoints. We also find a reference in the old records that Maharajadhiraj Bahadur of Burdwan suggested to the Government in 1908 that a sanatorium should be established for the benefit of members of the poor middle classes suffering from TB and other diseases, and himself offered a contribution of Rs One lakh towards its expenses. Sir Andrew Fraser, the Lieutenant Governor of Bengal, sympathized with the scheme and appointed a committee to consider it. The Committee tentatively selected Shimultala as the most suitable site for the proposed sanatorium, and had a plan and an estimate of cost prepared. Apart from the land, the cost of the building and equipment was estimated at Rs 1,85,000, and maintenance charges at Rs 14,000 per annum. Major Deane and Rev Hearn suggested Hazaribag, and Major Calvert suggested Kalimpong, as likely places for the sanatorium treatment of pulmonary TB.[39] In 1909, however, it was decided by the Government that the financial position did not permit of the project being given effect to and it was accordingly dropped.

Therapeutic Intervention: The Birth of a Clinic

In 1918, a young medical student from Bengal fell a victim to pulmonary TB in London and was sent back home for treatment. Unfortunately, he did not survive; but it was at his instance and at the suggestion of his physician, Dr B. C. Roy, that he made a bequest of his property for the establishment of a TB sanatorium in Bengal, or failing such an institution, the investment of the property by Calcutta University for the purpose of founding a scholarship for research in TB. This benefactor was Sri Provash Chandra Ghosh. The property bequeathed, amounting to Rs 1,75,000, made over to Calcutta Medical Aid and Research Society (CMARS). CMARS opened the first TB hospital in Bengal at Jadavpur, with four patients, in the year 1923.[40]

Origin and Growth of the Tuberculosis Association of Bengal

By the beginning of the 20th century, it was believed by the medical fraternity in Bengal that TB was chiefly spread by intimate personal and family contact, and that a multiplicity of interacting causes, such as ignorance, poverty, low hygienic standards of living, inadequate and bad housing, adverse industrial condition, unfavourable social environment, and some specificities of cultural geography tended to operate in determining the incidence of disease in a community. The task of checking the spread of such a ubiquitous disease, it was believed, would be stupendous without state aid. But the matter of starting the Tuberculosis Association of Bengal for the study and prevention of TB was rather an accident than the outcome of a long-thought-out plan.[41]

Early in November 1928, two American ladies took Dr A. C. Ukil to see another American lady who was suffering from advanced lung TB, and who died within a few days under very tragic circumstances. The pathos and tragedy of her life made such an indelible impression on one of the

ladies, Mrs Campbell Forrester, who had previous anti-tuberculosis training that she made up her mind to work for the cause. On 28 November
1928, she invited half a dozen men and women to confer on the problem
of tuber prevention in the province. A committee was soon formed with
the Governor of Bengal as President, and Dr C. A. Bentley, the Director
of Public Health, as its first Chairman. This American lady became its
first Honorary Secretary and organizer, and soon mobilized a band of
earnest workers to help in furthering the scheme. The Association was
founded in January 1929.

Even by the 1930s, it can be noticed that a province, with a population of
4.6 crore, could boast of only one TB hospital with 139 beds.[42] A scheme for
establishing a climatic sanatorium for the province was formulated in 1935.
A Government Committee was set up to select a suitable place, and the
entire capital expenditure of the scheme amounting to about Rs three lakh
was obtained from a Marwari philanthropist. The Committee unanimously
selected a site in the Kalimpong hills, but for some reasons not adequately
explained, the Government cold-shouldered the scheme. But a small beginning had been made by the authority of the CMARS in establishing in 1937
a small sanatorium for non-pulmonary and convalescent pulmonary cases
at Kalimpong, in the Darjeeling district, with a provision of 25 patients.

In 1946, the country's needs for health management were assessed
by the Bhore Committee and subsequently by the Mudaliar Committee. But at that time, the TB problem as a public health problem was
ignored. With Independence, in the late 40s, there was a realization that
large areas of the country were deprived of basic health services. Though
the development plans of this period were extensive, appropriate, and
interrelated, Bengal, by the 1950s, could boast of a provision of 2,550
beds for more than 40,000 tubercular patients. Of these, Kanchrapara
TB Hospital housed 275 beds and still another 250 beds were earmarked
for TB patients migrated from East Bengal.[43] Subsequently, the National
Tuberculosis Programme (NTP) and other health programmes were
initiated. The NTP was formulated in 1961 by the National Tuberculosis
Institute (NTI), which was established for this purpose. The programme,
based on a large number of studies, was to serve the community by
providing diagnostic and treatment facilities throughout the country,
through government health services. But in the mid-1970s, due to several
socio-political compulsions faced by the country, the achievements of
the NTP fell far from expectations.[44]

TUBERCULOSIS AND SUBALTERNITY

One can argue that TB reflects in microcosm an inverse relationship between the hygienic and sanitary standard of a people and the disease incidence. When this standard sinks at the bottom, the body resistance of the population is also lowered, and the incidence of the disease tends to reach its nadir. This expresses itself more acutely in the occurrence and spread of infectious diseases. Of these, TB is perhaps more intimately related to the social and economic condition of a people than others. We know today that every infectious disease is a matter of contestation between the soil or body resistance and the virulence and numerical strength of the disease, the germs, or seeds.

In the West, one of the most important social factors behind the high TB mortality rate during the last century was the rapid rise in urbanization.[45] In Sweden, during periods of intense migration to a town, the TB mortality rate increased. In general, the TB mortality rate increased during the 1870s, and subsequently decreased slowly. There is a clear indication that pulmonary TB was the greatest killer in the poorer areas, and particularly so in the areas of the poor houses. Where the negative factors, like poor housing, sub-standard nutrition, poor hygiene, followed in the wake of a rapid industrialization, the towns with a high proportion of industrial workers were hit much harder, especially those located in areas with a generally high TB level.

By the beginning of the 20th century, Indian doctors used to believe that the following factors usually contribute to lowering of the body resistance—(a) Unhealthy home conditions, which include an insanitary home and its surrounding, and unhealthy habits of the inmates; (b) Impure air; (c) Dust, dirt, and dang; (d) Absence of sunshine; (e) Defective and insufficient dietary, especially with regard to fats, protein, and vitamins; (f) Defective dietary during infancy and childhood; (g) Defective school hygiene; (h) Unhealthy occupations; (i) Incidence of certain infectious diseases, especially those involving the lungs, for example, influenza, pneumonia, repeated respiratory catarrh, malaria, diabetes, *kalazaar*, asthma, and so on; (j) Drink indulgence, and; (k) A bad economic and social environment.[46] If an individual, it was argued by the 20s of the last century, whose body resistance had been lowered by one or more of the above causes was exposed to a source of contagion, that is, an individual who was discharging tubercle bacilli to the exterior, he was himself infected by repeated inhalations of tubercle infected dust or sputum.[47] TB, it was concluded, was a 'disease of civilization', which was prevalent chiefly in thickly populated and inadequately housed towns and cities with a bad sanitary environment. Tubercle bacilli, it was argued, did not exist everywhere; they existed in places where there were open cases of TB. It was spread to villages by people who went back to the country after being infected in towns, the usual endemic spots, where they had come in quest of business, situation, money, or study.[48]

This observation has been further corroborated by more recent researches all over the globe. A sample survey, for instance, was conducted in January-February 1968, in the railway colonies of West Bengal, to determine the 'Sociological Tuberculogenic Factors' that were responsible for the growth and spread of TB in the population. The sample studied was found to be representative of the general population. The trend and behaviour of disease was dependent on the relevant standard of living (separate colonies were built for officers, upper subordinates, and other categories with wide difference in social conditions), working conditions, habits, and social evils such as alcohol consumption and *ganja* (illicit drug) smoking. The incidence of disease was more rampant amongst the low-paid categories and was inversely related to the group's income.[49]

It has been observed that most of the TB cases in rural community in India were at least conscious of the symptoms of the disease, about three-fourths of them seemed worried about their sickness, and about half of them actively sought treatment for their symptoms at rural medical institutions.[50] Traditional wisdom ordained that TB occurring in an individual had always been an interruption in life—physically, psychologically, and economically as well as socially. Indeed, when the diagnosis was first divulged to a patient seemingly having an ordinary cough and/ or fever, a sudden psychological trauma did occur. Even today there are plentiful conceptions in public minds. Tuberculosis causes social stigma and results in adverse psychological reactions.[51] It also entails a higher degree of neuroticism and psychosexual disturbances.[52] Many patients have guilt feeling, helplessness, loss of self-esteem, apathy, and jealousy towards others due to interaction of complex psychological factors. During hospitalization, s/he may react emotionally to the illness in a way, which may be fatal during the first episode of the illness.[53]

A number of factors—cultural, social, political, economic, and technical—seem to have informed the nature of society's response to

TB. In 1997, a study was conducted at the Rajan Babu TB Hospital in New Delhi to find out the emotional problems encountered by hospitalized patients.[54] Out of 550 patients, 300, or 60 per cent, were in the age group of 20–40 years, comprising of 366 (73.2 per cent) males, 306 (61.2 per cent) illiterates, and only 16 (3.2 per cent) educated up to higher secondary. Socio-economic profile was that 60.4 per cent of the patients came from upper lower middle class, 12.8 per cent from lower middle class, and 6.4 per cent from upper middle class. No patient belonged to upper class. The results revealed that 59.6 per cent patients lost their self-esteem, which is the borderline of depression, followed by 16.3 per cent with apathy towards the world, and 15.9 per cent had the desire to commit suicide. The loss of self-esteem was found to be more prevalent among those in the age group of 30–50 years (60.53 per cent), while the desire to commit suicide was more common in older age groups. With regard to emotional reactions of self-avoidance of social gathering, 310 (63.5 per cent) patients said that they avoid going to the parties themselves. This trend was more common among those in the age group of 20–40 years (61.9 per cent). Feeling of loneliness and of being ignored by the family members was experienced by 12.5 per cent of respondents.

LIVING IN THE SHADOW OF DEATH: SOCIAL RESPONSE TO TUBERCULOSIS

While the medical history of diseases such as TB has been fairly well documented, the patients' experience hasn't been. The mythologies of consumption, created by such literary figures as Keats and Kafka, Chopin and Thomas Mann conveyed the impression that consumption was experienced as something beautifully tragic. However, once the bacteriological theory was gradually accepted, the new understanding of the condition as contagious and communicable routinely worked to stigmatize patients, particularly the poor. 'TB is a good respectable disease', noted Henry Sewall, a Denver physician, in 1904, 'if you have money, but without it, it is a mean low-down business'.[55] While interrogating TB and social experience of illness in American history, Sheila M. Rothman approximates it as living in the shadow of death.[56] In Britain, perceptions of the character of TB changed between 1940 and 1970, following the application of new medical technologies and investigative methods in the diagnosis and tracing of the disease. Recent writings conclude that the new techniques replaced the old romanticized image of TB as a disease of youth with one centred on children and the old.[57] People of Ghana have had a general superstitious belief as also a negative perception that TB is caused by witchcraft.[58] More recently, however, the government officials are exhorting to do away with such beliefs and resort to more scientific treatment—to eat fruits and vegetables and take balanced diet to improve their nutritional status, and to keep their environment clean to avoid infectious diseases. All these shifts suggest that diseases change names, they change meanings, and they even change culture as well.[59]

Coming back to our specific study area, one can notice that in the historical trajectory of tubercular disease in India, little inter-faith dialogue did exist between the patient and the physician. The parties concerned hardly switched sides. The patient had his own notion of the disease, informed by certain value-laden cultural specificities. And the doctor had his own project of therapeutic intervention, premised on the recently discovered technique of recovery. The society, on its part, believed that its rigorously idealized self-image of TB was about to be subverted by the technology-driven intervention; a veritable re-run of the way in which the systematizing claims of science once circumscribed the authority of the church during the smallpox, cholera, and plague epidemics in eastern India.

In fact, mere mention of the word 'tuberculosis' caused widespread public alarm, and people in general would fight sight of a tubercular patient. People would therefore take utmost care not to get it divulged and try hard to conceal the disease. Vomiting blood was believed to be the surest indication of contacting TB, and members of the family vowed not to let the patient spit in public.[60] They would even insist on the attending doctor to keep it as a closely guarded secret. When a member of a family fell victim to TB, the course of action left to his kin generally followed two extremes—they would either confine the patient in a room, severing all ties with the outside world, for fear of social stigma, or allow him to roam freely, hobnob with neighbours, throwing all therapeutic precautions to the wind. Worse still, parents would hardly hesitate to marry off a tubercular maiden to a healthy groom, and a tubercular widower would delight in procuring a healthy bride. And the result was predictable. It remained no longer a problem, private and personal; it overtly became public and started eating into the vitality of the society as well. The nature of social stigma also more often than not tends to reflect gender roles.

Oral evidences tend to indicate that TB-related stigma is worse for female patients than it is for males, sometimes resulting in divorce or separation.

An earning member of a family, if contacted tubercular disease, would not even be allowed by his kin to take leave of the job for fear of falling income, nor would he/she be allowed to recuperate at a sanatorium apprehending that the neighbours would sense the ailment and impose a social boycott. Rwitwik Ghatak's celluloid marvel *Meghe Dhaka Taaraa* is a case in point. Neeta, the sole earning member of the family contacted TB, but she dragged on without proper treatment until when her condition worsened beyond recovery she was sent off to a sanatorium much against her will. Ghatak demonstrates forcefully how the hegemonic familial culture of the Bengali middle-class was built upon a system of exclusions that very conveniently distanced it from the ailing individuals stigmatized by a rigid disease perception.

Even in more recent time, when people fall ill, decisions about treatment becomes a huge priority in the troubled household. Symptoms of the disease and their severity are sought to be assessed and the likely cause of the illness speculated upon. Culture-driven knowledge about disease causation is weighed against knowledge about the Western-derived approaches applied at the local clinics. A decision about the likely cause of the ailment is reached that directs people either to the traditional or biomedical sectors, or to a particular specialist practitioner. Ethnicity and minority status also informs decisions about where people seek treatment. When marginalized people feel excluded from services, for example, if the staff and most of the users in a clinic speak a different language, members of the minority group are more likely to avoid that service.[61] When alternative choices are limited, factors relating to exclusion tend to reduce the overall demand for services and increase the burden of disease. For the very poor, migrants, and internally displaced people, choice between service providers might be a luxury, and affordability is often the crucial factor in decisions as to whether to seek treatment at all.

Not unlike most of the countries in the East, access to primary health services, the critical link between individuals with symptoms of TB and the treatment programme, is limited by systemic barriers for many individuals in India. Patients' narratives indicate that they do not generally reveal their disease to their family members for fear of being separated from others; female patients are scared to tell their disease to their husbands and mothers-in-law for fear of rejection; workmen hide their disease from their employers for fear of being sacked; having known about the disease, the husbands leave out with their children and start living with other women; even after cure patients are not allowed to do household work.[62] Examinations of the histories of patients in the treatment programme for TB reveal that a significant number of the patients in the lowest economic strata experienced delay in diagnosis even after they entered the primary health care system. Indian socio-cultural stigma of TB contributes to abandonment of treatment as also inordinate delay in seeking professional care. Even their own families abandon them to their fate, homeless and helpless. Thus, social stigma might be experienced as an overt social exclusion, that is, enacted stigma, or an anticipation of it, that is, felt stigma.[63] Individuals, who seem to withdraw electively from treatment, or fail to seek treatment in a timely manner, are often characterized within Indian biomedical practice and research by negative stereotypes—alcoholic, irresponsible, inherently possessing poor judgement, and so on. TB patients, not unlike many other tradition bound society, are less respected within the community; neighbours think that people who acquire TB through drinking and smoking are getting what they deserve.[64] But we need to understand that 'social' diseases—diseases characterized by a high correlation to poverty—require social responses through social engineering, and not just medical policing.

NOTES

1. Chakrabarty (1990:376).
2. Benedict (1997:722–24).
3. Rogers (1909).
4. Entin (1995).
5. Brandt (1987).
6. Rothman (1994)
7. Burris (2000:1168–71).
8. The present author has of course attempted one such study, *Malarial Fever in Colonial Bengal, 1820–1939: Social History of an Epidemic*, Calcutta, 2002.
9. Klein (1972); Arnold (1986, 1988, 1993); Nicholas (1981).
10. Harrison and Worboys in M. Worboys and L. Marks (eds) (1997).
11. Cave (1935:142–52).
12. Ryan (1992).
13. Entin (1995).
14. Cited in M.A. Entin, 'Romance and tragedy of tuberculosis: Edward Archibald's contribution to the surgical treatment of pulmonary tuberculosis', *The Canadian Journal of Plastic Surgery* (1995,Vol. 3, No. 4. p. 213).

15. Narayan (1975:40–4).
16. Ewart (1882:335).
17. Ibid., *op. cit.*
18. Webb (1848).
19. Morehead (1856:394).
20. Morehead, *op. cit.*, pp. 394–419.
21. Lankaster (1920:11).
22. Ukil (1926:215–16).
23. Lankaster *op. cit.*, pp. 11–72.
24. Rogers (1919: 200).
25. Ukil, *op. cit.*, p. 217.
26. *Report of the Health Officer for the City of Calcutta, 1922.*
27. Ibid.
28. Rogers (1925).
29. Ibid., p. 44, *op. cit.*
30. Ibid.
31. Ibid., p. 45, *op. cit.*
32. Harris (1908: 41).
33. Ibid., p. 41, *op. cit.*
34. Ibid., *op. cit.*
35. Ghosh (1857:23).
36. Rogers, *op. cit.*, (1925:45).
37. Ukil (1938:525).
38. 'Gleanings from the Calcutta Post-Mortem Records: II. The Incidence of Tuberculosis Disease in Bengal', Rogers, Leonard in *Indian Medical Gazette*, February 1909.
39. Ibid., p. 526, *op. cit.*
40. Ibid., p. 527, *op. cit.*
41. Ibid.
42. Ibid., p. 536, *op. cit.*
43. *Chikitsa Jagat*, Volume 26, No. 11, pp. 415–16.
44. Narayan (1975:40–4).
45. Bi (2003).
46. Ukil (1926).
47. Ibid., p. 230, *op. cit.*
48. Ibid., p. 231, *op. cit.*
49. Khan S. U. 'The railway and the social aspects of tuberculosis', National Conference on Tuberculosis and Chest Diseases, 26th session, Bangalore, India (3–5 January 1971:312–16).
50. Banerjee (1965:103–6).
51. Dubey, Bhasin, and Bhatia (1998:30).

52. Dubey, Bhasin, and Bhatia (1999:680).

53. Geetakrishnan, Pappu, and Roychowdhury (1988:83–98).

54. Dubey, Bhasin, and Bhatia (2000:65–69).

55. Roy Porter, Review of Sheila M. Rothman's, *Living in the Shadow of Death: Tuberculosis and the Social Experience of Illness in American History* in *Medical History*, 1995 July; 39 (3), p. 384.

56. Rothman (1994).

57. Hardy (2003: 535–56).

58. 'TB patients urged to do away with superstition', *Business Ghana*, Ghana, 19 April 2006.

59. Golden (1997:600–5).

60. Ghosh (1363:16–20).

61. Jones and Williams (2004:156–61).

62. Jaggarajamma *et al.* (2008:183).

63. Scamber (1998:1054–5).

64. Moller and Erstad (2007:103–19).

12 Delivering the 'Murdered Child'

Infanticide, Abortion, and Contraception in Colonial India

INDIRA CHOWDHURY

INTRODUCTION

In what ways could we characterize the 'exchange' of medical ideas within the colonial context? The interaction and exchange between Indian medical systems has been historically debated and problematized.[1] However, there have been very few attempts to look at the larger ideological issues that frame such interactions and exchanges. This chapter treats abortion and birth control as the twin sites of 'exchange' of medical and colonial ideologies. By analyzing the debates around infanticide and abortion in 19th century India, and later within birth control propaganda in the 1930s and 1940s, this chapter attempts to map processes of criminalization of social practices and bodily functions, as processes that are marked by the colonial encounter. In 19th century India, debates about infanticide and criminal abortion developed within juridical, missionary, and medical discourses. A domain of knowledge was thus created about sexual practices and bodily functions of Indian women that from its inception based itself on the multiple discourses about the lack of morality among Indians. This chapter demonstrates how this domain was redeployed within Planned Parenthood agendas for India in the 1930s and 1940s.

Focussing on two contrasting moments when 'abortion' and the issue of infanticide surface in the Indian context—the 19th-century criminalization of abortion and 20th century propagation of birth control—I analyse a range of sources—19th century Bengali pamphlets about widow remarriage, abortion and childbirth, juridical notes on criminal abortion, missionary descriptions, along with later sources from the 1930s and 1940s—reports of population and birth control conferences and articles from *Marriage Hygiene* which was edited by A. P. Pillay. In India, even as birth controllers like Edith How Martyn, Magaret Sanger, and A. P. Pillay focussed on 'medicalizing' the domain of birth control, they shaped and reinforced a 'hygienic' concept of sex which was also perceived as an essential characteristic of adjustment in marriage. It is within such a context that discussions of abortion surfaced, taking on an altered guise whenever it resurfaced within such discourses.

ABORTION AND INFANTICIDE IN 19TH CENTURY INDIA

Writing a description of Indian diseases and pathology in 1848, Allan Webb, Professor of Descriptive and Surgical Anatomy at Calcutta Medical College, began the section on 'The Pathology of Generations' of his book *Pathologica Indica or the Anatomy of Indian Diseases*, with a discussion of idolatry. The discussion that followed, though extraordinary in the context of a treatise avowedly on the pathology of diseases, was nevertheless not unusual. After a description of what he pronounced to be the worship of 'gross representations of the male and female organs' at Elephanta, Ellora, and Rajpootana, Webb went on to justify the inclusion of such a discussion in the context of disease. The immoral practices and practices of 'devil worship' that were rampant in India were, according to Webb, closely tied, not only to a range of diseases but also to the characteristic infirmity of body and mind that Indian women were susceptible to. In Webb's words—

'Nor are these considerations irrelevant to a full understanding of the pathology of the female organs of generation in this country; since many of their most serious lesions, result from vicious institutions or practices connected with this very idolatry, so fatal to that only safeguard of chastity, purity of mind'.[2]

Webb went on to state that—

Perhaps, no country on earth has immolated so many new-born infants as India, nor has any race of mankind more generally practised the abominable act of murdering children when yet in the womb of the mother. The art of producing abortion and all its long train of evils, at once subverting both the order of nature and the end of being, is but too openly practiced even now. Whilst the strong arm of a humane Government has done much to cleanse the land from the foul stain of child-murder, it has not been able to reach this more common and secret practice of abortion, as many of the preparations in the museum sufficiently attest, and also that the death of the unfortunate mother is no uncommon result of this crime which in other instances leads to hopeless sterility.[3]

If Webb's description has the ring of familiarity to it, it was only because the same story had been repeated many times over within numerous discourses of colonialism. My point here is not to reiterate the already well-known story of Orientalism, but to push it further and investigate the making of a peculiar epistemic culture that created a picture of India where 'depravity' and moral character of Indians could be used to account for everything from rituals, social practices, and physiological characteristics.

Webb's was not an isolated example within the 19th century European medical fraternity in India. Writing *A Manual of Medical Jurisprudence for Bengal and the North Western Provinces*, in 1856, Norman Chevers, MD and Secretary to the Medical Board, Fort William, Calcutta, accounted for criminal abortion by including in his analysis the lack of 'true morality' and the presence of 'vigilant control' in Hindu society over 'the conduct of females'. Offering a prevalent sociological analysis of the situation, Chevers maintained that the two reasons why widows were particularly susceptible to immoral behaviour was the prohibition of widow remarriage and the fact that most widows were 'compelled to rely upon uncertain support of their relatives'. Criminal abortion was a natural consequence of such social arrangements and therefore, it was to be expected, as Chevers reiterated, that 'great crimes should be frequently practised to conceal the results of immorality'.[4]

Chevers' assumptions about the relationship between 'native' depravity and the frequent occurrence of abortions did not draw on medical statistics but on the testimony of the missionary William Ward. Citing Ward as his 'informant', Chevers reported that at least 10,000 children are murdered in the womb every month in Bengal.[5] The mode of describing bodily functions, pathology, and diseases of the 'natives' in terms of the moral rather than the physiological was, by the late 19th century, being adopted by Indians themselves as a mode of explaining their own social reality. Thus, a conceptual framework that was adopted by the Europeans to render the culture of the 'other' intelligible was transformed into one that explained the world of the colonized. Post-colonial studies of colonialism and the history of medicine has not paid adequate attention to this singular phenomenon by which a new domain of knowledge about sexual practices of the colonized was created; a domain which blurred the boundaries of the moral, the social, and the physiological.

In order to contextualize the creation of this domain of knowledge about sexual practices, let me turn briefly to Ward's own description of the social life and moral beliefs of the Hindus which was amplified into a pathology of the bodily functions of Indians within the literature of colonial medical jurisprudence. The Hindus, according to William Ward, lacked in 'solid virtues such as integrity, humanity, truth and or generosity'.[6] Writing his four-volume commentary *A View of the history, literature and religion of the Hindoos*, between 1817–20, Ward wrote that moral corruption was rampant not only among men, who, influenced by the example of their lustful god (Krishna) frequented houses of ill-fame, but also among women who routinely practiced infanticide—

> In the family of a single kooleenu bramhun, whose daughters never live with their husbands, it is common for each daughter to destroy a child in the womb annually; this crime is also very prevalent among widows, so numerous in this country. The pundit who gave me this information, supposes that 10,000 children are thus murdered, in the province of Bengal every month!!...He said that the fact was so notorious that every child in the country knew of it; and that the crime had acquired an appropriate name, petu-phela, viz, thrown from the belly; pet-phelanee is also a term of abuse, which one woman often gives to another.[7]

My reason for invoking William Ward's description is to demonstrate how the creation of this domain of knowledge about sexual practices and bodily functions included from its very inception, multiple discourses about the lack of morality among Indians. The missionary as well as colonial discourses on the lax morals of the Hindus induced, as I have argued elsewhere, a nationalist response that tended to claim that while Indians did have a glorious past, their moral and physical weaknesses were of recent provenance and provoked by the changes brought about by colonialism. By the late 19th century, such charges surfaced fairly frequently and in all realms. This chapter then, is about the ways in which a certain domain of knowledge about Indian sexual practices came to be hegemonically established within a colonial framework and how this domain implicitly incorporated selected information about Indian culture from the diverse epistemological networks that colonialism had put in place. Finally, this chapter is also about the ways in which this domain was transformed with the ushering in of population control as a mode of government.

The period to which these medical descriptions belong, is also a period of social reform in Bengal. In his second proposal on the introduction of widow remarriage, Vidyasagar had lamented the reluctance of his countrymen to bring about this much-needed social reform, which he had taken great pains to show, was permitted by the *Shashtras*. Aware of the sexual exploitation of widows, he presented remarriage as a possible solution to the problems faced by widows who helplessly, 'shed all anxieties about right conduct and out of sheer public shame commit abortions'.[8] Far from being a moral condemnation, Vidyasagar's proposal attempted to outline the plight of helpless widows. What Vidyasagar makes amply clear in his proposal is that the issue of abortion was linked with the issue of illegitimacy and fear of social expulsion rather than an intrinsic moral infirmity in the widows.

THE IMPACT OF CRIMINALIZATION

In his own lifetime, Vidyasagar was to witness the failure of the Widow Remarriage Act of 1856 to achieve a better life for the child widows of Bengal. Nor did the legalization of widow remarriage put an end to abortions. By 1860, the British had sought to contain the problem by introducing Act XLV of the Indian Penal Code, with the following sections—

> Sections 312, 313, 314: Causing miscarriage, causing miscarriage without woman's consent, death caused by an act done with intent to cause miscarriage.
>
> Section 315: act done with intent to prevent child being born alive or to cause it to die after birth p. Section 316 Causing death to a quick unborn child by an act amounting to cupable homicide. Section 317 Exposure and abandonment of a child under twelve years by parents or persons having care of it.
>
> Section 318 intentional concealment of birth by secret disposal of dead body of a child whether such a child die before or after or during its birth.[9]

The criminalization of abortion resulted in the creation of a vigilant and powerful group of civil surgeons who were now obliged to file medico-legal returns annually. Some of them, like J. D. M. Gribble, Civil Surgeon of Madras, felt the need to voice a word of caution about 'natural abortions' which were very common (citing the evidence of Mr Whitehead's 2,000 pregnancies as being one in seven); apart from which, he went on to state—unmarried women were 'more liable to suffer from natural abortion than the married one' as the former will necessarily 'conceal her condition and often undertake heavy work which the 'married woman having nothing to conceal would not undertake'.[10] It was far more usual, however, for most medico-legal reports to emphasize criminality. Reporting on the extent of criminal abortions, between 1870–72, Robert Harvey, Surgeon in the Bengal Army wrote—'Three hundred and seventy-eight cases of were investigated during the three years, 132 of which were fatal…. A few of the cases may have been examinations of women suspected of infanticide, but the bulk were cases of abortion or miscarriage, actual or alleged involving a criminal charge'.[11]

These systematic reports give us details of the mechanical means and 'home remedies' used to bring off an abortion, although sometimes external violence was resorted to—kneading of the womb—to procure abortion. There are also descriptions of perforation of the uterus and the peritoneum by the introduction of a branch of *Lal chitra* into the womb along with a common household seasoning, asafoetida or *hing*, which often resulted in unsuccessful abortions, gangrene, and subsequent death of the woman.[12] Traditional abortifacients such as juice of the *madar* plant, carrot seeds, unripe pineapple with salt, ginger, garlic, tamarind, used in combination with several roots, seemed to have non-fatal results. There were several cases of death caused by the use of arsenic and borax.

'NATIVE' TRADITIONS, COGNITIVE ENSLAVEMENT, AND REFRAMING THE ABORTION DEBATE

The details of such returns, however, throw little light on the traditional means employed by the 'native' *dhais* (midwives). The legal and institutional framework, thus introduced to track this criminal practice, granted no space for a different epistemology. Harvey concluded—'[These cases]…are probably, for the most part, the work of inexpert practitioners, while many of the non-fatal cases where nothing but the fact of recent abortion could be spoken to were probably examples of criminal abortion brought on by *dhais* and others concerning whose mode of proceeding we know little or nothing'.[13]

Within the parameters that rendered abortion a cognizable criminal offence, traditional knowledge of the dhai had no legitimacy. The
emphasis on abortion and its association with traditional medicine
resulted in a peculiar configuration—the traditional knowledge of the
dhai, and traditional medicine for female disorders were both reduced
to knowledge of abortifacients.[14] What was completely ignored was the
fact that traditional medicine saw menstruation as central to women's
bodily functions.[15] Menstruation was not only central to an understanding of female disorders, the unhealthy retention of menstrual blood was
often seen as a result of the disturbance of *vata* and usually dealt with by
the use of purges.[16] Indeed, the process of criminalization of abortion
set in motion the publication of inventories of abortifacients by 'native'
doctors. Harinarayan Bandyopadhyay, Assistant Surgeon at Kandee
Charitable Dispensary, published one such catalogue in 1875, calling it
'Gurbini-Bandhab', literally, 'Friend of the Pregnant woman' with the
English subtitle: 'A Treatise on Abortion to which are added symptoms
of Pregnancy'. The contents of this treatise was earlier serialized in the
Bengali journal *Chikitsha-Darpan*. The purpose of this publication, the
Preface asserts, is social reform—'The description of evil practices is the
only way of achieving social reform. I will consider my task a fulfilled if
the Reader learns the contents that have been communicated here and
devotes himself to bringing the wicked to book'.[17]

Harinarayan emphasized the criminal nature of such practices, and
refused to grant any epistemological recognition to traditional ways of
healing—he claimed, before offering a detailed list of abortion practices,
that these sometimes brought on abortion and proved fatal for women,
while at other times, seemed to have no effect at all. His attempt to catalogue 'native' practices was consistent with colonial arguments against
abortion. Hardly surprising therefore, that Harinarayan too should
cite William Ward's passage on abortion in Bengal as providing a 'true'
understanding of what must have been part of his own experience of
contemporary social reality. Harinarayan's attempt characterizes the
consequences of what Vivek Dhareshwar has described as 'the long ap-
prenticeship with the West'.[18]

Not all social reformers demonstrated Harinarayan's 'cognitive en-
slavement', to use Akeel Bilgrami's phrase.[19] I shall discuss one essay
by a social reformer which characterizes an attempt to account for the
prevalence of abortions in colonial India in terms that are both different

and complex. The author of this 18-page long article that appeared in the influential Bengali journal *Arya Darshan*, Vidyaratna Kshetramohan Sen Gupta (1846–1918) was trained in Sanskrit and later became Assistant Editor of the same journal. One of the most accomplished political and economic analysts of his time, Kshetramohan's article entitled 'Bhrun-hatya, Shishu hatya nibaraner upay ki? Parityakta shishuder ke raksha karibe?' ('How can we prevent abortion and infanticide? Who will protect the abandoned children?')[20] was published nearly 20 years after the legislation on widow remarriage and 15 years after the Indian Penal Code was put in place.

At the very outset, Kshetramohan rules out the correlation between poverty and abortion. Since, abortions, he argues, are not uncommon in Europe. Referring to India's colonized status, he states with biting sarcasm—'In the country of barbarians, there are no poor people. Everyone is equal there...'.[21] 'Moreover, poverty takes on a different connotation in countries that have liberty and autonomy; therefore, in Europe, poverty is often the cause of abortions'.[22]

In a lengthy analysis of the social system in ancient India, Kshetramohan argues that men and women could legitimately exercise their emotional and sexual needs as there existed different forms of marriages. Since children born out of such relationships were not treated as illegitimate, therefore, having laws against abortion or infanticide served no purpose. In more recent time, Kshetramohan argues, distorted social beliefs have created a complex situation where the issue of legitimacy has attained an overwhelming importance. 'Social reform began to consider the life of our ancestors as unworthy of respect. So all the Pandavas were disgraced because of their birth. Bhisma came to be seen as a bastard. What wonderful reform! A youthful child widow could no longer accept a young man as her husband'. 'Naturally', Kshetramohan concludes, 'abortion and infanticide increased'[23]). Furthermore, these distorted social beliefs were also responsible for the continuation of the exploitative practice of *kulin* polygamy and contributed to the de-recognition of practices such as widow remarriage—

Before long, society began to worship those distorted beliefs. Such notions brought infanticide and abortion into society. Soon the king's law —which functions as a cohort of such distorted social beliefs could do nothing about such 'murders' and created an exacting penal code to punish these offenders, as a result the penal code took control of the offender's life and the penance far outweighed the sin.[24]

Kshetramohan also analyses the causes of female infanticide in Rajasthan and correlates it to the simultaneous existence of a dowry system and poverty. The only Rajput ruler who attempted to address the dowry system was Jaisingh but no other ruler attempted a similar reform.[25]

Kshetramohan goes on to present a comparative analysis of ancient and medieval societies. He quotes from the Koran Mohamed's warnings against infanticide but points out that this is not the same as abortion for social pressure.[26]

> History tells us that prior to the spread of Christianity many countries had no laws against abortion or infanticide. Perhaps the ancient rulers had realized that no matter how tough the law, no crime disappears until the root cause of the crime is wiped out. The Greeks, Romans and Jewish people had recognized that abortion and infanticide were the greatest of misdeeds which is why the practice of abandoning the child became more prevalent than abortion or infanticide.[27]

During the reign of the first Christian emperors in Rome, there were no laws against abortion or infanticide. Instead, the state had orphanages for abandoned infants. But numbers of abandoned infants increased as the root causes were never addressed; laws were passed that made the abandoning of a child punishable—death sentence for abortion and infanticide, and life imprisonment for abandoning an infant. To quote Kshetramohan—'When there was death sentence for abortion and infanticide and life imprisonment for abandoning an infant and over and above that disgrace, ignominy, torture of family, why should a mother then not kill her child? Why should she not bury it alive or throw it in the ocean?'.[28] Within the framework of Kshetramohan's analysis, the spread of Christianity in the world was responsible for the establishment of orphanages for abandoned children by monasteries.[29]

Kshetramohan concluded his analysis with an elegiac address that targeted the 'civilized Europeans' for failing to engage with the root causes of the problem—

> Why is a secret love affair considered sinful? Does the recitation of a few lines from the Bible, or mantras chanted before the sacred salgram stone or the chanting of a few lines of Hebrew amount to matrimony? No amount

of holy water will make you pure if you harbour poison within. If the meeting of two hearts is not considered a marriage, then change your system of
marriage!...You are blind to your own flaws and do not see the harm you
are doing to society. Society is suffering because of you. You need to be
banished from this society![30]

Kshetramohan's analysis of why European attempts to reform social
practices in India had failed points towards a social domain which
operated within a separate epistemic domain. Cutting to the heart of the
matter, Kshetramohan pointed out that making abortion a cognizable
offence would not stop the problem of infanticide since the question was
intrinsically linked with question of marriage and legitimacy. Within
the moral-epistemological domain created by colonialism, the diverse
systems of marriage encountered in India were all non-sacramental
practices and, were all, therefore, characterized as 'immoral practices'.
The disciplinary measures that were put in place by the colonial state
can be seen as part of what Michel Foucault has called the disciplinary
mode within which the 'governmental apparatus' is developed.

GOVERNMENTALITY, SEXUALITY, AND A FRAMEWORK OF ANALYSIS

This is also an appropriate moment to link Foucault's idea of the
emergence of 'governmentality' to his ideas about sexuality, as I find both
useful in providing a useful conceptual framework of analysis. Indeed,
Foucault's notion of 'governmentality' has been seen as fuelling Indian
debates about the size and characteristics of the Indian population.[31]
However, I would like to revisit the notion in order to outline the ways it
could be used as an analytical tool. Foucault tells us that the emergence
of population as a domain of governance made it possible to re-centre
the notion of economy. The phenomenon of population revealed that it
had its own regularities, its rate of deaths and diseases. Prior to this, the
art of government was conceived in terms of the 'management of the
family' on a larger scale. However, the emergence of the phenomenon
of population rendered the family from a model of government to a
privileged segment from which information about sexual behaviour,
demography, and so on, could be acquired in order to govern. The
ultimate end of government now became the welfare of the population it
governed, the improvement of its conditions, its health and longevity, and
so on. Sovereignty, discipline, and government then began to function

as three modes which targeted the population.[32] Within colonialism, the disciplinary mode and the mode of governmentality functioned at times simultaneously and at other times, one mode predominated over the other. The setting up of the disciplinary mode within colonialism involved a complex move that involved a scrutiny of sexual and bodily practices of the colonized by the colonizers. This mode was put in place through the emergence of what Foucault has called the *scientia sexualis*.

Michel Foucault in his *History of Sexuality, Volumes I and II*, has distinguished between two oppositional categories of sexual knowledge—the *ars erotica* and scientia sexualis.[33] These two forms are brought into place by very different cultural norms. Contemporary applications of Foucault's analysis of sexuality often misses the point that he was trying to make—that scientia sexualis was a product of the Christian West put in place by a set of norms very different from non-Western, non-Christian societies.[34] It was for this reason that when Foucault attempted to look for sexuality in ancient Greece, he could not find it. What he found instead were four separable but related domains—that of pleasure, dietetics, domestic economics, and erotics or the love of the boys. I would like to present here the provocative argument that in colonial India, it was scientia sexualis that provided the framework through which 'native' sexual and other bodily practices were processed. As a result, the domain of experiential knowledge of the body, its pleasures and functions that were known and accessible to Indians in different terms, was replaced by a different epistemic domain that tended to interpret experiential knowledge through laws of what was permitted and forbidden.[35]

Indeed, my reason for dwelling at length on the essay by Kshetramohan Sengupta was to illustrate the fact that there were, perhaps, other modes of understanding social and bodily practices which was gradually being replaced through an interpretative framework of laws that authorized or prohibited 'native' practices. The latter epistemic domain soon came to dominate and led to a differentiation and hierarchization between bodily pleasures, bodily management, and useful and legitimate sexual knowledge. The latter belonged to the 'modern' sphere of birth control while the former was relegated to the 'ancient' and baser realm of erotic pleasure, its excesses, and consequences.

I shall now turn to the 20th century propagation of birth control in India to demonstrate how the early 20th century attempts to gain legitimacy for contraception, eugenics, and population spoke of sexual practices as part of family hygiene endorsed by the practitioners of Western medicine. By mid-century, when arguments for the legalization of abortion came to be articulated, abortion not only had to be 'rescued' from the outlawed domain of 'native' medical practices for the modern practitioner of Western medicine, but also had to be salvaged as a procedure offered to married women for eugenic reasons.

OF NATURAL APPETITES AND ARTIFICIAL CONTRACEPTION

Researchers who have looked at the emergence of birth control agendas in the Indian context have often concentrated on the emergence of reproductive sexuality or the related issue of eugenic maternity.[36] Scholars have also delved into various ways in which advocates of birth control contended with Gandhi's opposition to their cause.[37] The puzzling disappearance of the discourse on abortion is hardly accounted for. This section of my chapter will attempt to account for the apparent disappearance of the issue of abortion by focussing on the early discourse on birth control as it attempted to validate its existence in India.

In his influential book *Sex Problem in India*, in 1927, N. S. Phadke argued for the recognition of the sexual appetite as natural as 'eating, drinking or sleeping'.[38] Pitting his opening argument against Gandhi's articles advocating continence and responsibility that appeared in 1925 in *Young India*, Phadke argued that since 'certain consequences of the sexual act arise' even after 'the exercise of reason and moderation', the 'contention that a man must accept all consequences of each act is itself ridiculous' (NSP, 245–6). An examination of Phadke's arguments for the use of artificial birth control for eugenic reasons is revealing for the attention it draws to the relationship between the knowledge of indigenous contraceptives and illicit sexual relations. Phadke asserts that 'illicit intercourse' exists in Indian society just as it exists elsewhere. However, people in such relationships had no access to 'scientific contraceptive' knowledge. The indigenous knowledge of contraceptives originates in ancient Aryan medical treatises, apart from which several remedies were devised during the Mogul reign, on account of the 'luxurious and sensual habits of the Mohamedans'. This knowledge, Phadke alerts us, still exists among 'quacks' whose 'virulent medicines, chemicals or herbs' are aimed at 'producing abortion' and not at rendering 'pregnancy impossible' (NSP, 256–7). Phadke's point about sexual urges as 'natural appetites' falters when it encounters indigenous contraceptives. He, therefore, shifts the argument to contrast 'scientific contraceptives' and 'virulent herbs and chemicals' on the one hand, and modern 'preventive measures' and indigenous abortifacients on the other.

Phadke's contrast had a significant resonance within the discourse on birth control. The modern scientific methods of prevention of conception was promoted by all birth controllers and arguments about methods were presented in terms of safety, efficacy, and cost. By contrast, indigenous contraceptives were identified with abortifacients. Norman Himes in his *Medical History of Contraception* quotes P. K. Wattal's article 'The Population Problem in India', based on the 1901 Census Report, that—

'Among the tea-garden coolies of Assam means are frequently taken to prevent conception, or to procure abortion'.[39]

While Himes mentions both prevention of contraception and abortion, by the mid-1930s, abortion when mentioned as a possibility within the context of population control, was rarely prescribed, as the existing Indian Penal Code invariably cast its long shadow over such references. In his Presidential address in the Family Hygiene Section of the All India Population Conference in Lucknow in 1936, V. R. Khanolkar argued against the feasibility of abortion as a birth control measure in the following manner—

The flow of a river can be stemmed somewhere along its course, the birth of children can be checked somewhere along a complex physiological process. For example, it might be proposed to accomplish it by a method which was not unknown in the countries to the east and west of us, and was prevalent in our own country in times of famine and misery. This was infanticide or destruction of children soon after birth. The destruction could be effected...during the period of gestation itself by induced abortion. Under our present day conditions, though both these methods are often practised, they could not advocated, *for obvious reasons*, as feasible methods. [Emphasis mine][40]

Abortion as a means of birth control was viewed as a cognizable offence and hence it could not be recommended for *obvious reasons*. The focus on women's health was yet to emerge and if it did, it concentrated on the health of the married woman. Indeed, within debates of population control and birth control, the focus remained resolutely on the family as a reproductive unit. Abortion was viewed mainly as the termination of an illicit and illegitimate pregnancy that was often the plight of unmarried women and widows and hardly found a place within this discourse. When it did, it was firmly expunged. Marie Stopes, who applied her understanding of the lives of English working-class women to the poor Indian woman in her pamphlet '*Constructive Birth Control for Indian Women*', in 1935, found the issue of abortion worth addressing. Speaking to the poor Indian woman, she said—

> ...very often it happens that you 'get caught' and you know that the baby you feared might come has already begun...and you may try to do a desperate thing to get rid of the baby before it has 'gone too far'. Your neighbours or some old woman you know may tell you various dodges which they have tried, and which may get rid of the beginnings of a baby, and perhaps you try one after another; but either it may have gone too far; or in that way you may be strong, and you may find that the little unwanted baby continues to grow within you and comes to birth alive, but not all it might have been.[41]

As I have discussed elsewhere, this expanded version of Stopes's pamphlet would remain unpublished.[42] Indeed, Stopes's discussion of abortion in the context of working-class marriages was explicitly stated by her collaborator in India as one of the reasons for not publishing the pamphlet. Returning the manuscript to Stopes in December 1935, Mrs Pearson Powis wrote— 'I have it on the authority of leading medical man that abortion is not practised by Indian women except among those who are forbidden sexual intercourse, e.g., widows and unmarried women. Hence page two, three and four would only give offence'.[43]

Stopes's focus on the married woman's demand for abortion, although considered perfectly legitimate by most of her contemporaries, was not perceived as an acceptable or even a justifiable right for women in the early 20th century. The married woman became the main focus of attention within the twin discourses of birth control and eugenics. The widow and the prostitute who resorted to the criminal practice of abortion were ousted from the discourse of birth control. As the discourse of birth control became increasingly medicalized, it also disallowed access of contraceptive knowledge to unmarried women and widows.

THE MEDICALIZATION OF BIRTH CONTROL IN INDIA

As I have attempted to demonstrate in an earlier section of this chapter, the necessity of introducing methods of birth control in India was first articulated by members of Eugenics and Neo-Malthusian societies. The link between 'voluntary' limitation of births and population control, as we saw in Phadke's account, was also related to the establishment of medical authority in a bid to oust the 'quacks' who administered and sold abortifacients. Concern about the burgeoning population of India as validated by the 1931 Census of India (with a total population of 279.0 million) was articulated in several quarters. As 'the issue of population acquired a new prominence in thinking', questions about the limitation of births came to the forefront and the dissemination of birth control advice through medical officers in Presidencies such as Madras, was perceived as a feasible official measure.[44] Around the same period, the birth control movement in India underwent an interesting shift.[45] While the European and American women birth controllers, such as Margaret Sanger, Edith How-Martyn, and Marie Stopes were not medical women; there was in India a strong appeal to medicalize contraceptive advice. This was carried out through the organization of training sessions in contraceptive techniques for medical students from India and the colonies.

Speaking at the International Conference on Birth Control in Asia held at the London School of Hygiene and Tropical Medicine, in 1933, Edith How-Martyn placed before the panel, chaired by Harold Laski, a few practical measures for the dissemination of contraceptive information—

'...we appealed to two organizations — the Indian Women's Conference and the Indian Medical Association — to grant us one or two days at the end of their annual conferences for the consideration of the subject: the Indian Medical Association to consider contraceptive technique and the Women's Conference, the sociological and the mother's side. Both organizations have replied favourably'.[46]

Reporting on her 'Great Indian Tour' that lasted 12 weeks, the journal of the Eugenics Society, *The New Generation*, quoted her interview to the *Times of India* where she 'exploded the theory that India, as a whole, was opposed to birth control'. Elaborating on the basis of her experience she said—

'I have addressed altogether seventy meetings in about a score of cities and towns during my recent tour, and the opposition has been insignificant, though these meetings have been attended by men and women by all communities'.[47]

In an editorial written about her visit in his journal, *Marriage Hygiene*, A. P. Pillay wrote that while he appreciated the importance of training doctors for the dissemination of birth control information, How-Martyn's enthusiastic 'labour of love', was perhaps unrealistic in the conclusions it drew—

> We cannot, however, share her conclusion that there was practically no opposition in India. Recently in the Council of State was moved a modest resolution on the subject...which was negatived. The organised opposition came from the enlightened British members of the Government. Similar resolutions hitherto brought before the Provincial Councils and Municipal Bodies met with more or less the same fate.[48]

In subsequent visits, both How-Martyn and Margaret Sanger sought out medical and women's organizations rather than officials from administrative units of the government. Their interactions with women's groups such as the All India Women's Conference (AIWC) were to prove exhilarating. For both How-Martyn and later Margaret Sanger, the enthusiasm with which the 1935 resolution on birth control was passed at the Trivandrum All India Women's Conference, was a sharp contrast to their experience in USA and Britain. Writing about her 10-week tour of India, Ceylon, Burma, and Malaya in 1936, Margaret Sanger wrote—'All the dubious and dismal prognostications as to the religious objections of Hindus and Mohamedans have proven false in my experience. As in other countries, the opposition came from the Roman Catholics and in India this weak opposition was expressed by foreign-born priests and a few Eurasians'.[49]

In her speech at the 10th AIWC conference in Trivandrum in 1935, Margaret Sanger argued that birth control would solve the problems of ever-increasing population, poverty, and the high infant and maternal morality.[50] During her visit, Sanger also lectured on contraception at the Indian Obstetrics and Gynaecological Congress held at Madras in January 1936. During her visit to India in 1935–6, Sanger travelled '10,000 miles, visited 18 cities and addressed 64 meetings, and met the leaders of public opinion such as Nehru, Gandhi, Tagore, Sarojini Naidu the Maharaja and Maharani of Baroda, the Dewan of Mysore and the Maharani of Travancore'.[51] The future action, Sanger concluded, would depend on 'medical and official direction'.[52]

The emphasis on medical training in contraceptive techniques remained the focus of How-Martyn's second tour of India in 1937–8. Her presence also enabled the AIWC to focus its birth control resolution at that year's Nagpur Conference on medicalization. To quote—

This conference believes that it is the duty of medical departments and local authorities to take immediate steps to put an end to the advertisement and sale of birth control remedies by quacks which ruin the health of women in many cases. It appeals to medical departments and municipalities to educate men and women in birth control methods, from the point of view of their ill health, mental weakness and economic considerations. Such clinics should be specially opened in labour areas.[53]

The medicalization of the birth control agenda in India was perceived as a way of providing it with legitimacy as well as authority. Such a move also reinforced a 'hygienic' concept of sex which was also an aspect of 'a well-adjusted marriage'.[54] In India, the process of medicalization of contraceptive advice resulted in the creation of several birth control clinics which advised mainly married women. It also resulted in sex education classes as well as demonstration classes that were open to men and women. The demonstration classes organized by A. P. Pillay in 1934 allowed the 120 students, most of whom were from the medical profession, to practise the fitting up of the diaphragm pessary on a woman who was 'hired for the purpose'. 'The greatest difficulty', Pillay wrote, was to find a bacteriologically "clean" woman'.[55]

Demonstration classes as well as the medicalization of birth control affected only the elite section of Indian society. The woman hired for the demonstration class would not be a learner-participant in such classes but a 'specimen', whose body would be used to inscribe the lessons of birth control.

The single-mindedness with which birth controllers embraced this new agenda, the passion with which they medicalized the domain resulted in an emphasis on 'marriage hygiene', population control, and fit progeny and family limitation. There were only oblique references to abortion. In a radio talk given in Bombay on 30 November 1935, Sanger spoke of birth control as a 'means to prevent' and 'not to destroy'. Thus, setting up 'abortion' as the hidden adversary of birth control, Sanger assured her listeners that birth control did not 'mean to interfere with life after it had begun'.[56] For both Sanger and How-Martyn, the focus remained on population control agendas and on birth control propaganda for healthy and satisfactory marriages. Although How-Martyn did raise the issue of abortion in her agenda note before her first visit to India, she articulated it in terms of an issue for married people.[57]

The domain that remained outside of the notion of a healthy family continued to harbour the infanticide and the quack and the abortionist.

As Dr Ruth Young of the Women's Medical Service and Director of the Maternity and Child Welfare Bureau wrote in 1935, the optimism about the success of birth control was baseless. The first erroneous belief, Young pointed out, was that 'women were crying out for birth control. While they did desire release from 'perpetual childbearing and the misery which so often accompanies it,...that is not synonymous with the desire for birth control'. More importantly, Young also pointed out that '...the vast majority know nothing whatever about it [birth control] in the modern sense though they may have a nodding acquaintance with the Indian counterpart of the professional abortionist'.[58]

Ruth Young's contentious attempt to relocate the story of birth control in India as a less successful one, forced the reader to admitting the persistence of the surreptitious and the illegitimate—by acknowledging the outlawed 'traditional' abortionist and the quack. The abortionist, the 'native' dhai and the even the 'native' *vaidya* remained peripheral to the concern of the birth controllers.

When the question of legalization of abortion was first raised at the International Conference on Planned Parenthood in Bombay in 1952, it was broached in medical terms as well as within the legitimate sphere of family 'hygiene'. H. S. Mehta argued for decriminalization of abortion so that qualified medical doctors could offer it scientifically. Moreover, he argued, if 'the practice of abortion were treated as a scientific technique... it would lead to a considerable research in the use of new drugs and new methods'. Scientific research would also direct the re-examination of the repertoire of the traditional abortionist because, Mehta argued,

'It is quite possible that in India several herbs and concoctions are used to procure abortion which, if scientifically analysed and studied, may prove to be extremely useful and perhaps economical'.[59]

Mehta proposed that abortion be offered when pregnancy endangered the life of the mother, when a woman was the victim of rape and incest, and for eugenic reasons, when it could be 'reasonably assumed that whether one or both parents would hereditarily transfer to their offspring mental disease, idiocy or any grave defect of some other kind'.[60] The story of the arrival of modern techniques of birth control to India now came to be narrated alongside arguments for the legalization of abortion. The plea for decriminalization included medical and scientific reasons. Indeed, as Geetanjali Gangoli has demonstrated, when the Medical Termination of Pregnancy Bill was discussed, most members of Parliament supported it, articulating recognition of 'failure of contraception' as a reason for abortion, completely disregarding the idea that the failure of contraception could also be seen as loss of a woman's control of her body.[61] As arguments for the legitimization of abortion were articulated, the Indian Penal Code that incriminated the 'native' abortionist and the Indian woman who resorted to infanticide or the use of abortifacients became an obstacle for practitioners of Western medicine as well. As is evident from eugenic arguments about healthy progeny, only married women came to be included in discussions about the decriminalization of abortion. This was not unexpected as the family remained in focus in all arenas of social control as we shall see in the following section.

POPULATION CONTROL AND THE INDIAN FAMILY

Birth controllers like Sanger, How-Martyn, and Stopes faced enormous opposition from the Church and the State in their own countries. In India, although the colonial state did not create a family planning or population control policy, birth control propaganda faced very little opposition on social or religious grounds. On the contrary, birth control was greeted with enthusiasm by the middle classes and perceived as a need by the working classes. Birth control, however, had developed abroad mainly as an oppositional discourse to the Church and the State. Therefore, in India, it began the process of identifying its 'adversary' within the social practices of marriage and family. The emergence of population control as a field of government intervention in 20th century colonial India saw the emergence of the family in a dual role—it was identified as the adversary against which the discourse of birth control set itself up, at the same time, it was also the privileged segment which provided statistical information about sexual behaviour, demography, and so on, of the inhabitants of the state.

The Census of 1931 brought forth a burgeoning literature on data analysis. In 1934, G. S. Ghurye published an analysis of the fertility data, in the Census data, and came to two disparate conclusions. First, he lamented that the fertility data presented in the Census ended up supporting a popular eugenic belief 'that our population is being replenished from the poorer stocks than from the better'.[62] His second conclusion focused on the Hindu practice of child marriages and stressed that a campaign for raising the woman's age at marriage had to be simultaneous with a campaign for control of birth.[63]

Unhappy with the 'defective' Census data of 1931, Ghurye took up a different sample for analysis in a subsequent paper entitled 'Marriage and Widowhood in India, A Study of a Middle Class Sample of 3,400 Marriages' which he presented before the first All India Population Conference at Lucknow, in 1936. The Indian middle class family had become a problem on several counts—the effects of early maternity on reproduction, the short duration of birth intervals, on one-third of the sample, and the high percentage of young childless widows for whom remarriage was out of the question. A large proportion in the last category had their 'sex-life completely smothered when they are of tender age', while the childless among them had 'no object in life on which they could centre their repressed impulses in a sublimated form'.[64]

In 1935, *Marriage Hygiene* also presented an analysis by K. K. Bhattacharya of Calcutta, on 'The Present Day Matrimonial System and its effects on the Sex Life in Bengal'. Bhattacharya examined what he termed the rigid social system that has led to 'unbalanced' marriage practices. The vile matrimonial system was responsible for the 'loss of sexual balance between a healthy man and a healthy woman'. Besides, it indirectly resulted in the 'prevalence of abortions' at places of pilgrimage (because widows were not allowed to remarry). The practice of kulin[65] polygamy too, the author argued, created 'disharmonious marital sex relationship resulting in unsatisfied sex-hunger which expressed itself in various morbid physiological and psychological states'.[66]

The creation of this 'hygienic' domain of legitimate sexual practices could only be achieved if the contemporary system of marriage were purged of what Bhattacharya labeled as 'sexual imbalances' that were inevitable in child marriages, on account of the differences in age, education, and ability to contribute to domestic economy between the partners. Marriage as it existed was inadequately 'sexual'. For Bhattacharya—

> The ideal of the institution of marriage may be summarised thus: it affords facilities for both men and women of proper age to develop their sex function to the best advantage of the society which is enriched by the healthy progeny of sexually satisfied parents.[67]

Population control and the discourse on birth control created not only the idea of sexual compatibility but also the idea that sexual satisfaction of the parents as being responsible for the health of the offspring.

In addition, writers like Bhattacharya, himself a medical doctor, as well as other birth controllers, reinforced the idea that the lack of knowledge of birth control and sexual repression were mainly responsible for the sexual excess in society that expressed itself in infanticide, abortion, or venereal diseases.

The debates around population control and birth control in the 1930s brought about a re-centering of the 19th century domain of knowledge about the 'depraved' bodily practices of Indians. Within arguments for population control, the new focus turned to the Indian family as a re-productive unit and one over which the art of 'governmentality' could be practised. The Indian family and the institution of marriage were subjected to intense scrutiny and found to be lacking in the fundamental ingredients of sexual hygiene. The examination of the Indian family took several forms—on the one hand, the family provided data for under-standing the dynamics of the larger population, on the other, the analysis of social vices were shown to have originated from marriage and family system of Indians.

CONCLUSION

The Foucauldian framework enables us to read the conditions under which the interaction between the social and medical domains takes place under colonialism. As I have stated earlier, scientia sexualis provided the framework through which 'native' sexual and other bodily practices were processed. As a result, the domain of experiential knowledge of the body, its pleasures, and functions that were known and accessible to Indians in different terms, was replaced by a different epistemic domain that tended to interpret experiential knowledge through laws of what was permitted and forbidden. In 19th century India, this domain of knowledge about depraved Indian sexual and bodily practices was perceived as a domain of excess. The disciplinary mode predominated as the colonial state sought to bring under its control the aberrant practices of the 'native' system of medicine and its practitioners. In 20th century India, on the other hand, the emergence of a distinctive discourse on birth control and population control ushered in the era of 'governmentality'. Although a population policy was not put in place during the last decades of colonial rule, the medicalized discourse of birth control, eugenic concerns about the health of the population, its sexual practices, and its reproductive capabilities became a new object

for investigation and intervention, a mode which was later inherited by
the new nation-state. Three or four decades after independence, thanks
to the persistent efforts of the women's movement, the state began to
address issues of women's reproductive health within the birth control
practices it promoted. But that is another story.

NOTES

1. Arnold (1993).
2. Webb (1848:256–7).
3. Ibid., p. 260.
4. Chevers (1856:489).
5. Ibid., pp. 489–90.
6. Ward (1817–20:292).
7. Ibid.
8. Vidyasagar (1972:163–4).
9. Mayne (1876:266–9).
10. Gribble (1885:176).
11. Harvey (1876:295).
12. Chevers mentions that O'Shaughnessy had reported the use of the branch of this plant to occasion abortion. Chevers (1856:493).
13. Harvey (1876:307).
14. This is similar to the interpretation of the role of purges in Hippocratic gynaecology. See, King (1998:145–6).
15. See, Wujastyk (1998:154–5).
16. Valiathan (2003:503–10).
17. Bandyopadhyay (1875:Preface).
18. See, Dhareshwar (1998:211–31).
19. Bilgrami (2003:4160).
20. Kshetramohan Sengupta 'Bhrun Hatya, Shishu hatya nibaraner upay ki?' *Arya Darshan* Chaitra, (1875: 538–57).
21. Ibid., p. 543.
22. Ibid., p. 542.
23. Ibid., p. 556.
24. Ibid., p. 544.
25. Ibid., p. 548–9.
26. Ibid., p. 547.
27. Ibid., p. 550.
28. Ibid., p. 551
29. Ibid., p. 553.
30. Ibid., p. 555.

31. Arnold in Sarah Hodges (ed.) (2006).

32. Foucault (1991:100–02).

33. Foucault (1980:57).

34. My reading of Foucault is much indebted to Vivek Dhareshwar's current work, 'Normativity and Experience: The formation of Ontologically Peculiar Objects'.

35. For example, the christening of Vatsayana as the 'Machiavelli of Erotics' by Berriedale A. Keith and Herbert H. Gowen, quoted in Himes (1936:114–15).

36. See, Anandhi in John, Mary E. and Nair, Janaki (eds) (1998:139–66), and Hodges in Sarah Hodges (ed.)(2006).

37. Ahluwalia in Sarah Hodges (ed.) (2006).

38. Phadke (1927:243).

39. Wattal quoted in Himes (1936:122).

40. Khanolkar (1936:286).

41. Marie Stopes, 'Constructive Birth Control for Indian Women', this is an expanded version of her article of the same title published in *Marriage Hygiene*, 1, 2 November 1934. This version is dated 1935 and was unpublished. CMAC/PP/MCS/A 313.

42. See, Chowdhury (2002:214–42).

43. D. Pearson-Powis, to Marie Stopes, dated 29 December 1935, 3. BL 58576.

44. Arnold in Sarah Hodges (ed.) (2006).

45. See, Ramusack in Cheryl Johnson-Odim and Margaret Stroebel (eds) (1992:173–202).

46. Fielding (ed.) (1935:73).

47. 'Mrs How-Martyn's Great Indian Tour' in *The New Generation* (1935:41).

48. 'Editorial', *Marriage Hygiene* (1935:331).

49. 'Margaret Sanger in India: From the Newsletter of Margaret Sanger released by her in March', *Marriage Hygiene*, May, (1936:461).

50. 'Tenth All India Women's Conference', *Marriage Hygiene* (1936:326).

51. 'Margaret Sanger in India: From the Newsletter of Mrs Sanger', *Marriage Hygiene* (1936:462).

52. Ibid., p. 462.

53. Eileen Palmer's Travel Book, India Office Library and Records, MSS/EUR/D 1182/6.

54. For a comparison with the situation in America, see, Petchesky (1986:93).

55. 'Notes and Comments', *Marriage Hygiene* (1935:4).

56. 'What Birth Control can do for India: A Radio Talk by Margaret Sanger' in Eileen Palmer's Travel Book, India Office Library and Records, MSS/EUR/D 1182/62, p. 84.

57. Edith How-Martyn, 'A Practical Programme' *Marriage Hygiene* (1934) 1(2):123–4. This article was published on the eve of her first visit to India.

58. Ruth Young, 'Some Aspects of Birth Control in India' *Marriage Hygiene* (1935:39).

59. Mehta, 'Indian Law of Abortion: Suggested Reforms', *The Third International Conference on Planned Parenthood: Report of the Proceedings*, The Family Planning Association of India, Bombay, (1952:158).

60. Ibid., pp. 158–9.

61. Gangoli (1998:86).

62. Ghurye (1935:324).

63. Ibid., p. 326.

64. Ghurye (1936:266).

65. A high social class which enjoyed high ritual status in Bengal and were permitted polygamy.

66. Bhattacharya, 'The Present Day Matrimonial System and its effects on the Sex Life in Bengal', *Marriage Hygiene*, 2,1, August (1935:64–5).

67. Ibid., p. 65.

Select Bibliography

Ackernecht, Erwin H. 1967. *Medicine at the Paris Hospital 1794–1848*. Baltimore: The Johns Hopkins University Press.

Ahluwalia, Sanjam. 2008. *Reproductive Restraints: Birth Control in India, 1877–1947*. New Delhi: Permanent Black.

———. 2006. 'Power, Ideology, and Sexual Politics: Indian Middle Class Male Advocates of Birth Control in Colonial India 1920–1940', in Sarah Hodges (ed.), *Population, Birth Control and Reproductive Health in Late Colonial India*.

Ainslie, Whitelaw. 1826. *Materia indica or, some account of those articles which are employed by the Hindus, and other eastern nations, in their medicine, arts, and agriculture*. Volume II. London: Longman and Green.

———. 1813. Materia Medica of Hindoostan, and Artisan's and Agriculturarist's Nomenclature. Madras: Government of Madras.

Ainslie, W., A. Smith, and M. Christy. 1816. *Medical, Geographical and Agricultural Report of a Committee Appointed by the Madras Government to Inquire into the Causes of the Epidemic Fever which Prevailed in the Provinces of Coimbatore, Madura, Dindigul, and Tinnevelly during the Years 1809, 1810, and 1811*. London: Black, Parbury and Allen.

Akhter, R., A. K. Dutt, and V. Wadhwa. 1998. 'Health Planning and the Resurgence of Malaria in Urban India', in A. G. Noble, F. J. Costa, A. K. Dutt, and R. B. Kent (eds), *Regional Development and Planning for the 21st Century: New Priorities*, pp. 151–68. Ashgate, Aldershot: New Philosophies.

Alavi, Seema. 2007. *Islam and Healing: Loss and Recovery of an Indo-Muslim Medical Tradition*. New Delhi: Permanent Black.

Alborn, Timothy L. 1999. 'Age and Empire in the Indian Census, 1871–1931', *Journal of Interdisciplinary History*, 30 (1): 61–89.

Alter, Joseph S. 2005. *Asian Medicine and Globalization*. Philadelphia: University of Pennsylvania Press.

———. 2004. *Yoga in Modern India: The Body between Science and Philosophy*. Princeton: Princeton University Press.

———. 2000. *Gandhi's Body: Sex, Diet, and the Politics of Nationalism*. Philadelphia: University of Pennsylvania Press.

Anandhi, S. 1998. 'Reproductive Bodies and Regulated Sexuality: Birth Control debates in early twentieth century Tamilnadu', in Mary E. John and

Janaki Nair (eds), *A Question of Silence? The Sexual Economies of Modern India*, pp. 139–166. Delhi: Kali for Women.

————. 2003. 'The Natures of Culture: Environment and Race in the Colonial Tropics', in Greenough P. and A. Lowenhaupt-Tsing (eds), *Nature in the Global South: Environmental Projects in South and Southeast Asia*, pp. 29–46. Durham N.C.: Duke University Press.

Anderson, Warwick. 2002. 'Postcolonial Technoscience', *Social Studies of Science*, 32 (5–6): 643–58.

————. 1996. 'Immunities of Empire: Race, Disease, and the New Tropical Medicine', *Bulletin of the History of Medicine*, 70 (1): 94–118.

————. 1995. 'Excremental Colonialism: Public Health and the Poetics of Pollution', *Critical Inquiry*, 21: 640–69.

————. 1992. 'Laboratory Medicine as Colonial Discourse', *Critical Inquiry*, 18: 506–29.

Annesley, J. 1825. 'Observations on the Use and Abuse of Calomel' (Presented on 6 March 1824), *Transactions of the Medical and Physical Society of Calcutta*, i: 211–17.

Antoinette Burton. 1996. 'Contesting the Zenana: The Mission to make "Lady Doctors" for India, 1874–1885', *Journal of British Studies*, July: 368–97.

Appadurai, Arjun. 1996. *Modernity at Large: Cultural Dimensions of Globalization*. Minneapolis: University of Minnesota Press.

———— (ed.). 1986. *The Social Life of Things: Commodities in Cultural Perspective*. Cambridge: Cambridge University Press.

Armstrong, David. 2002. *A New History of Identity: A Sociology of Medical Knowledge*. New York: Palgrave.

————. 1995. 'The Rise of Surveillance Medicine', *Sociology of Health and Illness*, 17 (3): 393–404.

————. 1993. 'Public Health Space and the Fabrication of Identity', *Sociology*, 27 (3): 393–410.

————. 1983. *Political Anatomy of the Body: Medical Knowledge in Britain in the 20th Century*. Cambridge: Cambridge University Press.

Arnold, David. 2006. 'Official Attitudes to Population, Birth Control and Reproductive Health 1926–1946', in Sarah Hodges (ed.), *Population, Birth Control and Reproductive Health in Late Colonial India*, pp. 22–50. New Delhi: Orient Longman.

Arnold, David. 2005. *The Tropics and the Traveling Gaze: India, Landscape, and Science 1800–1856*. New Delhi: Permanent Black.

Arnold, David and Gabrielle Hecht. 2004. 'Colonialism, Decolonization and Development: Analytic Themes, Research Programmatics, and Collaborative Projects', Internet paper. Available at http://www.histech.nl/tensions/Projecten/

CC/Budapest/CD/Budapest/papers/themeworksh/CDAtheme.htm (Last accessed 28 June 2005).

————. 2001. 'Disease, Resistance, and India's Ecological Frontier, 1770–1947', in J. C. Scott, and N. Bhatt, (eds), *Agrarian Studies*, pp. 186–205. New Delhi: Oxford University Press.

————. 2000. '"Illusory Riches": Representations of the Tropical World, 1840–1950', *Singapore Journal of Tropical Geography*, 21 (1): 6–19.

————. 1999. '"An Ancient Race Outworn" Malaria and Race in Colonial India, 1860–1930', in Ernst Waltraud and Bernard Harris (eds), *Race, Science and Medicine*, p. 139. London: Routledge.

———— (ed.). 1996. *Warm Climates and Western Medicine*. Amsterdam: Rodopi.

————. 1994. 'The "Discovery" of Malnutrition and Diet in Colonial India', *Indian Economic and Social History Review*, 31 (1): 1–26.

————. 1993. *Colonizing the Body: State Medicine and Epidemic Disease in Nineteenth Century India*. Berkeley and London: University of California Press.

————. 1991. *Imperialism and Medicine in Bengal*. New Delhi: Sage.

———— (ed.). 1989. *Imperial Medicine and Indigenous Societies*. New Delhi: Oxford University Press.

————. 1989. 'Ecology and Cosmology of Disease in the Banaras Region', in Sandria B. Freitag (ed.), *Culture and Power in Benares: Community, Performance, and Environment, 1800–1980*, pp. 246–67. New Delhi: Oxford University Press.

————. 1988. 'Touching the Body: Perspective on Indian Plague, 1896–1900', in Ranajit Guha and Gayatri Chakravorty Spivak (eds), *Selected Subaltern Studies*, pp. 391–426. New Delhi: Oxford University Press.

————. 1986. 'Cholera and Colonialism in British India', *Past and Present*, 113: 118–51.

Aronowitz, Robert, R. 1998, *Making Sense of Illness: Science, Society, and Disease*. Cambridge: Cambridge University Press.

Askari, S. H. 1957. 'Medicines and Hospitals in Muslim India', *Journal of Bihar Research Society*, 43: 7–21.

Baber, Zaheer. 1998. *The Science of Empire: Scientific Knowledge, Civilization, and Colonial Rule in India*. New Delhi: Oxford University Press.

Bagchi, Amiya Kumar and Krishna Soman (eds). 2005. *Maladies, Preventives and Curatives: Debates in Public Health in India*. New Delhi: Tulika.

Baker, C. J. 1981. 'Economic Reorganization and the Slump in South and Southeast Asia', *Comparative Studies in Society and History*, 23 (3): 325–39.

Bala, Poonam. 1991. *Imperialism and Medicine in Bengal: A Socio-Historical Perspective*. New Delhi: Sage Publications.

Balfour, Francis. 1784. *Treatise on the Influence of the Moon in Fevers*. Calcutta: C.Elliot.

Balfour, Margaret and Ruth Young. 1929. *The Work of Medical Women in India*. London: Oxford University Press.

Bandyopadhyay, Harinarayan. 1875. *Gurbbini Bandhab: A Treatise on Abortion to Which are Added Symptoms of Pregnancy*. Kolkata: JP Ray and Co.

Bandyopadhyaya, Tarashankar. 1996. *Arogyaniketan* (English Trans. Enakshi Chatterjee). New Delhi: Sahitya Akademi.

Banerjee, D. 1965. 'India's National Tuberculosis Programme in Relation to the Proposed Social and Economic Development Plans', *Indian Journal of Public Health*, 9: 103–6.

Banerjee, Madhulika. 2009. *Power Knowledge, Medicine: Ayurvedic Pharmaceuticals at Home and in the World*. Hyderabad: Orient Blackswan.

Barnes, Barry. 1974. *Scientific Knowledge and Sociological Theory*. London: Routledge.

Basham, A. L. 1976. 'Practice of Medicine in Ancient and Medieval India', in C. Leslie (ed.), *Asian Medical System*, pp. 18–43. Berkeley: California University Press.

Basu, Amit Ranjan. 2004. 'Emergence of a Marginal Science in a Colonial City: Reading Psychiatry in Bengali Periodicals', *Indian Economic and Social History Review*, 41: 103–41.

Basu, Raj Sekhar. 2002. 'Medical Missionaries in a Native Indian State: The Case of the LMS in Travancore, 1866–1950', *Bengal Past and Present*, Calcutta Historical Society, 121 (232–233): Parts I–II.

———. 2001. 'Medical Missionaries at Work: The Canadian Baptist Missionaries in the Telugu Country, 1870–1952', in Deepak Kumar (ed.), *Disease and Medicine in India: A Historical Overview*, pp. 180–97. New Delhi: Tulika.

Bell, Heather. 1999. *Frontiers of Medicine in the Anglo-Egyptian Sudan, 1899–1940*. Oxford: Clarendan Press.

Bellemy, David and Andrea Pfister. 1992. *World Medicine: Plants, Patients and People*. Oxford: Blackwell Publishing.

Benedict, Carol. 1997. Book Review: 'The Modern Epidemic: A History of Tuberculosis in Japan', *Bulletin of the History of Medicine*, 71 (4): 722–4.

Bentley, Charles. 1911. *An Investigation into the Causes of Malaria in Bombay and the Measures Necessary for its Control*. Mumbai: Government Central Press.

———. 1910. *An Interim Report upon Malaria in the Southern Portion of the Island of Bombay*. Mumbai: Government Central Press.

Berberoglu, B. 1992. *The Political Economy of Development: Dependent Theory and the Prospects for Change in the Third World*. New York: State University of New York Press.

Bewell, Allan. 1999. *Romanticism and Colonial Disease*. Baltimore: The Johns Hopkins University Press.

Bhabha, Homi K. 1994. *The Location of Culture*. London and New York: Routledge.

Bhardwaj, Surinder M. 1981. 'Homoeopathy in India', in Giri Raj Gupta (ed.), *The Social and Cultural Context of Medicine in India*, Volume IV, pp. 31–54. New Delhi: Vikas Publishing House.

Bhargav, Raghubir Sahay. 1926. *Stethoscope*. Bulandshar: Author.

Bhattacharya, Deborah. 1984. 'Desire in Bengali Ethnopsychology', *Contributions to Asian Studies*, XVIII: 73–84.

Bhattacharya, Jayanta. 2009. 'The Knowledge of Anatomy and Health in Ayurveda: Colonial Confrontation and Its Outcome', *Eä-Revista de Humanidades Médicas and Estudios Sociales de la Ciencia Y la Tecnología*, 1(1):1–51.

———. 2004. 'The Body: Epistemological Encounters in Colonial India', in Vera Kalitzkas and Peter L. Twohig (eds), *Making Sense of Health, Illness, and Disease*, pp. 31–54. Amsterdam: Rodopi.

Bhattacharya, Sanjay, Mark Harrison, and Michael Worboys. 2005. *Fractured States: Small Pox, Public Health and Vaccination Policy in British India, 1800–1947*. New Delhi: Orient Longman.

Bhattacharya, Tithi. 2005. *The Sentinels of Culture: Class, Education, and the Colonial Intellectual in Bengal*. New Delhi: Oxford University Press.

Biswas, Arun Kumar. 2003. *Collected Works of Mahendralal Sircar, Eugene Lafont and the Science Movement (1860–1910)*. Kolkata: The Asiatic Society.

———. 2001. *Father Eugene Lafont of St. Xavier College, Kolkata and the Contemporary Science Movement*. Kolkata: The Asiatic Society.

———. 2000. *Gleanings of the Past and the Science Movement in the Diaries of Dr. Mahendralal and Amritlal Sircar*. Kolkata: The Asiatic Society.

Bhunt, E (ed.). 1938. *Social Service in India*. London: HMSO.

Bodding, Paul Olaf. 1986 (Reprint). *Studies in Santal Medicine and Connected Folklore*. Kolkata: The Asiatic Society.

Bontius, James (ed.), 1769. *An Account of the Diseases, Natural History, and Medicines of the East Indies*. London: T. Noteman.

Boonen, P. and Linden van der Sj. 2005. 'Case Number 33: About Being a Famous European and Suffering from Gout', *Annals of Rheumatic Disease*, 64 (4): 538.

Bose, Chunilal. 1930. *Food*. Kolkata: University of Kolkata.

Bose, Pradip. 2006. *Health and Society in Bengal: A Selection from Late 19th-Century Bengali Periodicals*. New Delhi: Sage Publications.

Boyd, Kenneth. 2000. 'Disease, Illness, Sickness, Health, Healing and Wholeness: Exploring Some Elusive Concepts', *Medical Humanities*, 26 (1): 9-17.

Bradford, Thomas Lindsley. 1970 (1895). *The Life and Letters of Dr Samuel Hahnemann*. Kolkata: Roy Publishing House.

Branca, Patricia. 1977. *The Medicine Show: Patients, Physicians and the Perplexities of the Health Revolution in Modern Society*. New York: Neale Watson Academic Publications, Inc.

Brandt Allan M. 1987. *No Magic Bullet: A Social History of Venereal Disease in the United States since 1880*. Oxford: Oxford University Press.

Briggs, Asa. 1961. 'Cholera and Society in the Nineteenth Century', *Past and Present*, 19 April: 76–96.

Brockway, Lucile. 1979. *Science and Colonial Expansion: The Role of the British Royal Botanic Gardens*. New York: Academic Press.

Bryce, James. 1796. *Account of the Yellow Fever, with a Successful Method of Cure*. Edinburgh: W. Creech.

Buckland, C. E. 1971. *Dictionary of Indian Biography*. New Delhi: Indological Book House.

Burnum, John F. 1993. 'Medical Diagnosis through Semiotics: Giving Meaning to the Sign', *Annals of Internal Medicine*, 119 (9): 939–43.

Burris, Scott. 2000. 'Contagion and Confinement: Controlling Tuberculosis along the Skid Road', *Journal of Health Politics, Policy and Law*, 25 (6): 1168–71.

Butler, B. 1829. 'On Public Health in India', *Transactions of the Medical & Physical Society of Calcutta*, IV: 121–56.

Bynum, W. F. 2000. 'Malaria in inter-war British India', *Parasitologia*, 42: 25–31.

Bynum W. F. and Roy Porter (eds). 1987. *Medical Fringe and Medical Orthodoxy 1750–1850*. London: Croom Helm.

Canguilhem, Feorges. 1978. *On the Normal and the Pathological*. Dordrecht: D. Reidel Publishing Co.

Carney, Judith A. 2001. *Black Rice: The African Origins of Rice Cultivation in the Americas*. Cambridge, Massachusetts: Harvard University Press.

Cave, A. J. E. 1935. 'Evidence of Incidence of Tuberculosis in Ancient Egypt', *British Journal of Tuberculosis*, 33: 142–52.

Chakrabarti, Pratik. 2010. 'Beasts of Burden: Animals and Laboratory Research in Colonial India', *History of Science*, XLVII: 125–52.

———. 2004. *Western Science in Modern India: Metropolitan Methods, Colonial Practices*. New Delhi: Permanent Black.

Chakrabarty, Dipesh. 1991. 'Open Space/Public Place: Garbage, Modernity and India', *South Asia*, 14 (1): 15–31.

———. 1990. 'Invitation to a Dialogue', *Subaltern Studies*, IV: 376.

Chatterjee, Partha. 1986. *Nationalist Thought and the Colonial World: A Derivative Discourse*. London: Zed Books for the United Nations University.

Chattopadhyaya, Debiprasad. 1977. *Science and Society in Ancient India*. Kolkata: Research India Publications.

Chaudhuri, K. N. 1985. *Trade and Civilisation of the Indian Ocean from the Rise of Islam to 1750*. Cambridge: Cambridge University Press.

————. 1978. *The Trading World of Asia and the English East India Company 1660–1760*. Cambridge: Cambridge University Press.

Chevers, Norman. 1856. *A Manual of Medical Jurisprudence for Bengal and the North Western Provinces*. Kolkata: Military Orphan Press.

Chisholm, Colin. 1795. *An Essay on the Malignant Pestilential Fever Introduced into the West Indian Islands from Boullam, on the Coast of Guinea, as it Appeared in 1793 and 1794*. London: C. Dilly.

Chopra, R. N. 1936. *A Handbook of Tropical Therapeutics*. Kolkata: Art Press.

Choudhary, B. K. 2008. *Tuberculosis in India: A Political Ecology Approach*. Saarbruecken: VDM Verlag.

Chowdhury, Indira. 2002. 'Instructions to the Unconverted: Marie Stopes, Indian Women and the Making of a Pamphlet, 1920–1955', *From the Margins*, February: 214–42.

————. 1998. *The Frail Hero and Virile History: Gender and the Politics of Culture in Colonial Bengal*. New Delhi: Oxford University Press.

Church, A. H. 1886. *Food-Grains of India*. London: Chapman & Hall.

Clark, James. 1797. *A Treatise on the Yellow Fever, as it appeared in the Island of Dominica, in the Years 1793-4-5-6*. London: J. Murray & S. Highley.

Clark, Thomas. 1801. *Observations on the Nature and Cure of Fevers, and of Diseases of the West and East Indies, and of America: With an Account of Dissections Performed in These Climates and General Remarks on Diseases of the Army*. Edinburgh: Bell & Bradfute.

Clarke, John. 1775. *Observations on the Diseases in Long Voyages to Hot Countries, and Particularly on Those Which Prevail in the East Indies*. London: D. Wilson and G. Nicol.

Cohn, Bernard S. 1999. 'The Command of Language and the Language of Command', in Ranajit Guha (ed.), *Subaltern Studies IV*, pp. 276–329. New Delhi: Oxford University Press.

————. 1997. *Colonialism and Its Forms of Knowledge: The British in India*. New Delhi: Oxford University Press.

Cook, Harold J. 2007. *Matters of Exchange: Commerce, Medicine, and Science in the Dutch Golden Age*. New Haven and London: Yale University Press.

Cooper, F. 1996. *Decolonization and African Society*. Cambridge: Cambridge University Press.

Cooper F. and A. L. Stoler (eds). 1997. *Tensions of Empire: Colonial Cultures in a Bourgeois World*. Berkeley: University of California Press.

Covell, Gordon. 1928. *Malaria in Bombay*. Mumbai: Government Central Press.

Crawford, D. G. 1930. *Roll of the Indian Medical Service 1615–1930*. London: Thacker & Co.

Crosby, Alfred W., Jr. 1986. *Ecological Imperialism: The Biological Expansion of Europe 900–1900*. Cambridge: Cambridge University Press.

———. 1972. *The Columbian Exchange: The Biological and Cultural Consequences of 1492*, Westport: Duke University Press.

Culler, Jonathan. 2001. *The Pursuit of Signs*. London: Routledge.

———. 1888. 'The Public Health in India', *Jr. of the Society of Arts*, XXXVI (February: 241–65).

Cunningham, J. M. 1884. *Cholera: What Can the State Do to Prevent It?* Kolkata: Government Printing Press.

Cunningham, A. and B. Andrew (eds). 1997. *Western Medicine as Contested Knowledge*. Manchester: Manchester University Press.

Cunningham, A. and R. French (eds). 1990. *The Medical Enlightenment of the Eighteenth Century*. Cambridge: Cambridge University Press.

Currie, James. 1809. *Examination of the Prejudices Commonly Entertained against Mercury as Beneficially Applicable to Most Hepatic Complaints*. London: J. M'Creery.

Curtin, Philip D. 1989. *Death by Migration: Europe's Encounter with the Tropical World in the Nineteenth Century*. Cambridge: Cambridge University Press.

———. 1984. *Cross-Cultural Trade in World History; Studies in Comparative World History*. Cambridge: Cambridge University Press.

Curtis, Charles. 1807. *An Account of the Diseases of India, as They Appeared in the English Fleet, and in the Naval Hospital at Madras, in 1782 and 1783; with Observations on Ulcers, and the Hospital Sores of That Country*. London: Longman and J. Murray.

———. *An Account of the Diseases of India*. Edinburgh: W. Laing.

Davis, Mike. 2006. *Planet of Slums*. London: Verso.

de Figueredo, John M. 1984. 'Ayurvedic Medicine in Goa According to European Sources in the Sixteenth and Seventeenth Centuries', *Bulletin of History of Medicine*, 58 (2): 225–35.

Deliege, Robert. 1985. *The Bhils of Western India: Some Empirical And Theoretical Issues In Anthropology In India*. New Delhi: National Publication House.

Denoon, Donald. 1989. *Public Health in Papua New Guinea*. Cambridge: Cambridge University Press.

Dey, Kanny Lal. 1866. *Hindu Social Laws and Habits Viewed in Relation to Health*. Kolkata: R. C. Lepage.

Dhareshwar, Vivek. 1998. 'Valorizing the Present: Orientalism, Postcoloniality and the Human Sciences', *Cultural Dynamics*, 10 (2): 211–31.

Drayton, Richard. 2000. *Nature's Government: Science, Imperial Britain and the 'improvement' of the World*. New Haven: Yale University Press.

Dubey, K. K., S. K. Bhasin, and M. S. Bhatia. 2000. 'Emotional Problems Amongst Hospitalized Tuberculosis Patients in Delhi', *Indian Medical Gazette*, 134: 65–9.

———. 1999. 'Impact of Tuberculosis on Sexual Relationship Amongst Hospitalized Patients', *Indian Practitioner*, 52: 680.

———. 1998. 'Psychological Reactions Amongst Patients, Their Family Members and the Community Regarding Hospitalized Tuberculosis Patients in Delhi', *Psychiatry Today*, 11: 30.

Dubey, Pandit Kali Charan. 1913. *Balakon Ke Poshanarth Avashyak Sikshayen*. Benares: Public Health Department, Municipal Board.

Dubos, R. and J. Dubos. 1952. *The White Plague: Tuberculosis, Man and Society*. Boston: Little Brown and Company.

Duncan, Andrew. 1794. *Medical Commentaries for the Year MDCCXCIII*. Volume VIII. London: G. C. & J. Robinson.

Dymock, W. 1884. *The Vegetable Materia Medica of Western India*. Mumbai: Education Society Press.

Eck, Diana L. 1983. *Banaras: City of Light*. New Delhi: Penguin Books.

Ehrenreich, J. (ed.). 1978. *The Cultural Crisis of Modern Medicine*. New York: Monthly Review Press.

Ehrlich, Paul and Robert Ornstein. 2010. *Humanity as a Tightrope: Thoughts on Empathy, Family and Big Changes for a Viable Future*. Maryland: Rowman and Littlefield Publishers.

Elgood, Cyril. 1970. *Safavid Medical Practice*. London: Luzac & Co.

Engelhardt, Ute. 2001. 'Dietetics in Tang China and the First Extant Works of Materia Medica', in Elizabeth Hsu (ed.), *Innovation in Chinese Medicine*, pp. 173–91. Cambridge: Cambridge University Press.

Ernst, Waltraud. 2002. *Plural Medicine, Tradition and Modernity, 1800–2000*. London: Routledge.

Ethirajulu Naidu, T. R. 1918. *The Ayurvedic System*. Chennai: Thompson & Co.

Ewart, Joseph. 1882. 'On Scrofula, Tuberculosis, and Phthisis in India', *Indian Medical Gazette*, 17: 335.

Fairchild, A. L. and G. M. Oppenheimer. 1998. 'Public Health Then and Now: Public Health Nihilism Vs Pragmatism – History, Politics and the Control of Tuberculosis', *American Journal of Public Health*, 88 (7): 1105–17.

Falck, N. D. 1776. *A Treatise on the Medical Qualities of Mercury*. London: B. Law.

Fanon, Franz. 1978. 'Medicine and Colonialism', in J. Ehrenreich (ed.), *The Cultural Crisis of Modern Medicine*, pp. 229–51. New York: Monthly Review Press, New York.

Faruqi, A. H. 1985. 'Tibb-I Shahabi: A Rare Medical Treatise of Tughlaq Period', *Studies in History of Medicine and Science*, 9: 35–42.

Fielding, Michael (ed.). 1935. *Birth Control in Asia: A Report of a Conference held at the London School of Hygiene and Tropical Medicine, November 24–25 1933*. London: Birth Control International Information Centre.

Filliozat, J. 1964. *The Classical Doctrine of Indian Medicine* (Translated from French by Dev Raj Chanana). New Delhi: Munshiram Manoharlal.

Fitzgerald, Rosemary. 2001. 'Clinical Christianity: The Emergence of Medical Work as a Missionary Strategy in Colonial India, 1800–1914', in Biswamoy Pati and Mark Harrison (eds), *Health, Medicine and Empire*, pp. 88–136. Hyderabad: Orient Longman.

Fleming, John. 1810. 'A catalogue of Indian medical plants', *Asiatick Researches*, 11: 1685–6.

Foster, W. D. 1959. 'The Early History of Clinical Pathology in Great Britain', *Medical History*, 3 (3): 173–87.

Foucault, Michel. 2003. *Society Must Be Defended: Lectures at the College de France, 1975–6* (Trans. D. Macey). London: Penguin.

———. 1991. 'Governmentality' (1978) in Burchell, Graham *et al*, (eds), *The Foucault Effect: Studies in Governmentality*, pp. 100–102. Chicago: University of Chicago Press.

———. 1980. *History of Sexuality: An Introduction*. New York: Vintage Books.

———. 1994. *The Birth of the Clinic: An Archaeology of Medical Perception*. New York: Vintage Books.

Fredriksen, S. 2002. 'Diseases are Invisible', *Journal of Medical Ethics: Medical Humanities*, 28: 71–3.

Fremantle, Francis. 1911. *A Traveller's Study of Health and Empire*. London: John Ousley Ltd.

Fryer, John. 1912. *A New Account of East India and Persia Being Nine Years' Travels 1672–1681*. (Edited with notes and introduction by William Crooke). London: The Hakluyt Society. (Indian reprint by Asian Educational Services, New Delhi, 1992).

Gadgil, M. D. 1935. 'Manav Sharir Ke Adhbhut Karya', *Saraswati*, 36 (3): 258–62.

Gaier, Harald C. 1991. *Thorsons Encyclopaedic Dictionary of Homoeopathy: The Definitive Reference to All Aspects of Homoeopathy*. London: Thorsons (An imprint of Harper Collin's Publishers).

Gaitonde, P. D. 1983. *Portuguese Pioneers in India: Spotlight on Medicine*. Bombay: Popular Prakashan.

Gandhi, M. K. 1949. *Diet and Diet Reform*. Ahmedabad: Navajivan Publishing House.

Gangoli, Geetanjali. 1998. 'Reproduction, Abortion and Women's Health', *Social Scientist*, 28 (11–12): 86.

Garcia da Orta. 1913. *Coloquios dos Simples e drogas he cousas medicinais da India*. (English trans. Clements Markham. *Colloquies on the simples and drugs of India*.). London: Henry Sotheran & Co.

Garg, Mahendulal. 1908. 'Plague-Tattva-Element of Plague', *Saraswati*, 9 (4): 208–10.

———. 1908. 'Rakt Brahman', *Saraswati*, 9 (11): 430–2.

Geetakrishnan K., K. P. Pappu, and K. Roychowdhury. 1988. 'A Study on Knowledge and Attitude towards Tuberculosis in a Rural Area of West Bengal', *Indian Journal of Tuberculosis*, 35: 83–98.

Ghose, Sharat Chandra. 1935. *Life of Dr Mahendra Lal Sircar*. Kolkata: Hahnemann Publications.

Girdavar, Babu Sannulal Gupt. 1922. *Stri Subodhini – Education for Women*. Lucknow: Newal Kishore Press.

Golden, Janet Lynne. 1997. 'Culturing Tuberculosis: The Multiple Meanings of Disease', Reviews in *American History*, 25 (4): 600–5.

Goldwater, J. 1972. *Mercury: A History of Quicksilver*. Baltimore: York Press.

Goodeve, H. H. 1837. 'A Sketch on the Progress of European Medicine in the East', *Quarterly Journal of the Calcutta Medical and Physical Society*, 2: 145.

Gourou, Pierre. 1966. *The Tropical World: Its Social and Economic Conditions and Its Future Status* (4th ed.) (Trans. S. Beaver, E. Laborde). London: Longman.

Gourou, Pierre and E. D. Ladorbe. 1953. *The Tropical World: Its Social and Economic Conditions and its Future Status*. London: Presses Universitaires De France.

Grant, Mark. 2000. *Galen on Food and Diet*. London: Routledge.

Gribble, J. M. D. 1885. *Outlines of Medical Jurisprudence for Indian Criminal Courts*. Chennai: Higginbotham and Co.

Grove, Richard. 1996. 'Indigenous Knowledge and the Significance of South West India for the Portuguese and Dutch Constructions of Tropical Nature', *Modern Asian Studies*, 30 (1): 121–43.

———. 1995. *Green Imperialism; Colonial Expansion, Tropical Island Edens and the Origins of Environmentalism*. Cambridge: Cambridge University Press.

Guha, Sumit. 2001. *Health and Population in South Asia: From Earliest Times to the Present*. London: C. Hurst & Co.

Guha, Supriya. 1998. 'From Dais to Doctors: The Medicalisation of Childbirth in Colonial India', in Lakshmi Lingam (ed.), *Understanding Women's Health Issues: A Reader*, pp. 145–61. New Delhi: Kali Publishing.

Gull, William W. 1853. *Report on the Morbid Anatomy, Pathology, and Treatment of Cholera*. London: Churchill Publications.

Gupta, B. 1976. 'Indigenous Medicine in Nineteenth and Twentieth Century Bengal', in Charles Leslie (ed.), *Asian Medical Systems*, pp. 368–78. California: University of California.

Gupta, Charu. 2001. *Sexuality, Obscenity, Community: Women, Muslims and the Hindu Public in Colonial India*. New Delhi: Permanent Black.

Gupta, Giri Raj (ed.). 1981. *The Social and Cultural Context of Medicine in India*, Volume IV. New Delhi: Vikas Publishing House.

Gupta, Prakash Chandra. 1968. *Makers of Indian Literature: Prem Chand*. New Delhi: Sahitya Akademi.

Guy, Attewell. 2007. *Refiguring Unani Tibb Plural Healing in Late Colonial India*. Hyderabad: Orient Longman.

Hacker, J. H. 1887. *Memoirs of Thomas Smith Thomson: Medical Missionary at Neyoor*. Travancore: The Religious Tract Society.

Haehl, Richard. 1971 (First published in 1922/23). *Samuel Hahnemann: His Life and Work. 2 volumes.* (Trans. from the German by Marie L. Wheeler and W. H. R. Grundy. Ed. by J. H. Clarke and F. J. Wheeler) New Delhi: B. Jain Publishers.

Haggett, P. 1990. *The Geographer's Art*. Oxford: Basil Blackwell.

Hahnemann, Samuel. 1979 (1843). *Organon of Medicine*. 6th ed. (Trans. by William Boericke). New Delhi: B. Jain Publishers.

Hall, Ruth. 1977. *Marie Stopes: A Biography*. London: Andre Deutsche Limited.

Hameed, Hakim Abdul. 1986. *Exchanges between India and Central Asia in the Field of Medicine*. New Delhi: Jamia Hamdard.

Hardiman, D. 2009. *Missionaries and Their Medicine: A Christian Modernity for Tribal India*. Manchester: Manchester University Press.

Harrison, Mark. 2009. 'Racial Pathologies: Morbid Anatomy in British India, 1770–1850', in Biswamoy Pati and Mark Harrison (ed.), *The Social History of Health and Medicine in Colonial India*. New York: Routledge, pp. 173–94.

———. 2005. 'Science and the British Empire', *Isis*, 96 (1): 56–63.

———. 2001. 'Medicine and Orientalism: Perspectives on Europe's Encounter with Indian Medical Systems', in Biswamoy, Pati and Mark Harrison (eds), *Health, Medicine and Empire: Perspectives on Colonial India*, pp. 37–87. Hyderabad: Orient Longman.

———. 2000. 'From Medical Astrology to Medical Astronomy: Sol-Lunar and Planetary Theories of Disease in British Medicine, c.1700–1850', *British Journal for the History of Science*, 33: 25–48.

———. 1999. *Climates and Constitutions: Health, Race, Environment and British Imperialism in India, 1600–1850*. New Delhi: Oxford University Press.

———. 1996. '"The Tender Frame of Man": Disease, Climate, and Racial Difference in India and the West Indies, 1760–1860', *Bulletin of the History of Medicine*, 70 (1): 68–93.

———. 1994. *Public Health in British India: Anglo Indian Preventive Medicine 1859–1914*. Cambridge: Cambridge University Press.

Harrison, Mark and Michael Worboys. 1997. 'A Disease of Civilization: Tuberculosis in Britain, Africa and India, 1900–1939', in M. Worboys and L. Marks (eds), *Migrants, Minorities and Health: Historical and Contemporary Studies*, pp. 93–124. London: Routledge.

Hartnack, Christiane. 2000. *Psychoanalysis in Colonial India*. New Delhi: Oxford University Press.

Harvey, Robert. 1876. *Report of the Medico-Legal Returns received from the Civil Surgeon in Bengal Presidency during the Years 1870, 1871 and 1872*. Kolkata: Central Book Press.

Hatcher, Brian A. 2000. *Idioms of Improvement: Vidyāsāgar and Cultural Encounter in Bengal*. New Delhi: Oxford University Press.

Headrick, Daniel R. 1981. *The Tools of Empire: Technology and European Imperialism in the Nineteenth Century*. New York: Oxford University Press.

Himes, Norman. 1936. *Medical History of Contraception*. Baltimore: Williams and Wilkins.

Hla, Ludu U. 1986. *The Caged Ones* (1958). (Trans. Sein Tu). Bangkok: Tamarind Press.

Hehir, Patrick. 1927. *Malaria in India*. London: Oxford University Press.

Hodges, Sarah (ed.). 2006. *Reproductive Health in India: History, Politics and Controversies*. Hyderabad: Orient Longman.

———. 2006. 'Eugenic Maternity', in Sarah Hodges (ed.), *Population, Birth Control and Reproductive Health*.

Hollen, Cecilia Van. 2003. *Birth on the Threshold: Childbirth and Modernity in South India*. Berkeley: University of California Press.

Houlston, Thomas. 1784. *Observations on Poisons and on the Use of Mercury in the Cure of Obstinate Dysenteries*. London: H. Reynell.

Hsu, Elizabeth. 2005. 'Tactility and the Body in the Early Chinese Medicine', *Science in Context*, 18 (1): 7–34.

Hume, J. C. 1977. 'Rival Traditions: Western Medicine and Yunani Tibb in the Punjab, 1849–1889', *Bulletin of History of Medicine*, 51: 214–31.

Hunter, W. 1891. *State Education for the People*. London: George Routledge and Sons.

———. 1836. 'Indian Hospital Reports', *London Medical Gazette; being a Weekly Journal of Medicine and the Collateral Sciences*, 28: 382–4.

Hutchinson, James. 1845. *Observations on the General and Medical Management of Indian Jails* (2nd edition). Kolkata: G. H. Huttmann.

Inkster, Ian. 1983. 'Aspects of the History of Science and Science Culture in Britain', in Ian Inkster and Jack Morell (eds), *Metropolis and Province: Science in British Culture, 1780–1850*, pp.11–54. London: Hutchinson.

Irschick, Eugene F. 1994. *Dialogue and History: Constructing South India, 1795–1895*. Berkeley: University of California Press.

Irvine, R. H. 1848. *A Short Account of the Materia Medica of Patna*. Kolkata: Military Orphan Press.

Jaggarajamma, K., Rajeswari Ramachandran, and Nirupa Charles. 2008. 'Psycho-social Dysfunction: Perceived and Enacted Stigma among Tuberculosis Patients Registered under Revised National Tuberculosis Control Programme', *Indian Journal of Tuberculosis*, Vol. 55, p.183.

Jaggi, O. P. 1981. *Indian System of Medicine*, Volume IV. New Delhi: Atma Ram and Sons.

Jameson, J. 1820. *Report on the Epidemick Morbus, as It Visited the Territories Subject to the Presidency of Bengal, in the Years 1817, 1818, and 1819*. Kolkata: Government Gazette Press.

Jeffery, R. 1988. *The Politics of Health in India*. Berkeley: University of California Press.

Jenkins, Mary. 1995. *Indian Interlude: A Surgeon in India, Derek Jenkins and the Place of Ghee – The Story of an Indian Village*. Aylesburg: Rakewell Limited.

Johnson, James. 1813. *The Influence of Tropical Climates, More Especially the Climate of India, on European Constitutions*. London: J. J. Stockdale.

Johnson, J. and J. R. Martin. 1841. *The Influence of Tropical Climate on European Constitutions*. 6th ed. London: S. Highley.

Jolly, Julius. 1977. *Indian Medicine*, 2nd ed. New Delhi: Munshiram Manoharlal.

Jones, C. and H. Williams. 2004. 'The Social Burden of Malaria: What are We Measuring?', *American Journal of Tropical Medicine and Hygiene*, 71 (Suppl. 20): 156–61.

Jones, Kenneth W. 1976. *Arya Dharma: Hindu Consciousness in Nineteenth Century Punjab*. Berkeley: California University Press.

Jordanova, Ludmila. 1995. 'The Social Construction of Medical Knowledge', *Social History of Medicine*, 8: 361–82.

Joseph, Jaques. 1987. *Rhinoplasty and Facial Plastic Surgery with a Supplement on Mammaplasty*, Stanley Milestein (Trans), San Francisco: J Norman & Co., 217–21.

Joshi, Sanjay. 2001. *Fractured Modernity: The Making of a Middle Class in Colonial North India*. New Delhi: Oxford University Press.

Kakar, D. N. 1988. *Primary Health Care and Traditional Medical Practitioners*. New Delhi: Sterling Publishers Private Limited.

Kakar, Sanjeev. 1996. 'Leprosy in British India, 1860–1940: Colonial Politics and Missionary Medicine', *Medical History*, 40: 215–30.

Kakar, Sudhir. 1982. *Shamans, Mystics and Doctors: A Psyhological Enquiry into India and its Healing Traditions*. New York: Knopf.

Kapila, Shruti. 2005. 'Masculinity and Madness: Princely Personhood and Colonial Sciences of the Mind in Western India 1871–1940', *Past and Present*, 187: 121–56.

Kaviraj, Vishgaratna Kunjalal. 1963. (Trans. and ed.). *Sushruta-samhitâ* (2nd edn), Volume ii. Varanasi: Chowkhamba Sanskrit Series Office.

Kawashima, Koji. 1998. *Missionaries and a Hindu State, Travancore: 1858–1936.* New Delhi: Oxford University Press.

Kazi, Ihtesham. 2004. *A Historical Study of Malaria in Bengal, 1860–1920.* Dhaka: Pip International Publications.

Kennedy, James. 1831. *The History of the Contagious Cholera; With Facts Explanatory of Its Origin and Laws of a Rational Method of Cure.* London: James Cochrane and Co.

Keswani, N. H. (ed.). 1974. *The Science of Medicine in Ancient and Medieval India.* New Delhi: Thompson Press India.

King, Helen. 1998. *Hippocrates' Woman: Reading the Female Body in Ancient Greece.* London: Routledge.

Kiple, Kenneth F. 1993. *History of Disease.* New York: Cambridge University Press.

Klein, Ira. 2001. 'Development and Death: Reinterpreting Malaria, Economics and Ecology in British India', *The Indian Economic and Social History Review*, 38 (2): 147–79.

———. 1972. 'Malaria and Mortality in Bengal, 1840–1921', *Indian Economic and Social History Review*, IX (2): 132–60.

Korner, T. W. 1996. *The Pleasures of Counting.* Cambridge: Cambridge University Press.

Kratoska, P., R. Raben, and H. Schulte Nordholt (eds). 2005. *Locating Southeast Asia: Geographies of Knowledge and Politics of Space.* Singapore: Singapore University Press.

Krishnankutty, Gita. 2001. *A Life of Healing: A Biography of Vaidyaratnam P. S. Varier.* New Delhi: Viking Penguin India.

Kumar, Anil. 1998. *Medicine and the Raj: British Medical Policy in India, 1835–1911.* New Delhi: Sage Publications.

Kumar, Deepak. 2007. *Science and the Raj* (2nd edition). New Delhi: Oxford University Press.

———. (ed.). 2001. *Disease and Medicine in India: A Historical Overview.* New Delhi: Indian History Congress and Tulika.

Kumar, Neelam (ed.). 2009. *Women and Science in India- A Reader.* New Delhi: Oxford University Press.

———. 1995. *Science and the Raj.* Delhi: Oxford University Press.

Kumar, Nita. 1988. *The Artisans of Banaras: Popular Culture and Identity, 1880–1986.* New Delhi: Orient Longman.

Lal, Maneesha. 2003. '"The Ignorance of Women Is the House of Illness": Gender, Nationalism and Health Reform in Colonial North India', in Mary P. Sutphen and Bridie Andrews (eds), *Medicine and Colonial Identity*, pp. 14–40. London and New York: Routledge.

Lal, Maneesha. 1994. 'The Politics of Gender and Medicine in Colonial India: The Countess of Dufferin's Fund, 1885–1888', *Bulletin of the History of Medicine*, 68 (1): 29–66.

Lall, Maikoo. 1896. *A Treatise on Cholera Fever and Small Pox*. Lucknow: Emerald Press.

Lambert, A. C. 1918. 'The Treatment of Amoebic Dysentery with Emetine and Bismuth Iodide', *British Medical Journal*, I: 116–18.

Langford, Jean M. 2002. *Fluent Bodies: Ayurvedic Remedies for Postcolonial Imbalance*. Durham, N. C.: Duke University Press.

Lankaster, A. 1916. *Report on Tuberculosis in India*. New Delhi: NAI.

Lannoy, Richard. 2002. *Benares: A World within a World – The Microcosm of Kashi Yesterday and Today*. Varanasi: Indica Publishers.

Latour, Bruno. 1987. *Science in Action*. Massachusetts: Harvard University Press.

Leach, Edmund. 1960. 'The Frontiers of "Burma"', *Comparative Studies in Society and History*, 3 (1): 49–86.

Leith, A. H. 1851–2. 'A contribution to dietetics', *Transactions of the Medical and Physical Society of Bombay*, 1: 114–27.

Leslie, Charles and Allan Young (eds). 1992. *Paths to Asian Medical Knowledge*. Berkeley: University of California Press.

Leslie, Charles. 1992. 'Interpretations of Illness: Syncretism in Modern Ayurveda', in Leslie, Charles, and Allan Young (eds), *Paths to Asian Medical Knowledge*, p. 197. Berkeley: University of California Press.

———. (ed.). 1977. *Asian Medical Systems: A Comparative Study*. Berkeley: University of California Press.

Lewis, L. 2000. *Empire State Building: War and Welfare in Kenya, 1925–52*. Oxford: James Currey.

Lewis, Michael. 2003. *Inventing Global Ecology: Tracking the Biodiversity Ideal in India 1945–1997*. New Delhi: Orient Longman.

Li, Shang-Jen. 2002. 'Natural History of Parasitic Disease', *Isis*, 93 (2): 206–28.

Lind, James. 1787. 'An Account of the Efficacy of Mercury in the Cure of Inflammatory Diseases, and the Dysentery', *London Medical Journal*, 8: 43–56.

Lindsay, A. K. 1829. 'Case of Lithotomy, performed by a Native', *Transactions of the Medical and Physical Society of Calcutta*, 4: 440–2.

Lloyd, G. E. R. 1990. *Demystifying Mentalities*. Cambridge: Cambridge University Press.

———. (ed.). 1978. *Hippocratic Writings*. London: Penguin.

Longmate, Barak. 1794. 'Curious Chirurgical Operation', *Gentleman's Magazine and Historical Chronicle for the Year MDCCXCIV*, 64 (2): 891–2.

Mabit, J. 1804. *Essai sur les Maladies de l'Armée de St.-Domingue en l'anXI, et principalement sur la Fièvre Jaune*. Paris: Ecole de Médecine.

Maclarty. 1796. 'History of a Case of the Epidemic Fever of Jamaica terminating successfully; in which a very large quantity of Mercury was employed, without any obvious Operation during the Fever', *Annals of Medicine*, 1: 328–33.

Maclean, Charles. 1810. *An Analytical View of the Medical Department of the British Army*. London: J. Stockdale.

MacLeod, R. and Lewis, M. (eds). 1988. *Disease, Medicine and Empire*. London: Routledge.

Macpherson, John. 1866. *Cholera in Its Home with a Sketch of the Pathology and Treatment of the Disease*. London: John Churchill and Sons.

Magner, Lois N. 1992. *A History of Medicine*. New York: Marcel Dekker.

Majumdar, G. P. 1935–6. 'Health and Hygiene', *Indian Culture*, II (1–4): 633–54.

Malhotra, Anshu. 2002. *Gender, Caste, and Religious Identities*. New Delhi: Oxford University Press.

Mandal, Panchanan. 1953. *Chithipatre Samajchitra* (A Picture of Social Life through Letters), vol. 2. Santiniketan: Viswa Bharati Press.

Manderson, Lenore. 1996. *Sickness and the State: Health and Illness in Colonial Malaya 1870–1940*. Cambridge: Cambridge University Press.

Manickam, Sundaraj. 1977. *The Social Setting of Christian Conversion in South India*, Weisbaden: Steiner.

Marks, Robert B. 2002. *The Origins of the Modern World: A Global and Ecological Narrative*. Lanham: Rowman and Littlefield.

Mason. George. 1873. *On the Surgery of the Face*. London: J. & A. Churchill.

Mayne, John D. 1876. *Commentaries on the Indian Penal Code (Act XLV of 1860)*. Chennai: Higginbothan and Co.

M'Cabe, James. 1825. *Military Medical Reports; containing Pathological and Practical Observations Illustrating the Diseases of Warm Climates*. Cheltenham: G. A. Williams.

McKeown, T. 1976. *The Modern Rise of Population*. London: Arnold-Heinemann.

McNeill, William H. 1982. *The Pursuit of Power: Technology, Armed Force, and Society Since A.D. 100*. Chicago: University of Chicago Press.

———. 1976. *Plagues and People*. Garden City, New York: Anchor Press.

———. 1963. *The Rise of the West: A History of the Human Community*. (Maps by Béla Petheö). New York: New American Library.

Mcphail, James M. 1906. *A General Survey: Medical Missionary Work in India* (A Paper read at the Calcutta Missionary Conference, 4 September 1905). Pakhuria, Manbhum: Indian Medical Missionary Association, Santal Mission Press.

Megaw, D. J. 1938. 'Medicine and Public Health', in E. Blunt (ed.), *Social Service in India*, p. 186. London: HMSO.

Mehta, H. S. 1952. 'Indian Law of Abortion: Suggested Reforms', *The Third International Conference on Planned Parenthood: Report of the Proceedings*, 158.

Metcalf, Barbara D. 1993. 'Hakim Ajmal Khan: Rais of Delhi and Muslim Leader', in R. E. Frykenberg (ed.), *Delhi through and Ages: Selected Essays in Urban History, Culture and Society*, pp. 186–202. New Delhi: Oxford University Press.

Metcalf, Thomas R. 1998. *Ideologies of the Raj*. Cambridge: Cambridge University Press.

Meulenbeld, G. J. 2001. 'Reflections on the Basic Concepts of Indian Pharmacology', in G. J. Muelenbeld and Dominik Wujastyk (ed.), *Studies on Indian Medical History*, pp. 1–16. New Delhi: Motilal Banarasidas.

———. 1999–2000. *A History of Indian Medical Literature*, 5 volumes, IA. Groningen : Egbert Forsten.

Meulenbeld, G. J. 1995. 'The Many Faces of Ayurveda', *Journal of European Ayurvedic Society*, 4: 1–10.

Mills, James H. and Satadru Sen (eds). 2004. *Confronting the Body: The Politics of Physicality in Colonial and Post-Colonial India*. London: Anthem Press.

Mines, Diane P. 1997. 'From Homo Hierarchicus to Homo Faber: Breaking Convention through Semeiosis', *Irish Journal of Anthropology*, 2: 33–44.

Mirza, Ismail. 1954. *My Public Life: Recollections*. London: Allen Unwin.

Mistry, Jerbanoo E. 1957. 'Association of Medical Women in India and its Fifty Years', *Journal of Association of Medical Women in India*, 45 (November): 107–27.

Moller, V. and I. Erstad. 2007. 'Stigma associated with tuberculosis in a time of HIV/AIDS: Narratives from the Eastern Cape, South Africa', *South African Review of Sociology*, 38: 103–19.

Morehead, Charles. 1860. Clinical Researches on Disease in India. London: Longman and Roberts.

Mukharji, P. B. 2009. *Nationalizing the Body: The Medical Market, Print and Daktari Medicine*. London, Anthem Press.

Mukhopadhyaya, Gananath Bhisagacraya. 1974. *History of Indian Medicine*, 2 volumes, 2nd edn. New Delhi: Munshiram Manoharlal.

Mukhopadhyaya, Girindranath. 1923–6. *History of Indian Medicine from the Earliest Ages to the Present Time*, 2 volumes. Kolkata: University of Kolkata.

Muraleedharan, V. R. and D. Veeraraghavan. 1995. 'Disease, Health and Local Administration: Madras City in Early 1900s', *Radical Journal of Health*, 1: 9–24.

Muthaiah, K. S. 1911. *Smiling Benares*. Chennai: Raithby Co.

Muthu, A. C. 1922. *Pulmonary Tuberculosis: its Etiology and Treatment*. Bailliere: Tindall and Cox.

Nair, Sunitha B. 2001. 'Social History of Western Medical Practice in Travancore: An Inquiry into the Administrative Process', in Kumar, Deepak (ed.), *Disease and Medicine in India: A Historical Overview*, p. 215. New Delhi: Tulika.

Nandy, Ashis. 1995. *The Savage Freud and Other Essays on Possible and Retrievable Selves*. New Delhi: Oxfrod University Press.

Neelmeghan, A. 1962. 'Medical Notes in John Ovington's Travelogue', *Indian Journal of History of Medicine*, VII: 12–21.

Neville, H. R. 1909a. *Benares: A Gazetteer*. Volume XXVI of the District Gazetteers of the United Provinces of Agra and Oudh. Allahabad: Government Press.

Newman, Charles. 1960. 'Diagnostic Investigation before Laennec', *Medical History*, 4 (4): 322–9.

Nicholas, R. W. 1981. 'The Goddess Sitala and Epidemic Smallpox in Bengal', *Journal of Asian Studies*, 41 (1): 21–44.

Nicholls, Phillip A. 1988. *Homoeopathy and the Medical Profession*. London: Croom Helm.

Nizami, Zafar Ahmed. 1988. *Hakim Ajmal Khan*. New Delhi: Publications Division, Govt. of India.

Nutton, Vivian. 1993. 'Humoralism', in W.F. Bynum and Porter Roy (eds), *Companion Encyclopedia of the History of Medicine*, p. 288. London: Routledge.

O'Rourke, Kevin H. and Jeffrey G. Williamson. 2002. 'After Columbus: Explaining Europe's Overseas Trade Boom, 1500–1800', *The Journal of Economic History*, 62: 417–56.

Ordi, Jaume, P. L. Alonso, J. de Zulueta, J. Esteban, M. Velasco, E. Mas, E. Campo, and P. L. Fernandez. 2006. 'The Severe Gout of Holy Roman Emperor Charles V', *New England Journal of Medicine*, 355 (5): 316-20.

Ormrod, David. 2003. *The Rise of Commercial Empires: England and the Netherlands in the Age of Merchantilism, 1650–1770*. Cambridge: Cambridge University Press.

O'Shaughnessy, W. B. 1844. *The Bengal Pharmacopoeia*. London: Bishop's College Press.

———. 1842. *The Bengal Dispensatory*. Kolkata: W. Thacker.

Otis, Laura. 1999. *Membranes: Metaphors of Invasion in Nineteenth-Century Literature, Science, and Politics*. Baltimore and London: The Johns Hopkins University Press.

Palit, Chittabrata and Achintya Kumar Dutta (eds). 2005. *History of Medicine in India*. New Delhi: Kalpaz Publication.

Palladino, Paolo and Michael Worboys. 1993. 'Science and Imperialism', *Isis*, 84: 91–102.

Pandey, Lalli Prasad. 1911. 'Malaria Ke Machhad–Mosquitoes of Malaria', *Saraswati*, 12 (2): 68–72.

———. 1908. 'Malaria', *Saraswati*, 9 (11): 492–4.

Pandey, Lochan Prasad. 1909. 'Manushya Ka Mastishka–Brain of a Human Being', *Saraswati*, 10 (5): 221–3.

Panikkar, K. N. 2001. *Culture, Ideology, Hegemony: Intellectuals and Social Consciousness in Colonial India*. New Delhi: Tulika.

Panikkar, K. N. 1992. 'Indigenous Medicine and Cultural Hegemony: A Study of the Revitalisation Movement in Keralam', *Studies in History*, VIII (2): 283–307.

Pati, Biswamoy and Mark Harrison (eds). 2009. *The Social History of Health and Medicine in Colonial India*. New York: Routledge.

———. 2001. *Health Medicine and Empire: Perspectives on Colonial India*. New Delhi: Orient Longman.

Pearson, M. N. 2001. 'The Portuguese State and Medicine in Sixteenth Century Goa', in K. S. Mathew, Teotonio R. De Souza, and Pius Malekandathil, *The Portuguese and Socio Cultural Changes in India, 1500–1800*, pp. 401–19. Lisbon: Fundacao Orient.

———.1995. 'The Thin End of the Wedge: Medical Relativities as a Paradigm of Early Modern Indian–European Relations', *Modern Asian Studies*, 29: 141–70.

Petchesky, Rosalind Pollack. 1986. *Abortion and Woman's Choice*. London: Verso.

Phadke, N. S. 1927. *Sex Problem in India*. Mumbai: Taraporevala Sons and Co.

Pollock, Sheldon. 2004. 'Introduction: Forms of Knowledge in Early Modern South Asia', *Comparative Studies of South Asia, Africa and the Middle East*, 24:19–21.

Porter, Roy. 2001. *A History of Public Health*. London: King's Fund Lecture.

———. 1999. *The Greatest Benefit to Mankind*. London: Fontana Press.

Power, Helen. 1996. 'The Calcutta School of Tropical Medicine', *Medical History*, 40: 197–214.

Prakash, Gyan. 2000. *Another Reason: Science and the Imagination of Modern India*. New Delhi: Oxford University Press.

Premchand. 1994. *Godan: A Novel of Peasant India*, 12th edition. (Translated by Jai Rattan and P. Lal). Mumbai: Jaico Publishing House.

———. 1923. *Nirmala*. Banaras: Saraswati Press.

Qaisar, Ahsan Jan. 1998. *The Indian Response to European Technology and Culture AD 1498–1707*. New Delhi: Oxford University Press.

Quaiser, Neshat. 2011. 'Science, Institution, Colonialism: Tibbiya College of Delhi 1889-1947', in Uma Das Gupta (ed.), *Science and Modern India: An Institutional History 1784–1947*, pp.523–61. New Delhi: Pearson Longman.

———. 2001. 'Politics, Culture and Colonialism: Unani's Debate with Doctory', in B.Pati and M. Harrison (eds), *Health, Medicine and Empire: Perspectives on Colonial India*. Hyderabad: Orient Longman.

———. 2000. 'Colonial Politics of Medicine and Popular Unani Resistance', *Indian Horizons*, April–June: 29–42.

Rahman, Abdul (ed.). 1982. *Science and Technology in Medieval India: A Bibliography of Source Materials in Sanskrit, Arabic and Persian*. New Delhi: Indian National Science Academy.

Rai, Madhav. 1947. *Dactory chikitsa*. Mumbai: Khemraj-Srikrishandas.

Raj, Kapil. 2006. *Relocating Modern Science: Circulation and Construction of Scientific Knowledge in South Asia and Europe, Seventeenth to Nineteenth Centuries*. New Delhi: Permanent Black.

Ram Bhishagratna, T. S. 1909. *In Defence of Ayurveda*. Cocanada: Author.

Ramanna, Mridula. 2002. *Western Medicine and Public Health in Colonial Bombay (1845–1895)*. New Delhi: Orient Longman.

Ramasubban, Radhika. 1988. 'Imperial Health in British India, 1857–1900', in R. MacLeod and Lewis Milton (eds), *Disease, Medicine, and Empire: Perspectives on Western Medicine and the Experience of European Expansion*, pp. 38–60. London: Routledge.

Ramusack, Barbara N. 1993. 'Embattled Advocates: The Debate over birth Control in India 1920–1940', in Cheryl Johnson-Odim and Margaret Stroebel (eds), *Expanding the Boundaries of Women's History*, pp. 173–202. Bloomington: Indiana University Press.

Ranga Iyer, G. S. 1927. *Father India*. London: Selwyn & Blount Ltd.

Ranger, Terence and Paul Slack (eds). 1992. *Epidemics and Ideas: Essays on the Historical Perception of Pestilence*. Cambridge: Cambridge University Press.

Rao, Ganapathi S. 1977. 'Dhanvantari Mahal', *Journal of the Tanjore Saraswati Mahal Library*, 30: I–IV.

Rao, Mohan. 2004. *From Population Control to Reproductive Health: Malthusian Arithmetic*. Delhi: Sage.

Ray, Kobita. 1998. *History of Public Health: Colonial Bengal 1921–1947*. Kolkata: K. P. Bagchi and Co.

Ray, Priyadaranjan, Hirendranath Gupta, and Mira Roy. 1980. *Susruta Samhita: A Scientific Synopsis*. New Delhi: Indian National Science Academy.

Roberts, Emma. 1838. 'The East India Vooyager', *Parbury's Oriental Herald and Colonial Intelligencer*, II (July to December): 245–52.

Rogers, Leonard. 1928. *The Incidence and Spread of Cholera in India*. Kolkata: Thacker, Spink and Co.

Rosenberg, Charles E. 1962. *The Cholera Years: The United States in 1832, 1849 and 1866*. Chicago: The University of Chicago Press.

Rothman, Sheila M. 1994. *Living in the Shadow of Death: Tuberculosis and the Social Experience of Illness in American History*. New York: Basic Books.

Roy, Mira. 2004. 'Āurveda', in Priyadaranjan Ray and S. N. Sen (eds), *The Cultural Heritage of India*, Volume iv, pp. 152–76. Kolkata: The Ramkrishna Mission Institute of Culture.

Roy, Rohan Deb. 2007. 'Mal-areas of Health Dispersed Histories of a Diagnostic Category', *Economic and Political Weekly*, xlii: 122–9.

Royle, J. F. 1837. *An Essay on the Antiquity of Hindoo Medicine*. London: William H. Allen.

Ryan, F. 1992. *Tuberculosis: The Greatest Story Never Told.* Bromsgrove, Worcestershire, UK: Swifth Publishers.

Samanta, Arabinda. 2002. *Malarial Fever in Colonial Bengal, 1820–1939: Social History of an Epidemic.* Kolkata: Firma KLM.

Sanskritayen, Rahul and Krishandev Upadhyaya (eds). 1961. *Hindi Sahitya Ka Vrihat Itihas, Volume-16: Hindi Ka Lok Sahitya.* Kashi: Nagari Pracharini Sabha.

Sanyal, Pulin Chandra. 1888. 'Vivaha Vichar (Consideration of Marriage)', *Cikitsa Sammilani (Union of Medicine),* 5 (1): 5–13.

Sarkar, Mahendra Lal. 1904 (1870). *A Sketch of the Treatment of Cholera.* Kolkata: Anglo Sanskrit Press.

Sarkar, Mahendra Lal. 1891. *Moral Influence of Physical Science being the Substance of a Lecture delivered at the Town Hall on January 7th, 1891, under the Presidency of His Honour the Lieutenant-Governor.* Kolkata: Anglo Sanskrit Press.

———. 1876. *On the Desirability of a National Institution for the Cultivation of the Sciences by the Natives of India (1872–76).* Kolkata: Anglo Sanskrit Press. This was also published in *The Calcutta Journal of Medicine,* 2 August 1869: 286–91.

———. 1870. *On the Physiological Basis of Psychology.* Kolkata: Anglo Sanskrit Press.

———. 1869. *Conferences upon Homoeopathy by Dr Jousset: An Essay on the Choice of Homoeopathic Remedies by M. Gallavardin.* (Trans. from the French by Mahendra Lal Sarkar). Kolkata: Anglo Sanskrit Press.

———. 1869. 'A Retrospect', *The Calcutta Journal of Medicine,* 2 (11, 12): 399.

———. 1868. 'Our Creed', *The Calcutta Journal of Medicine,* 1 (1): 2, 4.

Saunders, William. 1809. *A Treatise on the Structure, Economy, and Diseases of the Liver to Which is Added A More Particular Account of the Hepatitis of India.* London: William Philips.

Scamber, G. 1998. 'Stigma and disease: Changing Paradigms', *Lancet,* 352: 1054–5.

Schiebinger, Londa. 2005. 'The European Colonial Science Complex', *ISIS,* 96 (1): 52–5.

Schiebinger, Londa and Claudia Swan (eds). 2004. *Colonial Botany: Science, Commerce, and Politics in the Early Modern World.* Philadelphia: University of Pennsylvania Press.

Scot, H. 1817. 'Some Remarks on the Arts of India, with Miscellaneous Observations on Various Subjects', *The Ecclectic Repertory, and Analytical Review, Medical and Philosophical,* VII: 156–62.

Scott, William. 1824. *Report on the Epidemic Cholera as It Has Appeared in the Territories Subject to the Presidency of Fort St. George. Drawn up by the Order of the Government under the Superintendence of Medical Board.* Chennai: Asylum Press.

Sen, Gananath. 1943. *Āyurveda Parichay (Introduction to Āyurveda)*. Kolkata: Visva Bharati Granthalay.

————. 1916. *Hindu Medicine*. Chennai: D. Gopalacharlu.

Sengupta, P. C. 1970. 'Soorjo Coomar Goodeve Chuckerbutty: The First Indian Contributor to Modern Medical Science', *Medical History*, 14 (2): 183–91.

Sen Gupta, Nagendra Nath. 1901. *The Ayurvedic System of Medicine*. Kolkata: Keval Ram Chatterjee.

Sharma, Jagannarayandev. 1927. *Brahmacharya Vijnan – The Science of Celibacy*. Ajmer: Sasta-Sahitya-Prakashak-Mandal.

Sharma, Madhuri. 2012. *Indigenous and Western Medicine in Colonial India*. New Delhi: Foundation Books.

————. 2008. 'Debating Women's Health: Reflections in Popular Hindi Print-culture', *Indian Historical Review*, XXXV (II): 178–90.

Sharma, Nageshwar. 1969. 'Women in Magahi Folklore', in Sankar Sen Gupta (ed.), *Women In Indian Folklore: A Short Survey of their Social Status and Position*, p. 84. Kolkata: Indian Publications.

Sharma, Ram Narayan. 1912. 'Manushya Kya Cheej Hai? – What is Human Being', *Saraswati*, 13 (6): 301–4.

Sherring, M. A. 2002 (First published in 1868). *Benares: The Sacred City of the Hindus*. New Delhi: Low Price Publications.

Siddiqi, Tazimuddin. 1980. 'Hakim Ajmal Khan: A Champion of Indian Medicine', *Studies in History of Medicine*, 4 (3): 145–76.

Sigerist, Henry E. 1962. *Civilization and Disease*. Chicago: University of Chicago Press.

————. 1951. *A History of Medicine*. Oxford: Oxford University Press.

Simensen, J. 1988. *Norwegian Mission in African History, Vol. I, South Africa, 1845–1906*. Oslo: Norwegian University Press.

Singh, Suryabali. 1931. *Brahmacharya Kee Mahima – Glory of Celibacy*. Banaras: S. B. Singh & Co.

Sinha, J. N. 1991. 'Science and the Indian National Congress', in Deepak Kumar (ed.), *Science and Empire*, pp. 161–81. New Delhi: Anamika.

Sivaramakrishnan, Kavita. 2006. *Old Potions, New Bottles: Recasting Indigenous Medicine in Colonial Punjab (1850–1945)*. New Delhi: Orient Longman.

Smith, D. B. 1869. 'Early Records of Cholera', *The Indian Annals of Medical Science*, XXVII: 166–218.

Smith, Solvig. 1981. *By Love Compelled*. London: Salvationist Publishing.

Sokhey, S. S. and K. Shad (eds). 1947. *Report of the National Health Sub-Committee* (National Planning Committee). Mumbai: Vohra & Co.

Somervell, T. Howard. 1940. *Knife and Life in India: The Story of a Surgical Missionary at Neyoor, Travancore*. London: The Livingstone Press.

Spratling, Edgar J. 1902. 'The Physician as a Social Economic Factor', *Journal of American Medical Association (JAMA)*, 38: 1688–9.

Stewart, Duncan. 1835. 'Observations on the Fever which Prevailed at Howrah, during the months of June and July 1834', *Transactions of the Medical and Physical Society of Calcutta*, VII: 363–88.

Subash Chandran, M. D. 1998. 'Shifting Cultivation, Sacred Groves and Conflicts in Colonial Forest Policy in the Western India', in Richard Grove, Vinita Damodaran, and Satpal Sangwan (eds), *Nature and the Orient, the Environmental History of South and South East Asia*, p. 698. New Delhi: Oxford University Press.

Subba Reddy, D. V. 1957. 'Dar-us-Shifa Built by Sultan Muhammad Quli: The First Unani Teaching Hospital in Deccan', *Indian Journal of History of Medicine*, II: 102–5.

Subramanian, S. V. and V. R. Madhavan (eds). 1983. *Heritage of the Tamils Siddha Medicine*. Chennai: International Institute of Tamil Studies.

Tansukh, Rai Saheb. 1934. 'Bacchon Kee Bhisan Mrityu Sankya – High Death Rate of Children', *Saraswati*, 35: 407–15.

Taussig, Michael. 1993. *Mimesis and Alterity: A Particular History of the Senses*. New York: Routledge.

Tripathi, Ramakant. 1933. *Sachitra Injection Chikitsa Artharth Sui Kee Pichkari Duara Rogon Kee Chikitsa*. Mathura: Chetrapal Sharma– Sukhsancharak Company.

Trotter, Thomas. 1797. *Medicina Nautica: An Essay on the Diseases of Seamen: Comprehending the History of Health in His Majesty's Fleet, under the Command of Richard Earl Howe*. London: T. Cadell & W. Davies.

Trvelyan, Charles. 1838. *On the Education of the People of India*. London: Longman and Green.

Turner, Bryan S. 1992. *Regulating Bodies: Essays in Medical Sociology*. London: Routledge.

Turshen, M. 1977. 'The Political Ecology of Disease', *Review of Radical Political Economics*, 9: 55–60.

Twining, William. 1833. *A Practical Account of the Epidemic Cholera, and of the Treatment Requisite in the Various Modifications of That Disease*. London: Parbury, Allen & Co.

———. 1832. *Clinical Illustrations of the More Important Diseases of Bengal, with the Result of an Inquiry into Their Pathology and Treatment*. Kolkata: Baptist Mission Press.

———. 1835. *Clinical Illustrations of the More Important Diseases of Bengal*. Kolkata: W. Thacker.

Ukil, A. C. 1938. 'Anti-Tuberculosis Work in Bengal', *Indian Medical Gazette*, 73: 525.

Ukil, A. C. 1926. 'The Problem of Combating Tuberculosis in India', *The Calcutta Medical Journal*, XXI (5): 215–16.

Urdang, G. 1946. 'Pharmacopoeias as Witness of World History', *Journal of the History of Medicine and Allied Sciences*, 1 (1): 46–70.

Valiathan, M. S. 2003. *The Legacy of Charaka*. Hyderabad: Orient Longman.

Van De Graaf, R. C. 2009. 'Some Remarks on the Revival of Rhinoplasty in Europe in the Early Nineteenth Century', *Acta Otorhinolaryngologica Italica*, 29 (4): 226.

Varadarajan, Lokita. 2006. *Indo-Portuguese Encounters: Journeys in Science, Technology and Culture*. New Delhi: Aryan Books International.

Vickers, Andrew and Catherine Zollman. 1999. 'ABC of Complementary Medicine: Homoeopathy', *British Medical Journal*, 319 (23 October): 1115–18.

Visvanathan, Shiv. 1997. *A Carnival for Science: Essays on Science, Technology and Development*. New Delhi: Oxford University Press.

Wade, John Peter. 1793. *A Paper on the Prevention and Treatment of the Disorders of Seamen and Soldiers in Bengal*. London: J. Murray.

Waines, David. 1999. 'Dietetics in Medieval Islamic Culture', *Medical History*, 43: 228–40.

Walker, K. 1955. *The Story of Medicine*. New York: Oxford University Press.

Warner, John Harley. 1997. *The Therapeutic Perspective*. Princeton: Princeton University Press.

Warrel, David A. 2001. 'To Search and Study of the Secret of Tropical Diseases by Way of Experiment', *Lancet*, 358: 1983–8.

Watts, Sheldon. 1999. *Epidemics and History: Disease, Power and Imperialism*. New Haven: Yale University Press.

Wear, A. (ed.). 1992. *Medicine in Society: Historical Essays*. Cambridge: Cambridge University Press.

Webb, Allan. 1848. *Pathologica Indica or the Anatomy of Indian Diseases Based Upon Morbid Specimens From All Parts of the Indian Empire in the Museum in the Calcutta Medical College*. Kolkata: Thacker and Co.

Whitcombe, Elizabeth. 1995. 'The Environmental Costs of Irrigation in British India: Water Logging, Salinity, Malaria', in David Arnold and Ramachandra Guha (eds), *Nature, Culture and Imperialism Essays on the Environmental History of South Asia*, p. 257. New Delhi: Oxford University Press.

White, D. G. 2004. *The Alchemical Body*. New Delhi: Munshiram Manoharlal.

Whitehead, Judy. 1995. 'Modernising the Motherhood Archetype: Public Health Models and the Child Marriage Restraint Act, 1929', *Indian Sociology*, 29 (1–2): 187–210.

Williams, Raymond. 1960. *Culture and Society, 1780–1950*. London: Doubleday & Co.

Willson, D. Clarke. 1959. *The Story of Dr. Ida Scudder of Vellore*. London: McGraw Hill.

Wilson, H. H. 1825. 'Kushta, or Leprosy, as Known to the Hindus', *Transactions of the Medical and Physical Society of Calcutta*, 1: 27–8.

Wink, André. 1996–7. *Al-Hind: The Making of the Indo-Islamic World*. 2 volumes. Leiden: Brill.

Wise, T. A. 1860 [1845]. *Commentary on the Hindu System of Medicine*. Kolkata: Thacker and Co.

Woodbury (Jr.), Benjamin C. 1952. 'The Homoeopathic School of Medicine', *The Indian Homoeopathic Journal*, III (2): 145–70.

Worboys, Michael. 2000. *Spreading Germs: Disease Theories and Medical Practice in Britain, 1865–1900*. Cambridge: Cambridge University Press.

Worsley, Peter. 1982. 'Non-Western Medical Systems', *Annual Review of Anthropology*, 11: 315.

Wright, William. 1797. 'Practical Observations on the Treatment of Acute Diseases; Particularly Those of the West Indies', *Medical Facts and Observations*, 7: 1–25.

Wujastyk, Dominik. 2009. 'Interpreting the Image of the Human Body in Premodern India', *International Journal of Hindu Studies*, 13 (2): 189–228.

————. 2005. 'Change and Creativity in Early Modern Medical Thought', *Journal of Indian Philosophy*, 33 (1): 95–118.

————. 2004. 'An Argument with Medicine', *Friends of the Wellcome Library Newsletter*, 32: 6–7.

————. 2003. 'Indian Medical Thought on the Eve of Colonialism', *IIAS Newsletter*, 31 July: 21.

————. 2001. *The Roots of Ayurveda*. New Delhi: Penguin.

Yeoh, B. 1996. *Contesting Space in Colonial Singapore: Power Relations and the Urban Built Environment*. Singapore: National University of Singapore Press.

Zahuri, Hakim Abdul Wahab. 1966. 'The Nizamia Tibbi College, Hyderabad, Deccan', *Hamdard Medical Digest*, 4–6: 5–15.

Zimmermann, Francis. 2003. 'Bodily Humors in the Scholarly Traditions of Hindu and Galenic Medicine as an Example of Naïve Theory and Implicate Universals', in Glauco Saga and Gherardo Ortalli (eds), *Nature and Knowledge: Ethnoscience, Cognition, and Utility*, pp. 262–71. New York and Oxford: Berghan Books.

————. 1989, 'Terminological Problems in the Process of Editing and Translating Sanskrit Medical Text', in Paul Unschuld (ed.), *Approaches to Traditional Chinese Medical Literature*, pp. 141–51. Kluwer Academic Press.

————. 1987. *The Jungle and the Aroma of Meats: An Ecological Theme in Hindu Medicine*. Berkeley: University of California Press.

Zyzk, Kenneth. 1985. *Medicine in the Veda*. New Delhi: Motilal Banarasidas.

Glossary

acharyas	Indian preceptors
Anandakanda	The Root of Bliss
anna	unit of money, 1/16th rupee
antrikajvara	enteric or typhoid fever
Arka	distillation
bawarchi	chef
begaries	workers
bhindi	okra
bimaristans	hospitals
Brahmacharya	*celibacy?*
chaprasi	junior office workers who carry messages
dai	*indigenous mid-wife*
Dar-us-Shifa	House of Cures
dava	medicine
diwan	Chief Minister
dua	prayers
durwan	doorkeeper
Firangi roga	disease of the Europeans
goala	milkmen
Godan	Donation of a cow
granthikajvar	plague or bubonic fever
gupt rog	venereal diseases
Hakim al-Mulk	*Unani practitioner of the country (an honorific title)*
hing	asafoetida
jamini bimari	earthy disease
jivanu	micro-organism
kalajvara	kalazar, a disease
kalazaar	black fever
Kaliyuga	last of the four stages the world goes through as part of the cycle of yugas described in Indian scriptures

kaviraj	*Ayurvedic practitioner in Bengal*
kaviraji chikitsa	Āyurvedic treatment
krimi	microscopic organism
kulin	upper caste Brahmin
mahabhuta	five fundamental elements
maharatta	Maratha
mamlatdar	chief civil officer of the district
napunsaka	the third gender
nath siddhas	spiritual tantrics/yogis
nidana	treatment
nullah	drain
paharrees	hill men
parah	This worldly
pitta	bile
prasadhini	beautification
rasa siddhas	alchemists
rasa	nutritive juices
rasam	mercury
Rasashastra	medicine and alchemy
Rasavidya	alchemy
Rogarogvada	debate on illness and health
samhita	Treatise
samkranti	transmission of contagious diseases
Shashtras	sacred texts
sheetal vayu	cold wind
Siddha	the Tamil variant of Ayurveda
slesmakjvara	influenza
svasyantra	the respiratory tract
talati	village accountant (also kept records)
Todarananda	a 16th century encyclopaedic work
tridosha	the three humours
vaidya	Ayurvedic practitioner
vata	wind
vijnana	science
zamindar	landholder

About the Editors and Contributors

Sunil Amrith is Reader in Modern Asian History at Birkbeck College, University of London. He is the author of *Decolonizing International Health* (2006), and is currently studying the history of Tamil migration to Southeast Asia.

David Arnold is Emeritus Professor, Department of History, at the University of Warwick, UK. A founder member of the Subaltern Studies collective and a Fellow of the British Academy, he has written extensively on the history of modern India, including its medical and environmental history. His publications include *Colonizing the Body: State Medicine and Epidemic Disease in Nineteenth-Century India* (1993) and *The Tropics and the Traveling Gaze: India, Landscape, and Science, 1800-1859* (2005). His current research is on 'everyday technology' in India between 1880 and 1960, looking in particular at sewing machines, bicycles, typewriters, and rice mills.

Raj Sekhar Basu is Reader at the Department of History, University of Calcutta. He has published many articles on Dalit history in monographs and journals. He has co-edited two books along with Sanjukta Dasgupta, one on Dalit experiences, the other on Adivasi history. Currently he is working on the Dalit and Adivasi Conflicts in Ganjam in the nineteenth and twentieth centuries.

Jayanta Bhattacharya, by training a physician, has a PhD on Colonial Encounters in Anatomical Knowledge as Contained in Ayurveda and Modern Medicine. Currently he is engaged in tracing Indian medicine, with special reference to anatomical knowledge, through travelers' accounts during the seventeenth–nineteenth centuries. His works include—'The Body: Epistemological Encounters in Colonial India' in Peter L. Twohig and Vera Kalitzkas (eds), *Making Sense of Health, Illness and Disease* (2004); 'The Knowledge of Anatomy and Health in Āyurveda and Modern Medicine', *Eä - Revista de humanidades médicas & estudios sociales de la ciencia y la tecnología* (2009, 1:1–51).

Bikramaditya Kumar Choudhary is Assistant Professor, Department of Geography, Banaras Hindu University. He has extensively worked on urban problems especially on waste-pickers and health problems in India. He has several publications on these issues including a book titled *Tuberculosis in India: A Political Ecology Approach* (2008). His area of interest includes Health and Disease, Regional disparity, Urbanization and currently he is working on the issue of resource-conflict in India.

Indira Chowdhury is Scholar-in-Residence at the Srishti School of Art, Design and Technology in Bangalore. Her book, *The Frail Hero and Virile History*, (Oxford University Press, 1998) was awarded the Tagore Prize in 2001. She has set up several institutional and corporate archives including the Archives of the Tata Institute of Fundamental Research, Mumbai. Her book *A Masterful Spirit: Homi Bhabha 1909–1966* was released in June 2010.

Mark Harrison is Professor of History of Medicine and Director, Wellcome Unit for History of Medicine, at Oxford. He has published great deal on different aspects of history of medicine and public health in India and the tropics. His most cited works are *Public Health in British India: Anglo Indian Preventive Medicine 1859–1914*, (1994) and *Climates and Constitutions: Health, Race, Environment and British Imperialism in India, 1600–1850* (1999).

Deepak Kumar is Professor of History of Science and Education and Concurrent Professor, Centre for Media Studies, School of Social Sciences at Jawaharlal Nehru University, New Delhi. For more than three decades he has worked and published on different aspects of science and society interface in the context of British India. He is known for his work *Science and the Raj* (2nd ed. 2006).

Mridula Ramanna has authored *Western Medicine and Public Health in Colonial Bombay,1845–1895* (2003). She has contributed chapters on medical history to several edited volumes and has published articles in *Indian Historical Review, Economic and Political Weekly, Social Scientist,* and *Indica.* Her forthcoming publication is titled, *Health Care in Bombay Presidency, 1896-1930.*

Arabinda Samanta is Professor of History at the University of Burdwan, West Bengal. His work has been mainly on epidemics, medicine, and environment in colonial Bengal. His publications include *Malarial Fever* *in Colonial Bengal: Social History of an Epidemic* (2002); *The Revolt of 1857: Memory Identity History*, ed. (2009); *Locating Epidemics: Colonial Bengal, 1820–1939* (in press); *Life and Culture in Bengal: Colonial and Post-Colonial Experiences*, ed. (forthcoming). Presently he is working on Bone-Setters of Bengal.

Madhuri Sharma is a Junior Fellow at Nehru Memorial, Museum and Library, Teen Murti House, New Delhi, working on a project titled *Media, Medicine and Society in North India, c.1900–2000*. She is the author of *Indigenous and Western Medicine in Colonial India*, Foundation Books (2012). Her current research focuses on an analysis of medical advertisements in the period *c.*1900–2000 to frame the interconnections between medical practice, drug manufacturers, and the medical market in colonial and postcolonial North India.

Dhrub Kumar Singh teaches Modern Indian History at Department of History, Faculty of Social Sciences, Banaras Hindu University, Varanasi and his areas of interest include the history of Science, Technology, and Medicine.